Committee Worlds

Anthropology of Policy
Cris Shore and Susan Wright, editors

Committee Worlds

Governing Medical Research through Ethics in the Asia-Pacific

Rachel Douglas-Jones

Stanford University Press
Stanford, California

Stanford University Press
Stanford, California

Library of Congress Cataloging-in-Publication Data

Names: Douglas-Jones, Rachel, author.
Title: Committee worlds : governing medical research through ethics in the Asia-Pacific / Rachel Douglas-Jones.
Other titles: Anthropology of policy (Stanford, Calif.)
Description: Stanford, California : Stanford University Press, 2026. | Series: Anthropology of policy | Includes bibliographical references and index.
Identifiers: LCCN 2025025686 (print) | LCCN 2025025687 (ebook) | ISBN 9781503644274 (cloth) | ISBN 9781503644915 (ebook)
Subjects: LCSH: Forum of Ethics Review Committees of Asia and the Pacific. | Medical ethics committees—Pacific Area. | Medicine—Research—Moral and ethical aspects—Pacific Area. | Medical ethics—Pacific Area.
Classification: LCC R725.3 .D68 2026 (print) | LCC R725.3 (ebook) | DDC 174.2—dc23/eng/20250821
LC record available at https://lccn.loc.gov/2025025686
LC ebook record available at https://lccn.loc.gov/2025025687

Cover design: Ann Weinstock
Cover art: Adobe Stock & iStock
Typeset by Newgen in Brill 10.5/15

The authorized representative in the EU for product safety and compliance is: Mare Nostrum Group B.V. | Mauritskade 21D | 1091 GC Amsterdam | The Netherlands | Email address: gpsr@mare-nostrum.co.uk | KVK chamber of commerce number: 96249943

Printed and bound by CPI Group (UK) Ltd, Croydon, CR0 4YY

Contents

Acknowledgments

My parents tell a story about a friend of theirs, Peter, in Aotearoa New Zealand, someone who was bright but struggled to find good jobs. They were commiserating with him after another unsuccessful interview, going through the screening questions. To one, which read "Are you good at making decisions?", he had thoughtfully replied, "Yes. And no." His answer is repeated in moments of prime indecision in our family. Told with love for their indecisive friend, it is one of several formative starting points for my decades-long interest in how decisions are made. Books come from more influences than we can count, but in this one, I hope family will recognize themselves. I thank them all for their encouragement and support over the years.

This work began in Sri Lanka, through the hospitality of Prof. Vajira Dissanayake and Prof. Rohan W. Jayasekara and colleagues in the Human Genetics Unit (HGU) at the Faculty of Medicine, University of Colombo. I thank everyone there for the short eats and shared lunch breaks. It developed into something much larger because of the welcome offered by Prof. Cristina Torres, Atoy Navarro, and Prof. Juntra Karbwang-Laothavorn. Thank you so much for opening your networks and teaching me about your work.

The Economic and Social Research Council in the United Kingdom provided funding for this research, under the wider project *International Science and Bioethics Collaborations* RES-062-23-0215. Without this support, the research for this book would not have been possible. I thank the project members Adèle Langlois, Marilyn Strathern, Monica Konrad, Birgit Buergi, Achim Rosemann, Margaret Sleeboom Faulkner, and especially Bob Simpson and Salla Sariola, both of whom had formative roles in the making of this ethnography, through supervision, mentorship, and example. I thank Michael Carrithers, whose healthy skepticism served as a reminder to keep the stakes visible. I thank cohort peers at Durham, James Howard, Emilie Fairet, Carla

Handley, Megan Wainwright, Damien Boutillon, and David Henig. Thank you to research facilitators and coordinators Madeline Watt, Georgie Grace, and Kate Pedley, and to the IT University of Copenhagen's "Spark IT" fund for follow-up fieldwork funding in 2017 and 2018.

Along the way, Andrea Ballestero provided practical stepping stones, and Kaushik Sunder Rajan asked necessarily pointed questions about place and complexity of what I was allowing my interlocutors to gloss. Casper Bruun Jensen opened up academic futures in Denmark, and Brit Ross Winthereik built STS institutions from the ground up. Thank you both for these opportunities and the inspiration of Monitoring Movements. I thank Anja Marie Bornø Jensen, Ayo Wahlberg, and Maja Højer Bruun for their friendship, as well as all members of the Technologies in Practice group, particularly book pals Sunniva Sandbukt, Andy Lautrup, Katinka Schyberg, and Baki Cakici. Thank you to Erica Seruset-Borgstrom and Sally Atkinson for a decade of "no" consultancy. For the periods of focus needed to write, I thank Patricia Kingori and the much-missed Nina Hallowell for stays at ETHOX and the Big Data Institute, respectively. Thank you to Haiqing Yu, Atsuro Morita, and Courtney Addison for your incredible hospitality during my sabbatical. Rebecca Tapscott made herself a beacon for critical scholarship on ethics review, bringing together Sarah Babb, Adam Hedgecoe, Laura Stark, and myself at a time in the pandemic when such exchange was much needed. I thank my book buddy Sam Breslin for the mutual accountability and friendship, and three scholars whose own books lit the way, Susan Ellison, Lisa Messeri, and Nick Seaver, for encouragement at the right time. Ovnis and alfajores to Trin Rico, backyard chats to Catherine Trundle, and gudetamas to Jess Perriam.

As with any project in development over many years, there are a lot of people who have shaped it. My thanks to Sue Wright and Cris Shore, without whose encouragement and interest this book would not have been finalized, nor would I have returned to questions of ethics and integrity with new eyes. Peer review is a gift when readers push you toward clarity and make explicit their belief in you as an analyst and writer. My special thanks to the Policy Series' anonymous reviewers, and to Dylan Kyung-lim White and Justine Sargent at Stanford University Press who got me through.

Parts of this book have been reworked from prior publications. These include vignettes and arguments that appeared in previous forms in *Social Anthropology* ("A 'Good' Ethical Review," 2015), *Critical Public Health* ("Getting

Inside Ethical Review," 2019), *The Cambridge Journal of Anthropology* ("Building Capacity in Ethical Review," 2017, "Committee as Witness," 2021), *Medicine Anthropology Theory* ("Silent Mentors," 2017), and *Science and Technology Studies* ("Making Room for Ethics," 2017). My thanks to the special issue and journal editors who created the conversations to which earlier versions of these analyses have contributed.

H, you have seen this book from its beginnings. Thank you, across countries, time zones, and contracts, for being there the whole way through.

Introduction

In the summer of 2010, I was attending a training workshop on Good Clinical Practice and Research Ethics at Thammasat University in Bangkok. It was a little after noon, and trainers and trainees had spilled out of the dark lecture hall for lunch in the hot, tall glass atrium on the edge of campus. At that time, the building hosted the World Health Organization-Tropical Disease Research (WHO-TDR) Clinical Coordination and Training Centre for research activities in the Asia-Pacific region. Over baskets of lychees, Dr. Cristina, one of workshop's facilitators, was recounting to our lunch table a recent discussion she had had with a U.S. American academic, Dave. Dr. Cristina had been telling Dave about her work building a network of research ethics committees in the Asia-Pacific region, she said, working collaboratively to raise standards and ensure improved ethics review practices across the region. Dave had interrupted to ask: "How are you going to do a system when you don't have any laws?" Laughing, Dr. Cristina said she just told Dave, "Have you never heard of moral force?" "If a group of people believe something strongly enough," she said, to those of us gathered for the training, "you don't need laws. I think that is what we're doing here."

By that point, Cristina was well on her way to realizing her ambitions. Since 2004 she had been working as the coordinator of the Bangkok-based regional nongovernmental organization (NGO) called the Forum of Ethics Review Committees of Asia and the Western Pacific (FERCAP). Her world is one where people do believe strongly in the necessity and purpose of research ethics. Belief is necessary: The forum she led has been built from volunteer labor, hundreds of people working together to become more familiar with practices of ethics review. It was also necessary because at the time, few of the countries where she went to run workshops had established legislation or regulation for the protection of those who participate in clinical research.

As she put it herself that day, "We're not a human rights program, we're trying to create a duty-based ethics: If you don't do your duty then you're not a good professional. We're not working with patient groups. Our audiences are doctors, academics, regulators."

Cristina's network and their activities over the first quarter of the twenty-first century are the center of this book. Through them, I address the question of what it means to locate practices of ethics review—and the bureaucratic genealogies of committee work, decision-making, and ideas of science they embody—in the blurry-edged region that practitioners term the Asia-Pacific. The shift in focus prompts my book's driving question: What worlds does an ethics committee carry with it? Despite numerous accounts emerging from the era of clinical trials globalization and the international biomedical economy, we have few stories about what one of its key accompanying infrastructures, ethics review, looks like when *it* travels outside the U.S. (Stark 2012; Babb 2020), the UK (Hedgecoe 2020), or Europe (Jacobs 2022). Rather than building a series of national histories of bioethics or research ethics, in this book I narrate the work that the NGO Cristina works with does to build capacity in ethics review across the Asia-Pacific region. Looking closely at the growth of global infrastructures of biomedical research teaches us about the travel of the committee as a way of reasoning and making decisions about ethics in biomedical research. It also reveals the stakes. As critical policy scholars John Clarke, Dave Bainton, Noémi Lendvai, and Paul Stubbs observe, a series of questions unfolds around *how* policies move, including: "'Who and what makes it move?'; 'What happens as it arrives and settles in those 'elsewhere?'; 'What keeps it moving?'; and 'What happens to it as it moves?'" (Clarke et al. 2015, 1).

From time spent in meeting rooms, shadowing trainings and capacity building initiatives, I have followed ethics review to where it is made "local," a place Betsey Brada has shown us in her ethnography of global health is not only spatial but temporal (2023, 98). But it is crucial we do not imagine that ethics policies and practices move into emptiness. I follow ethnographer Tess Lea's proposal to consider an "ecology" of overlaid policies, that become "distributed, reproduced, instantiated, mystified, transacted with, and embodied across time and place" (2024, 1). Her invitation unsettles unidirectional causality, and offers an awareness of contingent policies interacting with one another. It is also well suited to the way practitioners themselves think about the ever-changing "ecosystem and context of [. . .] critical documents that layer on more detailed guidance or establish national or regional legal and regulatory policy" (Resneck 2025, 15). The backpack of acronyms and "living documents" practitioners live alongside in this book, with their overlapping names and eras, underpins ethics review as a material and social practice. By drawing on literatures at the intersection of anthropologies of policy and bureaucracy, global health and biomedicine, I tell a story of what ethics committee work and decision-making looks like as it is brought, by people like Cristina, to sites seeking both to host international clinical trials and those accelerating their own research environments, pushing to have their scientific researchers and publications recognized as part of "global science."

For the last forty years, researchers in anthropology, global health, and science and technology studies (STS) have highlighted how techniques of testing biomedical drugs and technologies often rest on the exploitation of longstanding global and colonial inequalities. They have consistently interrogated imbalances of power in the use of "other" bodies as sources and generators of scientific knowledge (Crane 2010; Merz 2021). This is especially true in the countries the World Health Organization classifies as Asia and the Western Pacific (often abbreviated in industry as APAC), out of which has come a strong body of research into the promise of the biosciences (Ong and Chen 2010; Ong 2016). In 2018, Wen-Hua Kuo described human research in East Asia—grouping Japan, Taiwan, Korea, and Singapore—"as both an advancement of medical science and one of the coming century's most promising 'industries'" (Kuo 2018, 2). At the same time, scholarship has shown the enrolment of science in national and cross-border competition (Sleeboom-Faulkner and Patra 2011) and their challenges (Wahlberg et al. 2021; Rao 2022). It is also the region that has seen the most growth in clinical trial activity since the turn of the century. The World Health Organization's Global Observatory on Health R&D, drawing on data from the International Clinical Trials Registry Platform (ICTRP),[1] visualizes figures of registered trials, noting that "in 2022 the number of trials registered in Western Pacific (12,337) was around 14 times higher than in Africa (861)" (WHO 2023). In what follows, I do not position the Asia-Pacific as a peripheral elsewhere for biomedical research: It is not inherently peripheral, and certainly neither singular nor undifferentiated. In shifting the empirical and narrative center of gravity of global research in health, both of major funding and of ethics, I make a move increasingly called for in the literature. Studying scientific ambition in India and China, for example, Joy Y. Zhang and Saheli Datta Burton ask scholars to acknowledge that analysis needs to shift from older models of "diffusion of norms from the centre to the periphery" (2022, viii) and turn toward "actors' perceived position of their unequal relations of epistemic power" (2022, ix). Starting with researchers' perceptions, Margaret Sleeboom-Faulkner foregrounds regulation "as an incentive for researchers to invest and engage in, sometimes, very complex and labor intensive, international science collaboration" (2025, 22). Theoretically, scholars in science and technology studies have wrestled with how to work with the Asian region as a "method" (Morita 2017). Acknowledging the pitfalls organizing thought around this imagined place, "Asia," and the way its "multiplicity keeps bursting out of any number of essentialist straitjackets" (Anderson 2017, 232), scholars working in the region ask how these pluralities "are being done in practice" (Lin and Law 2019, 131). To this first challenge, Warwick Anderson adds another, asking what it would take to regard this part of the world as "a site of theory making in STS, not just a space for data extraction or a place to which European concepts diffused" (Anderson 2017, 229). In this book, I build on Andrew Kipnis's arguments that a "robust anthropology needs more forms of comparative thinking than the culturally diffusionist arguments that derive from imagining a rampant globalization" (Kipnis 2008, 289), and bring them forward for an ethnography of ethics as bureaucracy.

Similar questions are being asked of the stories told of the "global" in global health. Is it a "straight swap" for words like "international," inviting ethnographies that depart from a tendency "to focus on institutions of western biomedicine that derive power and authority from past imperialisms" (Brazelton 2022, 2, 8)? Work in anthropology has tended to position such institutions, along with their imperial baggage, in ethnographic presents where Western biomedicine exists alongside more ways of knowing and being. Whether in the establishment of partnerships for HIV/AIDS treatment in Botswana (Brada 2023), the sustaining of "experimental infrastructures" of oncology in Uganda (Mika 2021, 24), or the everyday practice of medicine in postcolonial contexts, a critical, ethnographic interrogation of where ideas of health come from, and how they become institutionalized, is powerful. As Cristina Douglas and Barbara Pieta put it, current work is increasingly emphasizing the "political and historical embeddedness of RECs [Research Ethics Committees] both in more recently independent countries and in countries where they have a longstanding presence in histories of colonisation" (2024, 7). As is evident throughout the chapters of this book, I ask how to think of the committee as an organizational practice. By positioning this network as the outcome of collaborations between people from different countries in the Asia-Pacific I want to show the ways ideas and practices of research ethics travel across both regional and international borders. In conversation with accounts of global health, I study the expansion of research ethics by demonstrating that the power and authority research ethics committees seek is gained by drawing together the worlds around them with those carried by the committee.

I therefore take readers to research sites that, at the start of the century, were viewed as peripheral by multi-center clinical trial funders and from centers of ethics governance such as Brussels, Geneva, or the U.S. National Institutes of Health in Maryland. A pivotal 2001 report from the U.S. FDA's parent organization, the Department of Health and Human Services, entitled "The Globalization of Clinical Trials" noted that the U.S. FDA received "minimal information on the performance of foreign institutional review boards . . . it does not inspect these boards, nor does it tend to receive much information from the host countries of these boards" (Rehnquist 2001, ii). In addition to being produced in reports, peripherality is sometimes perpetuated by researchers who may have sought out scientific or ethics training in settings other than where they now practice their research. The healthcare ethicist Bridget Pratt, applying Ramón Grosfoguel's concept of "epistemic location" (Grosfoguel 2007, 213; cited in Pratt 2023, 632), observes that where one is "from" is not necessarily where one thinks from (see also Sariola and Simpson 2019, 16). As Zhang and Burton point out, a "one-way diffusion of science and its governing practices has always been a myth" (2022, viii); and, writing from their research in China and India, they suggest that today's "new generation of internationally trained researchers are no longer satisfied with simply 'selling their production capacity' to global science . . . [t]hey want to be recognised as equal partners" (2022, 155). These ambitions are sometimes caught up in what Aihwa Ong calls "a deep nationalist fervor in the race to be 'number one' in cutting-edge sciences, with its promise of a lucrative science-driven economy" (2010, 3). In collaborative universes populated with notions of partnership as an "affective ideal," an ideal that may "work to mask deeply unfair institutional arrangements"

(Kenworthy et al. 2018, 1; see also Jensen and Winthereik 2013), how do people push for equal epistemic treatment?

Through my fieldwork, as I watched the deepening establishment of Western-originating ethics bureaucracies, I also saw FERCAP's work held differences at bay without capitulation to forms of bioethics that essentialized. How these divisions are held in place is the political engine of this book, and what lies behind the question of what committee worlds carry with them. Building on Betsey Brada's ethnographic work in Botswana—which figures pedagogy as capacity building, and capacity building as dispossession (Brada 2023, 149)—I explore the pedagogies involved in FERCAP's way doing of "capacity building" in research ethics, a capacity building that originates within the region. How does what Paige West calls the "rhetorical strategy" of capacity building (2016, cited in Brada 2023, 150) organize sites of refusal, reinterpretation, and local sense-making of the premises embedded in bioethics stories—and review practices—from the United States and the UK?

Over the past two decades, workshops, networking events, fellowships, and certification schemes have taken place around the world to "develop capacity" in research ethics. According to the WHO Clinical Trials Forum, these have been decades during which the "global clinical trials ecosystem has gained in complexity and in cost and lost efficiency, while capacity development has stalled in many places" (Moorthy et al. 2024, 126). Often ephemeral, without institutional footing or funded through soft money, a social researcher seeking to understand research ethics capacity building will need to trace its patchwork history across defunct websites and out-of-date CVs. Without such work on the fleeting—or, rarely, enduring—lives of capacity-building initiatives, and work with committees themselves, we know little about the logics, principles, and standards to which recently formed ethics committees or their members hold themselves, or the challenges they face. We know little about what happens when newly trained ethics practitioners bring back experiences from courses and fellowships overseas. And we know less about the interaction between those forms of training and local environments.

In addition to asking what worlds committees create, in this book I also explore the normative question of where practitioners think ethics should be located. It is a question that reaches beyond biomedicine into the strained environments of science and technology regulation, professional standards and today's resurgence in codes of conduct. It is a question being continually asked on the frontiers of scientific development, where researchers and their institutions grapple with "responsible research and innovation" (RRI), "ethical legal and social issues" (ELSI), and Research Integrity (RI), designed to bring "society and science" into dialogue in the innovation pressure cooker. As research environments across the Asia-Pacific region become increasingly competitive, with pressures and incentives mounting on researchers to demonstrate national progress and publication (Svare 2020), it is also an ethical question of what kinds of research ethics processes are present, how they are resourced, and the kinds of roles they are able to take on within institutions. Throughout this book, people struggle with knowing where to convene discussions labeled as "ethical," and the committee—as it appears in this book—is a partial answer.

Ethics committees are one part of the wider health research infrastructure, split by Ayo Wahlberg and colleagues into distinct "spheres" of governance, such as national discussions, laws, guidelines and standards, committees, and the "ethical interaction" between patients and clinicians (2013, 294). I focus on the committee as a social device to which questions of research ethics have been delegated. The ethics committee adjudicates not only the acceptability of a given piece of research, but—in the narrative of its origins—holds together a sense of trust in science. As Adam Hedgecoe and colleagues have argued, "we need to see RECs in their context, as part of an international regulatory system" not as "individual, discrete bodies in which ethical debates are played out in isolation" (2006, 486). Yet doubts about in what and in whom ethics should be located linger in the anxieties where audit cultures bloom, where everyday bureaucratic realities meet national histories of research, ambitious new university research policies, and the global priorities of pharmaceutical companies. Led by the concerns of those for whom ethics is a voluntary calling and those for whom it is a job, my work explores the relationship between formalized bureaucratic ethics and the place of the ethical everyday, examining social technologies aimed at inculcating ethical behavior. I ask both what worlds come with the committee, and what worlds they meet. Following Cristina's forum and their activities, I trace the distinct genealogies of practice that alternately locate ethics in systems and in persons. Ethics, in this book, is an everyday bureaucratic exercise, but, seeping out through informalities, are pressures, prompts, and expectations that practitioners adopt newly ethical subjectivities, too. Through following these practices, I have come to ask whether one type of behavior—the conduct of clinical trials—can be governed through another: the ethics assessment of research proposals by a committee.

Committee Worlds

Looking at the question in institutional terms, the answer is yes. Committees of many types have held anthropological and scholarly interest throughout the twentieth century, and in the chapters to come, we follow the life of a particular kind of committee through the initial two decades of the twenty-first. Readers who sit on committees as part of their everyday academic duties may well struggle with them as a topic of scholarly curiosity. Introducing my work over the years has commonly led to one of two responses: either looks of horror (how could you survive that fieldwork?!) and an instant glazing over, or, more commonly, a fellow ethnographer's sudden outpouring of their frustrating experiences with "the ethics committee" (Shore 2024). Colleagues in the social sciences continue to write about their sense of "lack of epistemological fit between ethnographic methods and ethics review paradigms" (Bell and Wynn 2023, 537), which turns, sometimes, to "bad-tempered criticism and barely contained outrage" (Hedgecoe 2020, 16). Even if they have not felt their own projects stymied by committee, committee roles in academia and "meetings" (Schwartzman 1989; Brown et al. 2017) more broadly are often seen as distracting from the core tasks of teaching and research, despite their oft-powerful function in shaping the environments in which those activities take place. In Tess Lea's terms, anthropologists are "inside [bureaucracy's] accrued manifestations" (2021, 69), and it can be difficult to analyze our way alongside these all too familiar, and heavily affective, things called committees. In sum, it feels for many like a stretch to attempt to bring an ethnographic "openness of wonder" (Ballestero 2019, 199) to such committees and their worlds as ethnographic objects.

Yet this is precisely what I aim to do. My initial research questions on how (and why) ethics decisions were apparently being taken in the "same" way in different places led me to ask why it was that the *committee itself* had become the default form for making these decisions. When committees captured the anthropological attention during earlier eras it was because they were—are—sites of power. Whether focusing on political organization in eighteenth-century Cherokee politics (Gearing 1962) or questions of authority and engagement with British colonial administrators across Africa (Richards and Kuper 1971), the issues with which ethics committees struggle, and which I take to be of ethnographic importance, are shared with this body of earlier scholarship. When I explore the labor, deliberations, and compositions of ethics committees, I put them in conversation with anthropology's prior structural-functionalist preoccupations with order, social organization, social control, the mechanisms by which colonial policy could be implemented—often through existing forms of committees (Richards and Kuper 1971). Like Audrey Richards, Adam Kuper, and the authors in their edited collection *Councils in Action*, I also consider who is in these groups, their roles, and their record keeping, alongside themes of witnessing, scopes of authority, limits of enforcement, conditions of legitimacy, challenges of budget, as well as the speed and style of oratory involved in processes of decision-making. Reviewing Richards and Kuper's collection, Wendy James critiqued the narrowness of the focus on the council "as a mechanism for getting things done" and leaving "unanswered the more fundamental question of the sources of consensus, opposition and action within the societies examined" (1975, 120).

It is with James's critique in mind that I inquire after "worlds" that committees carry with them. I aim to examine the workings of the committee while at the same time keeping in view the wider research environments they have been created to serve. But like these earlier ethnographers I think there is still a lot to learn from close observation of the power and play of discussion and oratory. I share with them a curiosity about who gets to speak (chapter 4), how a committee is put together (chapter 3), and the relationship between committees and judicial bodies (chapter 5). These themes remain relevant to an analysis of how people try to make committee work *work*. To earlier themes, I add new scholarly sensitivities drawn from the anthropology of documents, policy and bureaucracy, audits, and standards, making it meaningful to reexamine both their form (Jacob and Riles 2007) and the affective, "emotive dimension" (Navaro-Yashin 2007, 79) of ethics. Ethics as a bureaucratic apparatus carries and is borne by a "social repertoire of stories," stories that matter for how it is engaged with (Sansone and Bonanno 2025, 5). Thus, in indirect conversation with these earlier works across the decades, this book aims to provide a current analysis of "the committee" as a form, upon which future work in the anthropology of policy can build.

In addition to committee-focused scholarship, there is also a growing field of sociological and historical work dedicated to research ethics committees. Since the publication of Laura Stark's *Behind Closed Doors* (2012), ethics committee deliberation has become a serious ethnographic object. Her historical research and observations of "Adams," "Greenly," and "Sander State" IRBs provided a glimpse into discussion dynamics in the United States in the 2010s, opening up the study of "evaluation as a social process" (Stark 2011, 250). For Stark, this meant the opportunity to "explore the practice of statecraft and to consider its effects on knowledge production" (2011, 250), as she was writing from an environment where "the state" was and remains an active actor in research governance. In speaking of IRB members assessment of risks and safeguarding of participants rights, her board members "say that they do these things because they are moral imperatives and also because they are the law" (Stark 2012, 9). A key element of what makes Stark's research compelling is that it adds IRBs to a broader consideration of what she terms "declarative bodies" (2011, 233) through whom state power is issued, along with "data-and-safety monitoring boards, funding panels, editorial boards and film rating committees" (Stark 2011, 233). When Sarah Babb, writing a decade later, frames contemporary American IRBs as "compliance bureaucracy," she highlights their character as "nongovernmental office that uses skilled staff—compliance professionals—to interpret, apply, and oversee adherence to government rules" (2020, 5). She is critical of the marketplace of compliance that has arisen. But, as I aim to show, "compliance" has different meanings in my material, with its orientation toward "international" norms and documents, and the anticipatiory character it takes on. Returning to my opening vignette, the question posed to Cristina by the American makes a little more sense. "How can ethics be done in the absence of law?" he is asking, starting from a point of perceived absence.

Through the arguments of this book, I extend existing literature on ethics review committees in a number of ways. First, I am not offering a national history. The ambitions, policies, and regulations of nation states are crucial: They contribute to motivations both for committees and researcher, and constitute historical reasons for collaborations. However, I am telling the story of an NGO that makes use of and positions nation states in order—I argue—to sustain its regional project. By positioning the national ("local") regulations of any given committee alongside "international guidelines," they enable a nonnational entity to exert pressure, through its members and its practices, on countries to introduce their own procedures. Second, my analysis engages literatures in development and global health otherwise absent from ethics review committee scholarship, to argue for the importance of studying how bureaucratic and managerial forms operate as vehicles for new forms of outward-facing legibility and institutional resources. Scholarship of ethics committees within the United States of America, the UK, and Holland has foregrounded expertise, democratic reasoning, and trust, themes I also address. But I draw these concerns out alongside and under the heavy complexity of institutional under-resourcing, national competitiveness, anxieties of exploitation, and ambitions of researchers and their institutions to be internationally legible within the global community of scientific research. Third, most members on research ethics committees in this book are researchers, academics, or clinicians, working at hospitals or universities. They are not the professionalized corporate taskforce of Sarah Babb's U.S. American compliance bureaucracy, nor are they Adam Hedgecoe's "de-institutionalized" research ethics committees of the UK's NHS (Hedgecoe 2012, 81). As we shall see, staffing is a matter for how comittees are resourced. Finally, it matters that the "unit" of the committee in this book is not uniform or constant. As I discuss, the NGO operates through abstraction, leaving its embeddedness in the hands of committee members. The names by which committees go indicate the different schools of ethics review—and parts of the world—to which they are oriented. They are part of radically different national research climates, with distinct ambitions and priorities. In 2012, Adam Hedgecoe warned against mistaking the problems and roles of committees in one setting for those in another, arguing that "the best critiques of ethics review will be those that avoid sloppy elision between different systems either by focusing on the problems of one particular system, or by comparative work that emphasizes difference and variation" (2012, 80). One indicator of the different traditions has been what they are called: Institutional Review Boards? Ethics committees? Research ethics committees? In this book, these names are not closely tied to practices. While the "institutional" may have almost wholly fallen out of the U.S. system from which it originates with the advent of commercial review boards, the acronym is used, sometimes by practitioners, interchangeably with ethics committee. I follow practitioners' usage, pointing out where the instability of committee names has significance for a committee's orientation toward the U.S. or the WHO.

The people in this book take up committee work as a form of organized ethical reflection on matters of biomedical concern. They do so in a novel landscape of research ethics work, one which, since the turn of the twenty-first century, has emerged internationally. One of my tasks is not only to convey this landscape and its stakes, but also to illustrate how the anthropology of policy and bureaucracy more broadly can learn from NGO activities dedicated to ethics committee labor and their bridging work between international guidelines and local practices. The researchers and committee members I discuss are responding to decades-old policy initiatives to improve capacities in both research ethics—and scientific research more broadly. Participants in my research have sat on countless committees, international meetings, and fora to describe into being futures for research ethics that better suit their settings. From its origins in the tumult of biomedical research scandals and the formalization of committee practices in the United States in the years after the Second World War, the ethics committee—known as an Institutional Review Board (IRB) in the U.S. and aligned countries—has become integrated into what it means to make "good science" (Thompson 2013). Good science is, in turn, written into policies that offer norms of practice.

Globalizing Research, Globalizing Ethics?

Multi-national research is part of understanding and controlling diseases of global importance. From malaria to cancer, diabetes to heart disease, obesity to dementia, randomized controlled trials (RCTs) remain a powerful technology upon which evidence-based medicine rests (Brives et al. 2016). But where I start this story of globalized research—and globalized ethics—matters. Two key documents are the 2001 "The Globalization of Clinical Trials: A Growing Challenge in Protecting Human Subjects," produced for the Office of the Inspector General at the U.S. Department of Health and Human Services, and the 2002 Nuffield Council on Bioethics report on "The Ethics of Research Related to Healthcare in Developing Countries," produced in the UK by an independent charitable body funded since 1991 through foundations and the UK's Medical Research Council. Both were published against a backdrop of tense questions about dual standards in research, particularly the use of placebos and what reference point should be taken for the standard of care following HIV trials in Uganda (Angell 1997). The debates that ensued catapulted bioethics forward as a discipline with "global" ambitions (Have and Gordijn 2013), critics arguing that "ethics" risked becoming the uncritical smoothing of the path of flows of global capital, or excessively burdensome, slowing or derailing multi-site clinical trials with an excess of "local" demands, adjustments, or conditions. Researchers began to ask what it meant to "export" bioethics models, and arguments have been made for ethics as a technology of imperialism (Angell 1988; Benatar 2002), suggesting that when committees make decisions based on or compliant with international principles, they are not taking "local" values sufficiently into account. Sometimes it is suggested that committees do this to attract research; at other times committees are cast as ignorant, ill-informed, corrupt, or simply for show. In a letter to the U.S. NIH, Edward K. Mbidde, chairman of the AIDS research committee on the Uganda Cancer Institute, "charged that it is 'ethical imperialism' for outsiders to dictate to Ugandan researchers and IRBs what sort of research is ethical or unethical for Ugandans to carry out on their own people" (Mbidde 1997, cited in Macklin 2001, 25; see also Simpson 2003). In 2000, the Declaration of Helsinki had just been revised for the sixth time, stating that placebos should not be used when a known standard of treatment exists; although, as anthropologist Adriana Petryna observed some years subsequently, "if the ethics were unambiguous, the regulatory weight of the declaration was not. Pharmaceutical companies, already expanding operations abroad and calculating the economic advantages of placebo use [. . .] were eager to learn from regulators about the legal enforceability of the declaration while finding ways to continue the placebo" (2007, 30).

"The Globalization of Clinical Trials: A Growing Challenge in Protecting Human Subjects," which laid out the "growth of non-U.S. clinical drug trials" and the U.S. "FDA's capacity to assure human subject protections in these trials," was in part a reputational concern (Rehnquist 2001, i). The report put as one of its top recommendations that worldwide capacity in research ethics be improved, suggesting a role for the U.S. FDA to "help inexperienced non-U.S. institutional review boards build their capacity" (Rehnquist 2001, 18). In its letter of response, dated August 14, 2001, a wonky photocopy of the agency submission reads: "Agency response. FDA strongly supports this recommendation but cautions that the agency currently has virtually no resources available for this activity" (Rehnquist 2001, 30). While "foreign data" had been used within applications to regulators since the 1980s, the 2001 report asks the U.S. FDA to "examine ways in which it can obtain more information about the performance of non-U.S. institutional review boards reviewing clinical trials that provide data" (Rehnquist 2001, 17) . The agency responds that it is "largely unaware of government or independent agencies that currently and comprehensively assess performance of non-U.S. IRBs in a way that would be meaningful to the assurance of human subject protection in studies submitted to FDA" (Rehnquist 2001, 30). The report recommends that the U.S. Office for Human Research Protections encourage voluntary accreditation, suggesting a collaboration between the U.S. "FDA, NIH, and others, [who] can help develop such a system internationally" (Rehnquist 2001, iii). The second possible starting point, the U.K's Nuffield Council on Bioethics report "The Ethics of Research Related to Healthcare in Developing Countries," emerged from the same moment, focused more on the bioethical discussion than the regulatory one. Its recommendation, in bold, is that "all countries should establish an effective system for the ethical review of research, which includes the establishment and maintenance of research ethics committees that are independent of government and sponsors in research" (2002, xvi). Not in bold, the following sentence argues that research should be reviewed both in the sponsoring country *and* the countries where the research would take place—the "hosts"—and points to sponsors of research as those who should commit funds to supporting the development of ethics committees.

Informative though both these documents are of concerns and desires at the time, as Anna Tsing has it, "there is no reason to begin a retelling of global connections in imagined world centers such as New York, Tokyo or Geneva" (2005, 271). The starting points closest to the action of this book are the inaugural 1999 and 2000 meetings of the Global Forum on Bioethics in Research (GFBR), whose "originally stated purpose was [. . .] to provide an open and transparent dialogue between delegates from the global north and south about the ethical challenges they faced" (Littler et al. 2014, 5). These were "series of colloquia designed to examine conceptual and practical challenges arising from cross-cultural research and to provide guidance in improving institutional capabilities in bioethics in the developing world" (Loff et al. 2001, 63). The careers of many of FERCAP's founding members originated in the 1990s within the networks of UNAIDS (Mathur et al. 2023, 18) and the tense discussions of how research should take place across unequal borders. For those gathered at the GFBR forum meeting in 2000, it was a valuable space since, as its participants put it, "until recently no platform existed for individuals from the developing world who are responsible for the ethical conduct of research in their countries, to engage in dialogue about how these issues might be approached in their own countries and in international collaborative research" (Loff et al. 2000).

In these choices of origin stories, the existence of FERCAP as a network to build capacity in research ethics review is a response not to a single specific technology—biobanking, stem cell research, gene editing—but to the expansion of research practices themselves across national borders, and the need to manage differences. But they are tied together. One of the key protagonists in this book, Juntra Karbwang, who was working in Geneva at the WHO at the time, co-authored a letter of response to the international "Globalization of Clinical Trials" report. In it, she and her co-authors suggest that "ten years ago it would have been awkward to speak of the globalization of clinical trials, let alone title a pivotal report with such an ominous (and promising) burden)" (Karbwang et al. 2001, 1). They note the U.S. Inspector General's Report's findings in "shortcomings of current oversight systems for human subject protections" and argue that any "the globalization of research requires a global approach to developing ethical review" (Karbwang et al. 2001). The subtitle of the letter is "defining policy through action." Action is the word that propels her, and many who had gathered at the GFBR meetings, over the next twenty years and throughout the chapters of this book.

Standards for Ethics

Coordinating clinical research is work made possible through standards. Ethnographers in anthropology and STS have followed processes of standardization across sciences and countries for decades, from Linda Hogle's ethnography of attempts to standardize organ donation processes (1995) to Ann Zimmerman's critical exploration of data reuse in ecology (2008). Decades of work have shown that standards allow for "the consistent coordination of people and things in ways that would be difficult to achieve on an ad hoc basis" (Timmermans and Epstein 2010, 83). But standards for *ethics*?

As my fieldwork progressed, I quickly discovered the centrality of standards in research ethics capacity building. Two initiatives put them front and center. The first was the publication of the *Operational Guidelines for Ethics Committees That Review Biomedical Research* (World Health Organization 2000) and two years later, its accompanying volume *Surveying and Evaluating*

Ethical Review Practices (WHO/TDR 2002). Juntra Karbwang, one of the letter writers introduced above, appears in the opening pages of both documentss as project manager, at the top of lists of international experts. The guidelines in *Operational Guidelines* were developed at a series of meetings in Chiang Mai, Thailand; Arusha, Tanzania; Bethseda, Maryland, U.S.; and Bangkok, Thailand, over the course of five months starting from August 1999. The second—connected—initiative was called SIDCER, or the Strategic Initiative in Developing Capacity in Ethical Review. As I introduce below, this initiative was funded initially through grants from the WHO's Tropical Disease Research (TDR) unit in 2001. It was envisaged as a parent umbrella to the newly formed FERCAP, and to four other regional fora: the Pan-African Bioethics Initative (PABIN), Foro Latino Americano de Comités de Ética en Investigación de Salud (FLACEIS), Forum for Institutional Review Boards in Canada and the United States (FOCUS), and the Forum for Ethics Committees in the Confederation of Independent States (FECCIS).[2] It was a hugely ambitious undertaking, but the stakes were high. In slides from the first decade of SIDCER's life, its "mastermind" (Chokevivat 2011, 9) Juntra would end with a cartoon and a quote. The cartoon, created by the British political cartoonist Steve Bell in 1999, depicts three somewhat monstrous figures and the caption "Run for your lives! It's the conservative ethics committee!!" (see Figure 1).

On Juntra's slides, the cartoon was set next to a quote from Jon Nicholl, then-director of the Medical Care Research Unit at the University of Sheffield in the UK. He had written an opinion piece in the *British Medical Journal* (BMJ) lamenting the impractical state of ethics approval in the UK. His closing line, reproduced by Juntra, read: "For ethics committees to have become barriers to ethical research, which could improve health care, is certainly immoral" (Nicholl 2000, 127). The statement echoed Edward Mbidde's concern in the aftermath of HIV transmission studies, that "sponsoring agencies might slow down or stop the trials because of the ongoing debate about how best to conduct them" (1998, 155). When Juntra put in her presentation, she enrolled it in a wider project of wanting to get ethics committees up and running, so that research could take place. In her own words,

> differences in standards of ethical review inhibited the progress of research, raised questions of fairness and threatened the protection of the dignity and rights of research participants at local, national and international level . . .

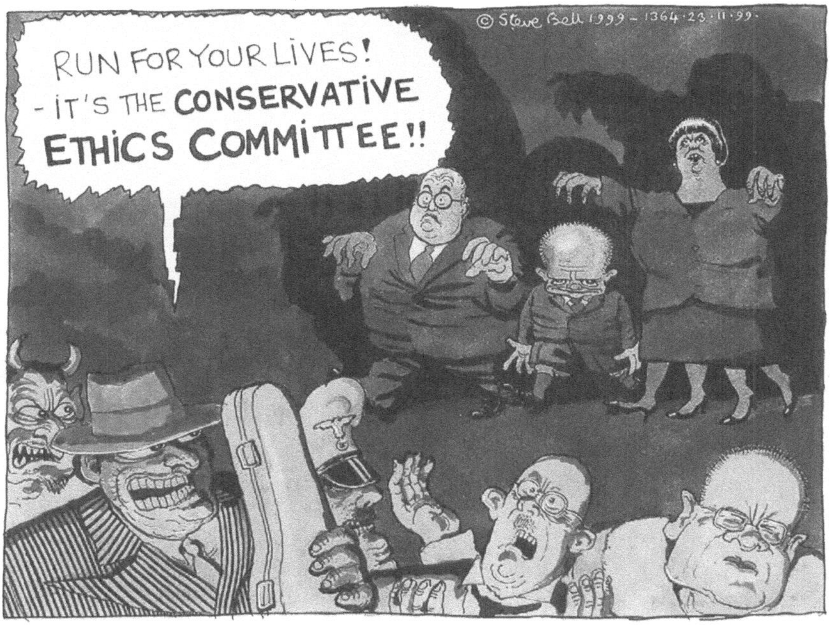

Figure 0.1. A cartoon used on Juntra's slides to convey the ethics of ethics committee work. Reprinted with permission. Copyright © Steve Bell 1999–All Rights Reserved.

> SIDCER was formed in 2001 to address these concerns by promoting responsible decision-making within countries and communities in which people, communities and values may be unfairly exploited. (Karbwang 2008)

The creation of standards for ethics has been done in the shadow of two powerful standardization regimes in biomedicine, both of which have also shaped the challenge of analysis in this book. The first is Good Clinical Practice (known by its acronym, GCP), an international harmonization effort in the 1990s to develop international guidelines for "more economical" use of resources. As its authors wrote, they sought the "elimination of unnecessary delay in the global development and availability of new medicines whilst maintaining safeguards on quality, safety and efficacy, and regulatory obligations to protect public health" (Molzon 2005). A note on the history and origins of GCP—a history not yet fully written[3]—is important both for the explicit values related in such declarations, and for the close relationship envisaged between ethics and science in GCP. It is described as both an ethical and scientific quality standard for the design, conduct, recording, and reporting of trials in which humans participate (ICH GCP 1996, 1). The authors offered readers the reassurance that

> compliance with this standard provides public assurance that the rights, safety and wellbeing of trial subjects are protected, consistent with the principles that have their origin in the Declaration of Helsinki, and that the clinical trial data are credible. (ICH GCP 1996, 1)

GCP was, at the outset, focused "on input by industry—the technical submission requirements for pharmaceuticals for human use" (ICH 2010, 2) and has continued to form a critical foundation for the mutual recognition of data across countries. "Compliance" with it makes data produced during research mutually available to regulators. It has, of course, had to change with the times. In 2015, commentators noted in an understated way that "a few technological changes that were unknown or in their infancy when the E6 Guidelines were issued include: the Internet, smart phones, electronic data capture, real time review of clinical data, drug development as a truly global enterprise, etc." (Widler et al. 2015).

It had a powerful reach: For Adriana Petryna, the ICH was a means of attracting pharmaceutical investment, and it created a push for countries to establish research ethics committees as part of compliance (2007, 31). While this is not a book about ICH-GCP, it is written in its shadow, and the themes that become salient are necessarily in conversation with sociological, socio-legal, and anthropological critique that has been leveled at the instrument over the years. For example, sociologists Kerry Holden and David Demeritt describe it as a "particularly effective form of standardization that allows scientific research to travel significant distances and still be relevant to dominant markets of the U.S. and Europe" (2008, 83). Michael D. E. Goodyear and colleagues have argued that "GCP is not an ethical code, but a procedural regulatory manual based on the regulatory framework of the U.S., Japan and Europe. Thus it is a description of existing procedures" (2009, 1559). And finally, the legal scholar Mark Flear, who has drawn attention to the "EU as an exporter of normative power through clinical trials abroad," points our gaze to how the narrowed form of "ethics," rooted in "consent and GCP," is "made marketable, that is, (re)shaped in ways that make them useful" (2014, 105).

The second standardizing technology casting its shadow in this book is the randomized controlled trial, or RCT. FERCAP has been building one of the core infrastructures that accompany this form of knowledge production, but it is important to remember that as a technology, the RCT continues to come under close critical scrutiny. Scholarship on the power RCTs hold over imaginations, with their "specialized focus on magic bullets" (Dumit and Sanabria 2022, 292), has been more vocal in recent years, and its limitations alongside projects of "alter-standardizing" better studied (Rosemann 2019). RCTs are not uniformly distributed or practiced: Some countries with whom FERCAP works have their own trials industry, while others may seek to become hosts, wanting to attract trials for their resources, contacts, and training opportunities as well as potential access to post-trial benefits and capacity building (Widger et al. 2022).

The standards that follow in this book are both aspirational and attainable, always shifting. They are without question, as scholars of standards have long argued, "infused with ethico-legal norms that are negotiated in spaces and that are always already both scientific and social" (Graham 2021, 263). But in the opening vignette, Cristina's invocation of the concepts "moral force" and "duty-based ethics" position herself and her organization along a different axis from techniques that rest solely on standards or bureaucractic virtues. Other things are happening here in this strained "cartography of pharmaceutical power and capital" (Aellah 2021, 70, drawing on Petryna 2009) where discussions of the intensified pressures of globalized research—including outsourcing, informed consent, group consent, undue inducement, the unfair proportion of risk to benefit, standards of care, the sharing of benefits, and biopiracy—take place. The question the American academic asked her betrays a sense of absence in the face of the project of "doing" a system: Where are the laws?

Guided by Cristina and her colleagues, I have sought to understand the ambitions, activities, and role of the Forum in research governance in the region they group as the Asia-Pacific. As scientists working in different countries enter into scientific collaborations (Wahlberg et al. 2013; Parker and Kingori 2016; Sariola and Simpson 2019) questions of research ethics, research infrastructure, and coordination arise. The Forum has aimed, since its inception, to systemize processes for research ethics. From its first meeting at the Royal Orchid Hotel in Chiang Mai, Thailand, in August 1999 (Chokevivat 2019),

FERCAP has grown into a network of over three hundred members, hosting an annual regional conference that brings together committee members from fourteen countries engaged in its work. Around the lunch table that April day, Cristina rested her project on the capacity to convince "important people," in the tacit absence of the "laws" sought by her interlocutor. The questions and chapters of this book stretch between the pole of enforceable legislation and that of moral force, examining the way ethics policies are interpreted and put into practice. They also stretch between that conversation and the present, where many of the countries in which FERCAP works have now adopted national guidelines and regulations focused on ethics review. The American academic, Dave, familiar with the legislative environment in the United States, was asking how ethical review could possibly operate in the absence of robust legislation: the force of the law. Cristina's response invokes another form of ethical practice, relationally and confidently built through the network of colleagues, peers, and friends convened around her, doing "capacity building" together.

In this book I bring the formalized, proceduralized shape that ethics has taken in contemporary medicine into conversation with critical perspective on genealogies of governance and standards. For anthropologists of policy, this means carving a path through scholarship on bureaucracy and cultures of audit, in a time when the limits to those forms of governance are being explored across disciplines. I have come to see that the tension pointed to by Cristina's conversation with Dave pervades numerous domains. The questions of the relationship between ethics and the law, and the difference between governing systems and governing selves, are far larger than ethics review committee work. Ethics committees are increasingly positioned at critical sites of scientific and technological advance, asked to assess both formal research occurring in hospitals and academic institutions, and newly formed to review research occurring in R&D spaces in industry (Sandler and Basl 2019; Friesen et al. 2021; Pater et al. 2022). But the pendulum swing between ethics as formalism and as everyday practice is particularly visible as committees travel to places where the implicit assumptions supporting the spread of audit are not given, and where audit itself is being reworked (Jensen and Winthereik 2013). As I studied the rapidly expanding network and traveled with its members to visit their committees, I came to better understand the models they were drawing from as they undertook their projects of capacity building.

Encountering the Forum through Collaboration

I first learned of the Forum that Cristina leads on my third day of fieldwork in Sri Lanka in March 2009. When I arrived with colleagues to the country's capital, Colombo, I was part of a UK research council grant on International Science and Bioethics Collaborations that sought to better understand the practical and conceptual implications of bioethical capacity building in international clinical trials and stem cell research. The "collaboration" of the project's title was critical, asking what happened when "discourses of development are reframed or replaced by those of collaboration, what kinds of socio-economic demands emerge and how are those formulated in the management of science across cultures" (Strathern et al. 2007). Answers emerging from that research have included a critical interrogation of the "collaborative impetus" (Konrad 2012, 8), a close analysis of the precarity of international collaboration in a "randomized controlled trial for the treatment of acute poisoning" in Sri Lanka (Simpson 2012, 154), and the "regulatory violence" at work across cultural, epistemic, economic, and power differences in regenerative medicine (Sleeboom-Faulkner 2025).

My colleagues Bob Simpson and Salla Sariola had worked with their local contact, Vajira Dissanayake, and set up a workshop with local speakers who would already be in town for the Sri Lanka Medical Association's annual conference, and together, they'd settled on the topic "Why Should We Be Concerned about the Ethics of International Collaboration" (Sariola and Simpson 2019, 145). In their discussion of the event, Sariola and Simpson review its overlaying of postcolonial critique, research extractivism, exploitation of vulnerability, and the local value of knowledge. For me, it was an intense entry point for fieldwork, its collaborative formation constituting what the anthropologist George Marcus (2008, 52) called a "para-site," a day of interests shared between us as researchers and our interlocutors. Dr. Hemantha, one of our Sri Lankan co-organizers, opened the morning session by speaking about collaboration from the point of view of his role as a member of an ethics committee. His tone was cautionary. He and his fellow committee members, he said gravely, "often only think of the positive side of collaboration, of all there is to be gained. We must never forget there is a negative side as well." He switched to his first slide. An image of shaven-headed women being paraded through the streets of Second World War France. "These women were collaborators," he said. Then: "I fear this. I fear this. If something goes wrong, we could be paraded around in the press. We have to be acutely aware we could be accused of colluding in exploitation. New colonialism, sweatshops."

The "parading" of an ethics committee member through the press was not unthinkable in Sri Lanka at that time. After the 2004 Boxing Day tsunami, both aid and research rushed to Sri Lanka's devastated southern coast, prompting public and heated debate about the ethics of disaster research and the absence (or controversial presence) of local research permissions (Sumathipala 2006; Citraningtyas et al. 2010). What kind of knowledge was being gained from and through these studies? Where were questions of ethics in disaster research? Appeals were made to journal editors to "insist on proof of ethics approval from the country where the data were collected" when papers were submitted (Sumathipala and Siribaddana 2005, 1419).

While research can bring financing, resources, materials, and training, it can also be extractive, oriented exclusively toward the priorities of external funders, and take data out of countries, with the resulting drugs never made available in the country where they were tested (Petryna 2007; Flear 2014). These are core issues of research ethics. So, while scientific and health research *can* be portrayed as an opportunity for increased exposure to the international economies of research, it may not always be so. Invoking the language of ethics is a powerful tool within this contested world where the question of research "for whom" lingers nearby: The *accusation* of unethical undertakings may be enough to stop research (Sariola and Simpson 2019). Dr. Hemantha's wariness of the "promissory term" (Brown 2015; Moyi Okwaro and Geissler 2015) collaboration contains the potential for this switch in collaborative meaning. Are the relations (and what they bring) welcome? Who decides?

Responding to both Dr. Hemantha's presentation and the theme of the workshop, Cristina stood to introduce the Forum of Ethics Review Committees of Asia and the Western Pacific, or FERCAP. Answering the question of "who decides," her presentation foregrounded the labor of ethics review committees. She presented FERCAP as a grassroots initiative originating in Thailand and run by volunteers, and outlined the reasons it had been set up. Large populations in China, India, Indonesia, Pakistan, Bangladesh, and Japan, she explained, represented vast markets for pharmaceutical products in development, and "we expect therefore that this area is going to be a site for different types of clinical trials." Anticipating clinical research arriving from well-funded sponsors, she pointed to ethics committees as those who stand between international researchers or pharmaceutical companies and local populations as the first—or only—mediating contact. In 2005, working with, and as the regional offshoot of, the public-private partnership called the Strategic Initiative in Developing Capacity in Ethical Review (SIDCER), her NGO had introduced a "recognition program," known colloquially as The Survey, to help newly established committees organize themselves, figure out how to operate, and fit in with certain international standards.

The kind of work Cristina was doing, particularly the Recognition Program, fascinated me. In contrast with the other presentations of the day, its scope went far beyond the single case study or dilemma. It represented an attention to ethics distinct from philosophical anxieties present in the books and articles I had been reading prior to beginning my field research. It dealt directly with convening meetings, deliberation, and the challenges of making international research happen. Was it bioethics? If not, what was it? Although over the next few years I took part in many more events like the one that day in Colombo, this first workshop touched upon the "fine line" walked by ethics committees in managing research collaborations, bringing into the light some of the anxieties experienced by committees that must not only evaluate a research proposal, but often do it from a "somewhere" that globalized science acknowledges as a site of data, but rarely as a site of its own ethical expertise. As colleagues and I observed at the time, the day brought the decisions of ethics committees *here* into sharp relief, risking being on the one hand "too restrictive [. . .] impeding scientific and economic development" or, on the other, showing "excess permissiveness," risking accusations of being "complicit in abuse, injustice or exploitation in research" (Simpson et al. 2010, 114).

Cristina became my guide in this research, and as a social scientist herself, she understood how and why the NGO might make an interesting object of study. She began her own academic career in history in the Philippines in the 1970s, followed by an MA in Asian Studies, and a PhD in Philippine Studies in Quezon City at the University of the Philippines Diliman (Ong et al. 2019, 3). Prior to her involvement in FERCAP, Cristina was well established at the University of the Philippines Manila, having started as an instructor in 1973 and being promoted to a full professorship in 1997. She became involved in research ethics committees (RECs) in the late 1990s as a social scientist who, her own words, "voiced out community concerns in a biomedical committee . . . there was no model to follow and we devised our own means to review clinical trials submitted to the committee" (Torres 2011, 43). In 2003, she embarked on a WHO-NIH Fogarty Bioethics Fellowship. In her telling, it was this time in the United States working for Western IRB, in Olympia, Washington, where her career developed in a new direction. Here, she met Juntra and was invited to become the FERCAP coordinator. Throughout my fieldwork, I witnessed the strengths of this perhaps unlikely collaboration between a clinical pharmacologist and a historian. Together, they made it through the long hours of travel, days of Survey schedules, and many, many meetings with a shared intensity for research ethics, similar sharply perceptive critique, a joy in the work, and ready laughter. Like Juntra, Cristina is firm in her knowledge and authority, and she is highly experienced. She delivers her critiques of committees with a lightness and encouragement, one sometimes laced with incredulity. While survey work was always serious business, it could also become funny that a committee had imported wholesale SOPs from a committee in the United States, complete with references to the Common Rule and HIPAA, the U.S. Health Insurance Portability and Accountability Act (1996). In Cristina's retelling of the discovery ("But your country is not governed by HIPAA!"), it was a moment of comedy rather than reprimand.

When we first met in Colombo, she had been leading FERCAP for five years, having been recruited by Juntra to take up the role. It involved months of travel, with some years with no more than two weeks in one place, and Cristina became known for the pasalubongs she would return to share with friends and colleagues in Manila. Realizing how substantial the role was becoming, she in turn had recruited Atoy Navarro, another historian from the Philippines, who worked alongside her in the Thammasat offices in Bangkok for many years, taking over the management of Survey coordination, trainings, and FERCAP publications. Atoy's deep knowledge of international guidelines and commitment to understanding histories of research in the Philippines meant he and Cristina have a shared perceptiveness of the social science dimensions of research ethics, foregrounding, in their terms, issues of access and justice as part of the administration of the network.

A Fieldworker Amongst the Auditors[4]

In the twelve months following, and at Cristina's invitation, I immersed myself in the network's activities. When I received an email from Cristina with an attached pdf document that outlined the network's upcoming Surveys, their dates and locations, as well as the trainings and workshops they had committed to run that year, I began to plan. I made an itinerary that allowed me to follow as many of the NGO's activities as my scholarship and budget allowed. While the network has its headquarters in Bangkok, Thailand, I joined activities across five different countries, showing up in hospitals and universities in Beijing and Guangzhou, Manila and Colombo, seeing offices and conference rooms, participating as a "foreign observer" or "local trainee" in workshops. I heard introductions to biomedical research ethics delivered over and over again, met hundreds of students for whom research ethics was an add-on to their existing biomedical trainings. I have a drawer of certificates of attendance, printed in color on glossy paper, adorned with the logos of SIDCER, FERCAP, WHO-TDR, the institution, and bordered with patterns.

During research, I kept some, though by no means all, of the hours that the Surveyors did, arriving on site by eight, not leaving until nine or ten at night. On days we finished "early" there would be homework: the review of a section of Standard Operating Procedures (SOPs). I would sit on hostel beds, going through the points one by one. Fieldnotes from such evenings read as alien poetry, and it is now difficult to recall accurately the state of mind that produced them: "Chapter Eight, Page 93: Inconsistency between 8.1 'special meeting' and 8.3 'emergency meeting'—or rather, is 'emergency meeting' a 'special meeting'?; Page 94, 8.3.3.2.2: Possible activities listed are inconsistent with the description of Scope. Page 97: Suggest logbook for phone calls." I would take these notes to the meetings the following day, and, wanting to make myself useful during Survey activities, I joined the teams who trawled through tall stacks of research protocols with translators, checklist in hand.

Understanding how FERCAP worked was ethnographically possible for three key reasons. First, I hold two "strong" passports, was not kept waiting for visas, and was affiliated with both a UK funder (with a fieldwork budget that allowed for considerable travel) and a UK university. These proximities smoothed access (Valdez 2023, 194). Second, English was the operating language of the network, and even while committee meetings were held and minutes produced in Thai, Mandarin, and Tagalog, the discussions, documentation, and evaluation all took place in English. The NGO's policy of encouraging committees to build expertise and documentation in their own languages resulted in translators being on hand for international surveyors, translators who also supported me during committee meeting observations. Third, this field site already had categories into which an ethnographer fitted, and that predated my presence: I could move through the field as a "foreign observer," sometimes taken to be an ethicist. While my presence was sometimes questioned with curiosity, it was rarely challenged with hostility or objection. I was sometimes assumed to be medically trained, some kind of expert in ethics, and occasionally a useful "international" dimension for the NGO. I could share with trainees (of all ages) a student status. Since I was surrounded by medical and academic professionals of different kinds, they understood what research meant, even if they did not always see how observing their classes constituted the kind of data collection they recognized. These professionals also published: Throughout this book, I draw on their scholarship—the self-documentation of the network as well as members' journal articles, blog posts, and presentations—to augment and support the findings of my fieldwork. There was a research ethics to studying research ethics. Several of the committees whose work I observed while part of studying the NGO reviewed my research proposal to study research ethics committees, creating loops of assessment whereby my research passed through under the assessment of the committees whose assessment procedures I wanted to get to know. While I was often studying "up," working with professionals with many forms of power, I was also dependent on committees' willingness to be observed *beyond* the observations they were already inviting through the NGO. Some asked me to sign NDAs about the protocols I would hear discussed and noted I should write this down, as evidence of their compliance with ethical practice.[5]

I combined an ethnography of a multi-sited NGO with an ethnography of audit, bureaucracy, and standards; to this I added ethnography at conferences, committee meetings, and close reading of documents in a field that produces many accounts of itself. While seeming to resemble increasing multi-sitedness of clinical trials, my fieldwork design was resolutely not one of methodological mimicry, with the imagined outcome being a larger sample size, more perspectives, resulting in a greater view on the "whole" work of the organization under study. Nor am I offering a quantitative "adding on" of sites to make up some purported whole. I followed FERCAP's work in the way that one might follow the life of an emerging technology or international science collaboration, inquiring into the work, motivations, and hopes of its members, tracing a system of knowledge. My ethnography is as much about observing trainings and conferences, and participating in the sociality that comes along with "building capacity" as it is observing committee meetings. Immersed in the participant observation role of surveying and critically assessing ethics review committees, I sometimes found it hard to stay an ethnographer and not slip wholly into the role of trainee auditor. While the topic of this book and the stakes held in mind by the people in it are both highly serious, there was also a lightness to the fieldwork. The people I talk about enjoyed one another's company and joked easily about bureaucratic work and its challenges. One evening in the spring of 2010, a Survey in Bangkok just complete, we were driven by our hosts to a canalside restaurant, and turned to the meanings of one another's names. Juntra, for the full moon on the day she had been born. Banana, meaning easygoing. "IRB is not banana," Cristina had responded quickly. No, replied the chair, casting a hand over our desserts of durian, mango, and the less loved jackfruit ice cream, "IRB is jackfruit!" So while I traveled to many different committees, the people I met became familiar as *they moved too*, conducting trainings, assessments, and meetings. I spent four months at the offices of the Colombo Medical Faculty Ethics Review committee, Sri Lanka, and for each of the subsequent fifteen committees with whom I had contact, I either observed their activities through the FERCAP Survey, met members at trainings, or sought interviews through contacts. The field-based research consisted of six months in Sri Lanka (March–July 2009, February–March and May 2010), resulting in contact with four committees; a month in Thailand (March–April 2010), largely interview- and workshop-based, contact with one committee; three weeks in the Philippines (April 2010), contact with three committees; three weeks in Taiwan (May–June 2010), contact with four committees; and just over a month in China (June 2010 and November 2010), contact with three committees. I returned to Bangkok in 2017, participating in the Surveys of a further two committees in Thailand and meeting up with many prior interviewees. In 2018, I attended the annual conference at the Chang Gung Memorial Hospital in Taipei. That year, over six hundred participants took part, from what FERCAP called their stakeholders: regulators, scientists, funders, industry representatives, educators, and, of course, committee members.

In social and cultural anthropology, PhD students and their supervisors "worry about the 'feasibility' of multi-sited projects" (Sunder Rajan 2021, 33), with reason. In addition to the time constraints of doctoral programs and complexities of language competence, there is concern for future employment prospects in departments organizing hiring by the "silos for scholarship" (Mitchell and Rao 2013, 135). Ethnography responds to the demands of its subjects. To a scaled imagination, it seems to be a challenge that its "problems"—think utopian deserts (Günel 2019), obesity (Yates-Doerr 2015), or climate adaptation (Vaughn 2022)—are "of global scale and complexity," while its method "in its very conception is oriented toward the local, the particular, and the contingent" (Sunder Rajan 2021, 1). In Ayo Wahlberg's terms, it is an "assemblage ethnography," responding to "a globalizing world where technocratic organization and technoscientific expertise continue to impact on and shape the lives of people everywhere" (Wahlberg 2022, 25). If I recount my fieldwork through the organizing device of a nation state, the impression is one of disjointedness. Yet—and this is crucial for conceptualizing both regional NGO work as an ethnographic site and understanding this particular network of people—I met the same people over and again, in remarkably similar looking offices in different countries, at different temperatures and times of year. Encounters with one facilitator spanned Colombo in March 2009, to Chiang Mai, Thailand, in November that same year; by March 2010 we were attending the same workshops in Chiang Mai, and the following month we met up again in Manila to review and assess an ethics committee in the Philippine capital. We saw each other again in Beijing, Shanghai, and Guangzhou for assessments of committees during June, then in November at the annual conference. When I returned to the field in the northern hemisphere summers of 2017 and 2018, we assessed committees in Bangkok together, and discussed recent developments like protocols for data sharing, the European General Data Protection Regulation (GDPR), and new software packages for supporting ethics review. Their work has continued, season after season, and I will catch photos uploaded to organizational Facebook pages, where small groups of smiling, tired people stand holding certificates at the end of long courses and conference days.

NGO members were and remain highly mobile, many of them scientists themselves (Sleeboom-Faulkner 2019). Since the normalization of digital conferencing technologies during the pandemic, there is even greater scope for holding meetings online, through the network's existing links. Speaking again with Cristina in the spring of 2025, I found her on Zoom, equipped with a professional stock image background of a generic minimalist living room.

The following day, she would be delivering another online training, this time "in" Indonesia, on the latest revisions of the Declaration of Helsinki (WMA 2024), the changes to ICH-GCP (ICH GCP 2025), and the new Benchmarking initiative of the WHO (World Health Organization 2023). Asking after my current employment—at the IT University in Denmark—she warmly invited me to present at the next FERCAP conference, to think of my new expertise as relevant to FERCAP members, now facing research applications based on synthetic data sets and AI landing on their desks. Relationships maintained through the ambient awareness of social media, along with return visits over the years, make for a "patchwork" of knowledge built from longstanding shared interests (Günel and Watanabe 2024, 135).

NGO Ethnography

Studying NGOs means "following." Recalling David Mosse's ethnography of "a joint government international NGO-private sector" project, Josiah Heyman suggests that the "dialectic between the narrative of a cohesive project and the reality of a multi-sited (geographically and socially) network of semi-incoherent voices, activities, and materializations" is needed for ethnographers to understand bureaucracy "as a life world and power process across many domains" (2012, 1275). In this book, I am less concerned with what this NGO is and more with what it does—its practices, processes, and context (Lewis and Schuller 2017; Pickering-Saqqa 2023). FERCAP has worked across countries, conducting surveys and trainings in Bhutan, Ethiopia, Indonesia, India, Japan, South Korea, Kazakhstan, Myanmar, Malaysia, Nepal, the Philippines, Sri Lanka, Taiwan, Thailand, and, until 2016, mainland China. In line with research on the practices of NGOs, in this book I am curious about *how* they do this. I agree with Steven Sampson that the anthropology of organizations has a lot to offer the study of NGOs—from the "pursuit of professionalism" (2022, 116) to the development of its own documentation, history, and techniques. I would add two seemingly separate dimensions: the presence of deep friendships, sustained by long hours and many years of common activity, and an appreciation of audit and its accompanying socialities. These literatures help me attend to the practical, organizational, and subtle mobility of the form research ethics takes in this book: This ethics has "a kind of institutional and conceptual penchant to create templates that pass virtually undetected across international frontiers" (Simpson 2012, 156).

Even if the organizational and managerial techniques I study are sometimes hard to pull to the ethnographic surface, that is not to say that FERCAP as an NGO has no struggles in crossing—or making—such international frontiers. Early in my fieldwork, emails circulated, bouncing between representatives of the pharmaceutical company Roche and university lecturers in Philippine universities, and on to philosophers: Who was FERCAP to "accredit" ethics committees? Questions arose about its sources of legitimacy (Lister 2003; Howell et al. 2020), as a nonstate actor. Through SIDCER, it had received funding from the World Health Organization's Tropical Disease Research (TDR) arm, itself financially supported by UNICEF, UNDP, the World Bank, and WHO. Early organograms showed a plethora of arrows pointing inward to a central bubble labeled "SIDCER" from other entities: the EFGCP (the European Forum on Good Clinical Practice), PATH (U.S. public-private), MFES (The Middleton Foundation for Ethical Studies), as well as PHRP, ICM, and Private Sectors IFPMA and WIRB (Western IRB). When SIDCER's launch was written up in *Nature Medicine*, the headline read "WHO and Industry Combine to Form Ethics Body" (Dickson 2002), specifying that "SIDCER hopes to attract money from the pharmaceutical industry through its trade organization, the International Federation of Pharmaceutical Manufacturers Association," whose officials argued that it would be "in the interests of the industry as a whole to secure a greater international recognition of the ethical reviews carried out in individual countries, as this would make it easier to persuade regulatory bodies in one country to accept the results of trials carried out in another" (2002, 645). WHO-TDR remained the primary source of FERCAP's support, and when that period of funding eventually ended, the network became self-sustaining through Survey and Conference fees. The question of who *should* be doing something like training or assessing research ethics committees has not vanished, but it has changed shape. For the period of my fieldwork as well as now, FERCAP was operating as a vehicle for "capacity building" across a range of highly diverse nation states. What were the contestations over epistemic authority, who should set the standards, and should they enable or constrain? Who should do this kind of recognition of committee work? While it has come to be agreed that governance over biomedical research is needed, the question of how it can be both effected and enforced varies.

As a study of policy, my work follows Tess Lea's tactics of policy ecology (2024), although I had no term for it at the time of my fieldwork. I entered the field with an interest in documents and decisions, but then I saw how much material conditions mattered. Lea's temporal dimension has come into view over the years I have continued to follow FERCAP. While its commitment to capacity building already gives the network a particular "vernacular timespace" (Bryant and Knight 2019, 35)—future making—the stories of research ethics past continued to saturate trainings and rationales for the need for committees in the first place. Few of these stories belonged to the places where trainees worked, something that FERCAP has sought to address (see chapter 8). This is a network of professionals who also publish, whose research I cite in this book, and whose key figures have been honored with Festschrifts and, sadly, obituaries, recalling their contributions to making the network over the decades (Kant and Mathur 2023, 224; Lea 2024, 4).

I have therefore not written a series of ethnographies of biomedical ethics in each of these *nation states*. Rather, as I discuss in chapter 1, I have foregrounded the work of the network as a *regional* forum. The nation state matters to this book. The countries where FERCAP works have radical differences in health systems, research needs, regulation, and law, as well as degrees of international collaboration and histories of research. By foregrounding the "human subject"—now the "human participant" (Resneck 2025, 15)—the network makes nation state a secondary question as it draws on and contributes resources—PowerPoint slides, guidelines, training initiatives, standards—to committees around the world. My research sites are where members of the network are, the places they make, and the people who work with them.

My chapters show Cristina and Juntra's leadership, expertise, and advocacy. There is a narrative risk of positioning these women as the "heroes" from whom all action flows. Their vision, energies, skills, expertise, and commitment are critical to understanding the network's activities. However, I take due warning from Joe Dumit and Emilia Sanabria's reading of science fiction author Ursula Le Guin. As she wrote, it is easy to tell hero-hunter stories and "hard to tell a really gripping tale of how I wrestled a wild-oat seed from its husk, and then another, and then another and then another, and then another" (Le Guin 1989, 165, cited in Dumit and Sanabria 2022, 292). Heroic ways of narrating lend themselves to "magic bullet" drug policies and research protocols. I do not want to replicate in my narration of the NGO and its work the heroism that Dumit and Sanabria critique: Neither FERCAP nor its work is a "magic bullet." Instead, I foreground Cristina and Juntra's expertise alongside their many colleagues—leaders and experts in their own right—who have constituted the Forum. These colleagues have built on FERCAP's techniques to further committee organization in their own countries, used its materials and formats to establish national fora for the discussion of research ethics, mentored and supported others, and encouraged other volunteers. Over the long years of networking and capacity building, they have sat together and wrestled seeds from their husks. Although their names do not appear in this book, they have been, and remain, crucial. As you read, they sit around committee tables, and the committee—being the product of a specific history of biomedical experimentation in Europe and North America—requires me to reconstitute what an ethics committee is from these new sites of its practice.

When I began my research, I had expected to do my fieldwork in Sri Lanka, working closely with committees across the country. Cristina's presentation that day—combined with the challenges of traveling and working in Sri Lanka during the intensification of conflict that came to mark the final months of Sri Lanka's civil war (Uyangoda 2010; Ganguly 2018)—made necessary a new set of locations for my exploration of capacity building in research ethics. My brief within the wider research project through which my study was funded was to study capacity building in ethics review, but also to examine the consequences of the fact that "most of the concepts and international regulatory principles in use continue to be derived from Western cultural values (Hess 1995, 2007; Nader 1996; Harding 2006)" (Strathern et al. 2007). Inspired by Cristina's talk, I thought that by following the capacity-building work of the FERCAP network, I could explore this statement empirically by studying how ethics committee work was being taught and promoted as a form of scientific governance, making the Asia-Pacific region into a distributed field site, and following practitioners on their long journeys to understand the challenges to which their work responds.

Capacity Building

Juntra was one of my key interlocutors and one of the women at the center of FERCAP's activities. Her career, featured in a 2024 *Women in Science* "storytelling showcase" (WHO 2024, 29–30), is an international patchwork of medical practice, global advisory roles, and academic positions in Thailand and Japan. After a BA in chemistry at Rosary College in Illinois, she earned her MD at South Western University in Cebu City, the Philippines, before continuing to a PhD at the University of Liverpool in the 1980s. From there, a combination of WHO advisory and academic positions followed, at WHO-TDR, Mahidol University in Thailand, and Nagasaki University in Japan. Juntra is a slight woman, fast moving, precise, and direct. She both thinks and speaks rapidly. Narrating how she moved into the world of ethics from her career in pharmacology, Juntra told me that "before," during her time as a researcher, she was happy when her papers were published. She spent years building an international research career, receiving TDR grants "to work on clinical pharmacology of mefloquine and artemisinin" (WHO 2024, 29). But that happiness, she said, was different from the pleasure she got from being involved in FERCAP: "I don't have grants to hand out, but I do have opportunities. When I see an opportunity for others, I connect them and give it to them. I don't feel like I'm working!" As we worked together over the years, I came to understand how her philosophy toward work combines her Buddhist outlook with a deep appreciation of quality management, attention to detail, and very high expectations of others. As much as she took satisfaction from her work, as a novice ethnographer, I was awed by the breadth of her knowledge, reach of her networks, precision of her expertise, and determination of her vision. At one point, she casually mentioned over lunch that I might write up my findings about FERCAP's work in the *New England Journal of Medicine*, a publication venue that was far beyond my imaginings, but well within hers. Her singular vision is present in SIDCER's founding documents, where the text describes plans for the new initiative: "SIDCER not only helps build in-country human subjects protection programs but is also a way to measure and provide accountability for the quality and effectiveness of ethical review worldwide" (Karbwang Laothavorn 2011, 11).

In a conversation we had early in my research, Juntra commented that during her work with the World Health Organization in Geneva, she had seen people *imagining* the issues they thought might be relevant in Vietnam, Cambodia, the Philippines, or India from their tables during in-house ethics review meetings. From these meetings, she had concluded that such committees simply did not have the knowledge to assess what would be acceptable locally. Geneva was too far away, too removed: "Review *has* to come from within the country," she told me. In a published opinion piece, she put it just as strongly: "It is no longer acceptable to overlook deficiencies in ethical review and rely on informed consent practices developed by researchers in very different cultures thousands of kilometers away" (Karbwang and Crawley 2007). Juntra's conclusion is a political critique of a landscape of intellectual and scientific power that would position good review *far* from the places where research will take place.

Similarly critical of flying visits and brief trainings, Nancy Kass, a health policy bioethicist at Johns Hopkins University in the United States, argued at the turn of the century that "short workshops cannot effect a sustained impact on their own [. . .] Without sustained local presence, it is unrealistic to imagine that ethics training ultimately will have much impact. And to state the obvious, it is both impractical and inappropriate for that role to be served by a transient professional from the outside" (Kass, cited in Eckstein 2004). Echoing Kass many years on, the medical anthropologist Claire Wendland, commenting on medical training workshops in Malawi, observes that "even when conducted locally, [workshops] are often designed and taught by consultants with little knowledge of epidemiological patterns of available infrastructure" (2016, 420). Looking at the impact of such events, scholars suggested that short-term training may reinforce existing disparities (Wagner et al. 2001; Shrum 2005; Ulrich 2011) or, as Wendland remarks, even be "dangerous" (2016, 421) within a landscape of "projectification" (Meinert and Whyte 2014).

For Juntra, review at a distance was not just inadequate; the current inequalities in review capacity were unjust. As a Thai researcher working in the WHO, she pointed out to her colleagues that when "Geneva" conducts reviews, "the power stays with Geneva." She explained that this left collaborating partners reluctant to try and seize the decision-making power to invite research into the country—and without the power to refuse projects they did not want. Her contention over many years that research review should (and could) take place in the countries where research took place led to questions from her Geneva-based colleagues: What evidence do you have, they asked, that this kind of ethical review is possible, in the countries where you work? There was an urgent need to create this evidence. Documents from the first meetings of the Global Forum on Bioethics in Research show an early focus on distributive justice and "fundamental questions of resource allocation, inter-country disparities, decision-making and balance of power" (Leng 1999). Participants noted that "since there is no standard law and practice in this regard for research conducted by all countries in the region, the meeting agreed to proceed with two matters: (1) to develop guidelines for the establishment of a research ethics committee; (2) to establish a regional research ethics committee forum and encourage each country to establish one" (Chokevivat 2019, 1145). Recalling the founding workshop in Chiang Mai, Thailand, in 2000, Vichai Chokevivat, the network's founding chair whose CV at the time included eleven years of rural medical practice in Thailand as well as many years of work in the Ministry of Public Health, wrote that

> we noted that working with government will be very difficult and very slow because of too much red tape. So instead of working with government, we chose to start from scratch and create our own organization starting with the participants of the seminar. (Chokevivat 2011, 7)

This origin story shows that FERCAP's foundation was not an "internationalization" of an existing NGO or a donor-driven initiative (Pickering-Saqqa 2023). The form of capacity building FERCAP chose was based on initiative and operations. While as an NGO it risked being seen as "weakening" or even replacing state-organized research ethics infrastructure (Bernal and Grewal 2014, 4), its members were well positioned in their own countries to use its existence to lobby for national change—something that they have done over the years. By, in its terms, "operationalizing," participants took hold of documentation that already existed and got on with the work of training new committees.

But which documents to choose? In Chokevivat's account above, it was Dr. Francis Crawley, a philosopher with longstanding expertise on research ethics, who used those five months between meetings to prepare "the terms of reference (TOR) for FERCAP" and made a first draft of what "became our *Silver Book*" (Chokevivat 2011, 7). The "Silver Book"—as I discuss in chapter 1—departed significantly from ethics guidance that existed and oriented itself in a promissory way to the future. Many of the Forum's most active members hope that they are working themselves out of a job and that capacity will, at some future date, be built. But the question then, as now, is what does "ethical enough" look like? And to what extent is this capacity building from *within* the region? Who, or what, is making whom ethical? To these questions, in this book I offer an ethnographic view on the different starting points of committees set up in countries with distinct regulatory landscapes, virtues of science, and histories of research. I do so with Tania Li's reminder to ask "how programs of improvement are shaped by political-economic relations they cannot change; how they are constituted . . . by what they exclude" (2007, 4). Instead of recounting national milestones, or imagining a landscape of compliance wherein progress is measured "in terms of the degree to which techno-rational systems of the West are imitated at the periphery" (Sariola and Simpson 2019, 10), I aim to ground both the "how" and the "why" of research ethics.

FERCAP's capacity building starts with people. Ethics appears as a solution to a failed science, an ethics of "research" whose practitioners, after the Nuremberg trials, cannot be entrusted to their professions or consciences. In Lea's terms, we need to listen for the "hauntings" within the practice, the "prior concepts, latent archetypes, moral imperatives and civic expectations" (2024, 3)—the unspoken atmospheres of what *could* happen if committees do not review. By attending to how FERCAP seeks to make particular types of people, I show, as the historian Steve Shapin does, "how and why people and their virtues matter to the making and the authority of late modern bodies of technological knowledge" (2008, 3). Shapin points out that in order to give an account of why personal virtue "*still matters*" he must also give an account of "why it is so widely said that it does not matter" (Shapin 2008, 11). This emphasis on personal virtues shifts us to the second side of the question: "how to get people to *do* things," with the emphasis on getting them to do something, what we tend to call governance. "Late modernity," writes Shapin, "is supposedly marked by the extension of impersonal means of control to ever new domains, ultimately bringing all of social life under the sway of impersonal reason" (2008, 9). He remarks that

> it would be convenient to be able to tell a story of linear transition from [. . .] a sacred to a secular world, from trust-in-familiar-people to anonymous trust in impersonal standards and faceless institutions; from virtue to institutional control as a solution to problems of credibility and authority. (2008, 17)

However, as his circumspect tone indicates, this is not the case. In the chapters that follow, I explore FERCAP's standardization agenda alongside its reliance on "familiar people," asking how the two successfully coexist. In distinguishing the work of FERCAP from a bioethics NGO, FERCAP's members pointed to guidelines "already there," arguing that the work they did was implementation, or *operationalization*. Researchers in public health and medical ethics have called for empirical research into how principles such as "autonomy," encoded into regulations, are actually applied (Pratt et al. 2014). But as I traveled with FERCAP, I became fascinated by the challenges of producing uniformity in different settings. What did such logics of standardization mean for research ethics? While the network was heavily emphasizing standards, they also spoke of their limits:

> Without a systematic approach to information gathering and capacity building, standards alone will not achieve greater protections for research subjects through independent and competent ethical review in all countries. Given the enormous complexity of cultural variations, national laws, and local medical and research practice local knowledge and local engagement are essential to develop ethical review. (Karbwang et al. 2001, 2).

On the one hand, the priority is to build ethics review capacity *precisely because* of the differences thought to inhere in local assessors. At the same time, standards, audit, and accreditation are cornerstone tools by which this work is advanced. Understanding this relationship as it has been written into FERCAP's work, between standards and "local"-ness, research for this book necessitated an archaeology of the ethics built into the *form* of an ethics committee: its prescribed, ideal composition; its accepted modes of reasoning; and its imaginaries of the democratic decision-making inherited from Euro-American models that give an ethics to ethics. It has also necessitated a deeper understanding of the ties between standards, accreditation, and quality assurance than I could ever have anticipated. As the anthropologist Kaushik Sunder Rajan reminds us in his study of policy harmonization and norm establishment in India, a Gramscian understanding of hegemony "involves a contestation for the 'common sense' of a society at a given moment in time" (Sunder Rajan 2017, 7); for countries seeking (or targeted by) norms and expectations of capacity-building initiatives, as always, the question is "capacity for whom?" (Mormina and Istratii 2021). Through observing contests over the epistemic authority given to committees, as well as trainings and conferences filled with anxieties about trust in science, I came to ask questions about authority, expertise, hierarchy, dialogue, and decision that exploded the bounds of the committee itself.

Structure of the Book

This book is divided into three segments, each of which is dedicated to areas of concern for capacity builders: training, practice, and futures. Linking international economies of biomedical research and the activities of new ethics committees, I start by exploring the *Standards and Subjects* emerging in efforts to train committees. We begin with "Networking a Region," to understand what a regional NGO is and what holds it together. I then take readers into its central activity with "The Hospitable Audit," which draws on stories from across the breadth of my multi-sited work, the hospitals and universities of Manila, the Philippines; Bangkok, Thailand; and Beijing, China. I detail how the surveying and auditing practices of the Forum foster a community of people who work for continuous improvement, wherein assessors must balance their standard-raising critique with kindness, friendship, and hospitality. When committees submit themselves to voluntary forms of assessment and accreditation, researchers quickly discover that establishing ethics review is a material practice, too. Often treated as a discursive enterprise, aspirational committees find the practical realities come to life: Forms must be designed and filled, physical space found for meetings, leaking roofs fixed, funds found for secretarial staff, and time carved out of schedules for training, reviewing, and meeting. The final chapter of this section, "Committees Immaterial," takes up the question of what the world looks like from this room, a room that keeps reconstituting itself in different sites around the world.

The book's second section, *Decisions and Models,* takes us into challenges of decision-making. Chapter 4, "Microcosming Models," looks at debates about the composition of the committee and traces the histories behind the roles given to each member. Each committee member's "role" is necessary for legitimate decision-making, but challenges arise as the logics of the committee encounter divergent political contexts. How a decision is reached in settings of intense professional vulnerability, hierarchy, and prestige while the ethics committee as a form contains egalitarian ideals is an ethnographic question. Chapter 5, "Dynamics of Decision," therefore examines decision-making in ethical review as political work. A decision is an ethnographically observable form of "social knowledge" demanding anthropological unpacking. Through a series of nationally distinct examples, we meet different forms of decision resolution—consensus, voting, or the chair's privilege. Managing ambiguity, the spaces of decision veer between formalistic and adversarial. Few ethics committees are open to observation, and this chapter draws on material gained while observing committees as a trainee auditor within the Forum's recognition program to explore the delicate question of how decisions arise, how they are communicated, and how they orchestrate their own authoritative voice.

In the final section, *Future Capacities*, I explore capacity building's forward momentum—a momentum that is full of promise (Douglas-Jones and Shaffner 2021). The presence of capacity-building enterprise implies a capacity yet to be developed. Chapter 6, "Ethics and the Law," follows comparisons made by critics and committee members alike that ethics review is—or should be—like a jury, exploring the analogy and its limits. Chapter 7, "Locating Ethics," details how, deep within the technocratic operationalization of ethics, some interviewees put their faith in the mechanisms of quality assurance and improvement, while others seek out a frame of "duty"—explicitly tying Kantian imperatives to regionally familiar Confucian norms. We arrive at questions of how capacity builders know their work is done. If capacity building's momentum carries them forward, how and when does that momentum run out? How do they know when capacity is built? What do the means selected to demonstrate progress, or even completion, teach us as observers? In "Dreams for an Ethics to Come," I bring forward the speculations and hopes of three practitioners for what its future might entail. Their decidedly forward-looking commitments to a different, better future are part of the work of bringing it into being. I take seriously these acts of speculation, both as revelatory in their own right and as illustrations that draw out the capacities envisaged for experimental worlds yet to come. Amongst these forms of technocratic dreaming exist visions of ethical subjectivity, narratives of conversion, and a belief in ethics. Bypassing the monitoring and auditing of the committee, the pendulum swings back toward ideas of scientific integrity, an integrity that responsibilizes the individual scientist and prefigures the policy-led institutionalization of integrity within the global project of science.

SECTION 1
Standards and Subjects

ONE
Networking a Region

The year before I began my fieldwork, FERCAP's annual conference was held in Bangkok, at the Rama Gardens Convention Center. I cannot describe it; I was not there. But the slides from the event circulated online in the years afterward and, more importantly, so did the ideas they contained. Researching the online digital footprint of capacity building, I read disembodied conference archives and found they took on a new lived form as committee members referenced them years later. One image returned repeatedly: Then chair of the SIDCER advisory board, the American anesthesiologist Dr. Greg Koski had spoken to FERCAP's gathered membership and described the international system of research as follows:

> The individuals and entities engaged in human research constitute a matrix of overlapping roles and responsibilities that together serve to ensure that the duties are satisfied. This matrix is like a finely woven silk cloth. A single broken thread causes a defect, a single defect spoils an entire cloth. A single hole can result in disaster, a single disaster can shred the fabric of trust. It is our duty to protect not just research subjects, but to protect the integrity of science itself. (Koski, 2008)

As one of the founding scholars of infrastructure studies Susan Leigh Star wrote, "power is about *whose* metaphor brings worlds together, and holds them there" (Star 1990, 52). When I heard Koski's 2008 metaphor repeated during fieldwork, and returned to it myself on slides downloaded years later, I saw how it had been crafted for and as a high stakes game, how it imbued each "single broken thread" with importance.[1] From even the smallest of "defects," he argued, the entire enterprise of science might be at stake. Koski was speaking from a position of having overseen "science itself," since in addition to his role on the SIDCER advisory board, he is also a former director general of the Office for Human Research Protections (OHRP) in the United States.

After the turn of the century, research on spatial mobility of the clinical trials industry, conducted primarily from the United States and Europe, showed an "outsourced world" (Petryna 2007, 21) whose scope and reach was vast but, as the twenty-first century began, was anxiously described as largely unknown (Sim and Detmer 2005). As discussed in the introduction, the growth of multi-centered clinical trials and contract research organizations (CROs) meant that not only was information being generated in many different places by many different people, but the sites of responsibility seemed vast and distributed. For sponsors, a "bioethics infrastructure" had "become an imperative because sponsors of research are becoming increasingly reluctant to choose sites where ethical review of research cannot be credibly assured" (Loff 2000, 1502). From a regulator's perspective, the challenge was only going to grow. As Fergus Sweeney, former Head of Compliance at the European Medicines Agency, put it, "wherever you sit in the world as a regulator, most of the clinical trials you receive in marketing applications . . . [are] taking place in territories outside of the jurisdiction of your regulatory system" (Sweeney 2011).

These developments brought unease for both regulators and wider research publics, rooted in anxiety that U.S. Americans might not trust "in science." They had reason not to. In 2002, reflecting the mood of the times, the U.S. magazine *Time* had run a front cover describing research participants as "Human Guinea Pigs," featuring a young blonde woman in a green hospital gown, caged, with a drip feed hanging from the bars (Lemonick and Goldstein 2002).[2] She is the test subject, caged, "trapped and bound by a rigid and demanding clinical research process," and claimed as the catalyst for two decades of subsequent patient engagement (Zuckerman 2022). Concern was not only for participants in research within the United States. Susan Reverby, whose historical research uncovered the "U.S.-sponsored inoculation study of sexually transmitted infections in Guatemala between 1946 and 1948" (Reverby and Moran-Thomas 2024, 564), was asked in a *Nature* interview what today's researchers could learn from the case. She replied: "Most U.S. drug trials are now conducted internationally. We have controls in the United States, but what's being done elsewhere in the world? . . . The lesson for today is the importance of institutional review boards, and of making sure that informed consent is really understood and applied in international trials" (Semeniuk 2010, 645).

To make sense of Koski's and Reverby's arguments for the need for ethics in a globalizing research world, in this opening section of the book I explore how FERCAP's activities emerged in a landscape of research change and heated debate. In this chapter, I introduce the Forum's version of networking and its main activities: the annual conference, its Recognition Program, and its trainings. I aim to make apparent how the network manages its "regionality" and the radical differences in histories and relationships to research that exist across it. I argue that this management is creative, narrative, and considered. To begin, I start with a counterfactual means by which networking could have been sought, namely through "Asian Bioethics." I show how the tensions within that could not meet the network's needs and introduce the kinds of networking it chose instead.

From a Single Broken Thread

The metaphor of research as a finely woven silk cloth is powerful, because it invokes both vulnerability and the need for coordination. Throughout fieldwork, people often told me that in the Asia-Pacific, "the system" for ethics, enforcement, and legislation "does not exist," and Cristina looked to the United States in contrast:

> In the U.S., they have money from government, and they have a system. Here, that system doesn't exist yet. The U.S. have a good system to check and balance. If the EC is not good, then they'll close them down. And funding will be stopped as well. Funding for that research, for the whole institution. You sign a Federal Wide Agreement (FWA) and it means you'll comply with all the regulations. So if you [the institution] don't support the EC, they'll be stopped, because you didn't comply. That's why it's so effective in the U.S.—they have control. If you're not compliant . . . they have a good system. In Asia, we don't have that.

These ideas of control and efficacy, the ability to "shut down" research, was something the U.S. Office for Protection from Research Risks (OPRR) had famously done in May 1999, when it "halted human research studies at Duke University Medical Center" (Institute of Medicine 2001, 29). Stories of the power of U.S. bodies such as the Government Accountability Office (GAO) to run a "sting operation" to test IRB performance also made their way to FERCAP conferences via delegates and their slides (Douglas-Jones 2019, 452). While these things were certainly true, in the United States, the landscape of IRBs is—and has long been—highly fragmented (Babb 2020). Cristina's view, looking toward the United States, is not necessarily a recognizable portrait for committee members there. Sociologist Sarah Babb, whose own experiences chairing a U.S. Institutional Review Board led to her book, argues that "our American IRB system is more profoundly decentralized . . . answerable to agencies that cannot engage in close monitoring, precedent-setting, or even regular policy updates" (2020, 7–8). The situation across the European member states has also been diffuse: Prior to 2022, trials in Europe were required to submit separately to each National Competent Authority (NCA) and ethics committee in each country to run European Medicines Agency (EMA 2022). There remain, as colleagues point out, "gaps in the ethical governance" of clinical trials in Europe (Bernabe et al. 2025).

Cristina's frustration was that few countries ran a "system" of committees, regulations, or standards. Few of the "spheres" or "layers" (Wahlberg et al. 2013, 295) of protection for research participants that she saw in other settings existed where she worked. Seen from her position as coordinator, few review processes were integrated into national health systems, and there were few national ethics committees. There were also few sustainable health research strategies and no standardized training of committees offered "in country." Yet the idea of a "system" was still motivating. Both practice and appearance mattered, as being seen to have sufficient capacity in ethics review was a prerequisite for attracting research, itself regarded as a means of increasing local competence and knowledge. With a greater number of trials conducted as "multi-sited" studies over the last two decades, sponsors and funders also look increasingly for sites with a certain degree of "capacity." Ethics has come to form an important part of this capacity, and its development is not always at the behest of governments or from public concern. In recognition of this, for the first decade of FERCAP's operation, the charge was placed with developing the capacities of committee members, who, as Cristina wrote, must "be convinced about the importance of their task for them to exert their utmost effort" (2011, 52).

At the outset, the problems were foundational. Writing up the 2000 Global Forum on Bioethics in Research meeting, held in Bangkok, attendees reflected that "if countries hosting collaborative research are to be full partners in the research process, it is crucial that they have their own capacity to conduct a thorough ethical review of research proposals. This may not be so simple, since *the precise elements that constitute capacity are not clear*" (Loff et al. 2001, 63; emphasis added). By the next year, work had been undertaken at international meetings to identify and evaluate problems. These findings made their way into a box in the 2001 U.S. Report on the "Globalization of Clinical Trials," titled "Some Weaknesses in Ethical Review Systems in Asia, Western Pacific, and Africa." The list ran as follows: "(1) Lack of procedures for reviewing the protocol and informed consent forms; (2) Lack of trained institutional review board members; (3) Insufficient resources; (4) Lack of monitoring systems; (5) Lack of quorum requirements for institutional review board meetings; and (6) Lack of independence" (Rehnquist 2001, 16). Next to this box, FERCAP appears as a newly formed entity, "a *network* for mobilizing resources, exchanging information and coordinating activities relating to institutional review boards. Among other activities, this forum facilitates training and education of members of ethics committees" (Rehnquist 2001, 16; emphasis added). Capacity building as a future-oriented exercise needs "lacks" to function, and from this clear list of "lacks," action could flow. The next question was whose task it should be to lead the action.

To speak in Koski's terms, Cristina's work has been to handle threads from which to make a cloth. The annual conference provided a forum—one that had previously not existed—in which members of committees can gather, raise concerns, share experiences, and learn from one another. As a commentator on the above debate said,

> In developing countries, we don't have laws and regulations. It is important that we advocate, so a regulatory authority can be set up. The initiative has to come from us. We cannot wait for [governments] to recognize the importance of an ethical regulatory system.

Members of FERCAP have not waited. Their work has been that of putting a "system" in place, but it is not primarily that of regulatory bodies, legislators, or guidelines. It has been concerned with the practice of research ethics, how committees establish themselves institutionally, and the standards to which they should aspire. But what has formed the basis of the training for practice? Where are the ideas drawn from?

Whose Ethics, Whose Bioethics?

At the beginning of my fieldwork, I thought of what FERCAP was doing as a part of a larger world of bioethics. The research project that had funded my fieldwork field was concerned with bioethics, and my own training in medical anthropology had sensitized me to issues that bioethicists also seemed to find interesting. As I sat through FERCAP's trainings, I listened to talks liberally peppered with stories claimed by the discipline of bioethics. However, many members of FERCAP do not define what they are doing as bioethics. About halfway through my 2010 stay in Manila, I got into a discussion with Leon, the chairperson of the committee I was visiting, about bioethics organizations and activities in the region. I had recently spent time in Bangkok, a visit that had included meeting up with bioethics staff at UNESCO's regional bioethics headquarters and talking about the Universal Declaration on Bioethics and Human Rights, adopted by all member states in 2005 (UNESCO 2005). Why was there so little overlap, I asked, between FERCAP's work and that of UNESCO, or other bioethics initiatives, like the Fogarty International training courses and the Global Forum on Bioethics in Research? There was a pause. I knew Leon was highly networked and had himself undertaken some of these international training courses. I gently reminded him that I was neither a bioethicist nor an auditor, and had no stakes in his reply. He opened up. In his view, it came down to the style of reasoning he'd observed in encounters with bioethics organizations: "Look, Rachel," he said, "in the moral dilemma approach, when something is resolved, they introduce another factor so another dilemma emerges. But research ethics needs to be solution oriented." At trainings he'd attended on bioethics ("the moral dilemma approach"), part of the exercise seemed to be based on extending and turning a problem around for consideration. He described a curriculum drawn up for a collaborative course between the University of the Philippines, Manila, and the Fogarty International Center on Bioethics:

> There was a lot of discussion. [Fogarty] wanted a course on "moral dilemmas" and they said it was a "skills" course! Doctors in the course said, "This is a never-ending discussion!" Suppose someone is run over by a car. Who is responsible? The driver. Suppose the pedestrian is drunk? Well, both. But say the driver . . . And you keep adding to the issue. It goes on and on. The medical doctors, they said, "There is no resolution to the issue!" That was the "skill" they learnt. It is a very different approach.

That bioethics was a "very different approach" to research ethics was a repeated sentiment throughout my research. This meant that engagement with explicitly "bioethics" networks was not a priority for FERCAP. Few considered this a great loss, since the attempts of certain FERCAP members to bring in bioethicists had led to blank faces and reportedly confused clinicians. Another interviewee illustrated for me the systems she implicitly understood to be at work in the region through an event involving American graduates from Harvard's Public Health Program on Ethical Issues in Global Health Research, Chinese bioethicists, and members of FERCAP. The difficulties arose from different disciplinary relationships to bioethics, she explained, making interactions with the Harvard fellows "complicated":

> Bioethicists in China, they are philosophers. So, they think we belong to one group. When you do training they put us together, with the bioethics lectures. We had a session on Standard Operating Procedures, management of Serious Adverse Events . . . and then the Chinese philosophy people talked about principles. They were talking about "there is no objective reality," the deconstruction movement. I know what it is, because I'm coming from a social science background. I've been exposed to these things at the University, about radical sociology, but can you imagine doctors listening to that! How can you tell which drug is more effective if there is no objective reality?! Meiji was doing the translation for me and I asked her what they were talking about and she shook her head and said, "I cannot translate this, I do not know how to." She is a very smart medical doctor. But she will just stop doing the translating and say, "I don't know how to translate that." Even she gets confused.

But the label of bioethics drove funds, particularly to cover the cost of attending international courses and fellowships. Even if brief, these courses could have significant impact: A 1997 WHO Fellowship taken by Vasantha Muthuswamy to the Kennedy Institute of Ethics, Georgetown University, for example, is credited as "the turning point of her professional life" (Kant and Mathur 2023a, 223), paving the way for her later role in FERCAP and as chairperson of the Forum of Ethics Review Committees of India (FERCI). In 2000, the U.S.-based Fogarty International Center of the National Institutes of Health started funding ethics training programs as "part of its wider commitment to strengthen research ethics capacity globally" (Pratt et al. 2014). Assessing the impact of these trainings, public health researcher Bridget Pratt and her colleagues in Australia interviewed Asia-Pacific graduates of the program, whose feedback highlighted the absence of cases from their home countries. The trainees they spoke to felt that non-Western approaches were "confined to units designed for this purpose and not incorporated into teaching in other subjects," while others said that they didn't "remember cases from Asia at all" (2014, 73). Yet researchers trained abroad in programs such as Fogarty's return to the region carrying ideas and assumptions about norms and "standards." The difficulty of this transition was picked up in the interviews conducted by Pratt and colleagues, who report that one trainee experienced at home "an animosity towards bioethics, a palpable animosity," while another faced opposition from senior consultants "because he studied in a Western country [and] they did not believe what he had learned was applicable" (2014, 76). More recent Fogarty initiatives in India, Malaysia, Myanmar, and Pakistan have aimed to address these limitations by creating master's programs "designed to meet [their] respective country's specific needs and challenges, offering in depth curricula that blend global best practices with local perspectives" (Gopalan et al. 2025, 7).

For some, an obvious response is to localize bioethical questions. Leo de Castro, a philosopher-bioethicist who served on the first FERCAP steering committee in 2000 and later as FERCAP's vice president in 2003, spent the late 1990s considering the problem of "Asian Bioethics." In an article asking whether there even is such a thing, he opens by considering what it would take for bioethics to be "Asian." He suggests two things: "Firstly, Asian bioethics must be peculiar (or contain features that are peculiar) to Asia. Secondly, Asian bioethics must be common to Asians" (1999, 227). Within the "region," however, he finds that difference "in bioethical thinking" proliferates. Referencing other scholars working on the challenge of an Asian bioethics, notably Ruiping Fan, he remarks that while they have identified "distinguishing features," scholars are also "quick to point out the variation in bioethical thinking *within* each region" (de Castro 1999, 229). He goes on to observe that the pursuit of a coherent Asian bioethics against "the alleged imperialism of Western concepts and bioethical principles" sets up a trap:

> In the attempt to characterize an Asian bioethics that is significantly different from Western bioethics, we can easily commit the mistake of universalizing (among Asians) a single Asian ethical perspective. (de Castro 1999, 234)[3]

So how is a boundary to be drawn around "Asia," and what happens in the drawing of this line? In order to create an "Asian bioethics," work must be done on generating a region, but the emergence of differences "within," and their suppression, complicates. As Leo de Castro asks, "how much peculiarity and commonality can there be?" (1999, 227). "Of what importance are the shared features," he asks, "if they do not amount to a unified theoretical system or a single coherent perspective?" (1999, 229). Soraj Hongladarom, a Thai philosopher who has long participated in bioethics symposia, struggles with the same framings as de Castro. Recalling an event on "Dialogue and Promotion of Bioethics in Asia," he comments that he said

> that there was no such thing as Asian bioethics because Asia was a very large continent containing highly diverse cultures, histories and traditions that made it very difficult, if not impossible, to find common elements that could define the "Asian" in Asian bioethics. (2004)

Foregrounding "Asian bioethics" in this way, commentators find it difficult to adequately "suppress" differences to create a sense of region, region here operating to equate sameness with geography. The framing forces them to grapple with the anthropologically familiar question of where "cultural differences" begin and end. De Castro tells us he is not the first to struggle: Prominent Hong Kong philosopher bioethicist Ruiping Fan (1997) "acknowledges that Buddhism, Taoism and Shinto have all combined to bring about variations in bioethical thinking from country to country, or from area to area" (de Castro 1999, 229). We are now not only dealing with countries, but transnational belief systems variously "combined."

Anthropologist Margaret Sleeboom-Faulkner argues that what is important for ethnographers (rather than philosophers) is how the notion of "(East) Asian Bioethics" is mobilized. Her analysis shows how it becomes a "vehicle" and "platform," how conferences and meetings allow the deployment of "techniques of replication: papers, speeches, reports, conference proceedings and feedback to universities and government departments" (2016, 22). She astutely observes that it also creates "outsiders." During a conversation with Cristina, I pushed the point about the relationship between bioethics and FERCAP's work. Sighing—because we had talked about this before—she put her hands in her lap, and asked me what the point of debating unresolvable differences could possibly be. "For us," she said firmly, "the guidelines are there. For us, what is more important is for us to be able to operationalize those guidelines. If a new issue comes up and they can incorporate it into the guidelines, we can follow it and start implementing." In her own writing, she has argued that FERCAP's approach

> has made it possible to operationalize the basic ethics principles of autonomy, beneficence, and justice in the review of health research and translate them into tools, such as checklists and assessment forms to assist the EC/IRB members in reviewing protocols, consent forms, and related documents. (2011, 49)

The language of implementation and operationalization reframes ethics as a part of a quality system: If research is unethical, it cannot be quality research. FERCAP's work is different from that of bioethics, argued Cristina, because it focuses on "the System" and the role of "stakeholders": "It's not about moral dilemmas. We say what's there and how we apply the ethics. Because that is what is lacking in Asia. The system. And we've established that niche."

So instead of mobilizing "Asian Bioethics" as a platform for commonality, Cristina is oriented toward the place of ethics review in the wider, global system of research. Her refusal of moral dilemmas and turn toward "quality" in operationalization resembles Joan Fujimura's definition of a "standardized package" (1992). Unlike the concept of boundary objects, used in the social sciences to describe contested objects around which people can collaborate while maintaining their independent interpretations (Star and Griesemer 1989), standardized packages are robust enough to change local practices, something upon which is clearly FERCAP's intent. As Fuijmura puts it, they are both "a theory and a standardized set of technologies" that together make it possible "to locally concretize the abstraction in different practices to construct new problems" (1992, 169, 179). But what does it mean to treat *ethics* as such a package, with attention to the politics of the differentiating work of standards and the technoscientific expertise needed for their efficacy?

A Networked Recognition Program

In 2000, there was no mechanism of finding out what committees, once established, were doing when they conducted a review. The task of deciding what a good review looks like is difficult, since ethics committees are "deliberative bodies charged with applying standards that are neither designed for nor typically capable of producing a single, objectively correct answer" (Lynch et al. 2022, 114614). The authors of the 2001 U.S. report *Preserving Public Trust* report rooted the need to inspect committees in Principle 7 of the Nuremberg

Code, asking how the emergent "system of protections be assessed in a reliable and valid way to ensure that it is effective, efficient and accountable—that 'proper preparations' have been made and that 'adequate facilities' have been provided to protect the experimental subjects of research"? (Institute of Medicine 2001, 23). While *Preserving Public Trust* was focused on piloting accreditation for committees in the United States, the ideas within it took new form in FERCAP's worlds.

After a few years of preparatory work, in 2005, Juntra used the platform that SIDCER gave her to design and launch a "recognition program" that would precipitate capacity building through assessing the reviewing work committees were doing. In addition to internationally sponsored multi-center clinical trials, committees in this book look at research proposals for regional trials as well as a wide range of medical studies including "investigator initiated" studies from device testing to epidemiology, population studies, and lifestyle interventions. Cases collected by the network, discussed in chapter 8, include pediatric studies, oncology research, genetic studies, psychiatric studies, social and behavioural research, traditional medicine research, and international health research (Navarro 2012, 3). But how they review them matters. Intended to be a set of operational standards used across SIDCER's five regions, the Recognition Program is known informally as "The Survey" and is today primarily implemented by FERCAP. Alongside the annual conference and training workshops, it constitutes the core of the network's capacity-building agenda and remains FERCAP's most intensive task. The Survey consists of a four-day in-person visit to the committee's "site"—language reminiscent of clinical trials monitoring. The first committees underwent recognition in 2005, submitting their operations for review according to a set of five standards. The first of these deals with the structure and composition of the committee, checking that the membership is appropriate both to the volume and the type of research the committee reviews. The second deals with Standard Operating Procedures, "for optimal and systematic conduct of ethical review." The third standard examines the completeness of the review process, concerning itself both with timely review and the procedure of reviewing "to protect the interests of research participants." The fourth takes up what happens after the review: the communication between the committee and the researcher, the duration of committee approval, and any follow-up procedures that will be required. The fifth and final standard concerns the committee's documentation and archiving practices, focusing primarily on their systematicity and timeframes. When committees are "recognized" at the annual conference of the Forum, it is for their "compliance" with seven different sets of *international* guidelines: the Declaration of Helsinki; the most updated guidelines from the International Council for Harmonization (ICH)'s Good Clinical Practice (GCP); the latest version of the Council for International Organizations of Medical Sciences (CIOMS); the 2001 and 2009 World Health Organization guidelines discussed below; their own Standard Operating Procedures (SOPs); and "Local Regulations" and Standards in Ethical Review. Recognition lasts three years, after which the Survey team must be invited back again.

The standards for the Survey were developed by a SIDCER working group who met in Olympia, Washington, in 2005, and was last revised into version 4.0 during the first year of the COVID-19 pandemic (Navarro et al. 2020). The original group included people with job titles such as Director of Quality Assurance, Internal Auditor, Quality Assurance Analyst, and Director of Regulatory Affairs, a composition of professions revealing of the priorities that went into the standards. They built on the World Health Organization's "Silver Book"—*Operational Guidelines for Ethics Committees that Review Biomedical Research* (2000)—a project Juntra had led a few years earlier, and developed

> because investigators in developing countries were conducting increasingly more research, but few people in these countries had experience setting up and running ethics committees. The existing international research ethics documents focused on ethical issues, not on how the ethical review committee should be staffed, organized or operated. (Rehnquist 2001, 27)

The shift from "ethical issues" to staffing occurred through "Standard Operating Procedures," known universally by their acronym, SOPs. SOPs embody the collision of quality assurance with clinical research. Two sources from the late 1990s prefigure the priorities of those involved in writing them. Writing in a special issue of the *Quality Assurance Journal*, Francis P. Crawley, the philosopher who assisted with FERCAP's founding terms of reference, argues that "since the product of ethical review is intangible, the structure of the review process becomes of paramount importance to the customer. The decision of an ethics committee *per se* eludes evaluation and makes a poor measure of quality. However, the organization and procedures of an ethics committee can be evaluated according to objective standards" (1997, 159). His summary is addressing Dr. Angela Bowen's contribution to the special issue, hence the presence of "customer" here, since Bowen was president of Western Institutional Review Board (WIRB), one of the largest and longest running commercial IRBs in the United States until its acquisition (Babb 2020, 69). For her part, Bowen stated simply that "we believe that quality begins with structure and that some structures are more conducive than others to the promotion of total quality assurance" (Bowen 1997, 161–62).

The use of the WHO's "operational" guidelines, with their focus on SOPs and committee practicalities, has not been without contestation. When researchers from across the region have undertaken fellowships in the United States and Australia, it has predominantly been courses in bioethics. These fellowships—as I show at various moments in this book—have not always led to practices that they could "bring home." But as FERCAP began to roll out its Recognition Program a philosopher associated with what they termed the "Harvard Group" circulated a complaint that the "guidelines of the WHO are a work for the typist, the clerk!" To him, Standard Operating Procedures failed to deal with actual ethical issues, avoided discussing principles, and were excessively procedural. The critique also carried judgment of those running courses and trainings in research ethics: How, asked some, could Cristina, with her PhD in the social sciences, contribute to building capacity in biomedical research ethics? Recalling the event more than a decade later, she explained that these critiques had hurt: From her perspective, research ethics *is* a social science. It is about people, understanding culturally appropriate methodologies, and of course it is also a lot of work. While we did not discuss it, the rumble of complaint from the philosopher carried a gendered denial of expertise, and more than a hint of disciplinary epistemic hierarchy. During my time with FERCAP, I saw Cristina brushing off clearly gendered doubt in her competence. In one conversation, she told me about "a philosopher" from Europe who had complained about her questions, and reported her as "incompetent" to her colleagues. In Cristina's telling, Juntra had, in solidarity, innocently asked him whether he though thought *all* professors from the Philippines were incompetent, knowing full well he had several collaborative projects in the country. Reportedly on the backfoot, he had muttered, "No, just this one," and dropped it. Many bioethicists are drawn from the famously gendered discipline of philosophy, which is replete with "small repeated incidents of disrespect, dismissal and misrecognition" (Bastian 2014, 222), like the one above, that lead to the production of an exclusive, well-policed "philosopher" identity. Cristina's experiences as "a social scientist who voiced out community concerns" on biomedical committees in Manila at the beginning of her career (Torres 2011, 43) will also have produced dissatisfaction with a form of discussion that, like philosophy itself, "excluded so many forms of experiences, lives, hopes and concerns from consideration" (Bastian 2018, 461). As she remarked simply, "I am under no illusion I am engaging the whole field of bioethics!" Turning away from the philosophical form of ethics and staying with practice, her aim was to "help countries help themselves" as they formalized their biomedical research arenas and engaged in international scientific collaborations.

Networking through Standard Operating Procedures

Recognition depends on having something to assess. The debates of the 1990s and early 2000s had led to deadlocks that set bioethicists against one another. FERCAP chose a different starting point. Standard Operating Procedures seem quite devoid of "culture," oriented at quality management and improvement. Perhaps unsurprisingly, a full history of Standard Operating Procedures is yet to be written, as they belong to the family of research topics that are "semi-cultural things that most people find quite dull" (Lampland and Star 2009, 11). But a brief cultural history shows how they come to play such a role in this book. In 1990, after decades of use in the military, manufacturing, and business, they formally became part of Good Clinical Practice Guidelines agreed on by the International Council for Harmonization. There, SOPs are defined as "detailed, written instructions to achieve uniformity of the performance of a specific function" (ICH GCP 1996, 8) and serve as a key measure against which monitoring can be carried out and noncompliance can be assessed. Committees are thus told that if they are operating without SOPs, they are in "major" violation of GCP. This kind of violation has the potential to render research data from its sites invalid. GCP auditors assess compliance, and in 2005, Beat Widler and Allan K. Johansen, former Roche quality assessment inspectors, presented joint findings of Roche GCP audits to FERCAP audiences at the annual conference. Longtime supporters of FERCAP's work, they brought their familiarity with GCP auditing, training, and compliance to help the organization see areas of "noncompliance" issues committees were facing. In 2005, the most significant of these was the absence of written procedures, namely SOPs.

And so, that year, members of FERCAP's steering committee created a draft template of SOPs for member committees. The template that has circulated amongst ethics review committees in the region had been added to, expanded, and modified according to national guidelines of the different countries, as well as their specific institutional arrangements. When I started my research with FERCAP, I found that they had spent the last few years emphasizing to committees the strict importance of SOPs. As a written record of the process, SOPs are capable of acting both as a description of what the committee does and as instruction for its practice. The Recognition Program's Survey pays a good deal of attention to how they are written, what they contain, their "consistency," language, and phrasing. One surveyor contrasted this new attention to the "old days" when documentation was lax. "Modeling is a good method," he said, "people join the survey, so it's moving even better." Cristina acknowledges that

> each ethics committee is unique, even if you copy the SOPs, something different comes out because you have different people, a different hospital. The composition is just like a person—just as each person is different, I have not seen two IRBs the same. I've seen over fifty. Every one is different from each other.

Templates and uniqueness exist in tension. In an interview with ClinPower News—a now defuct online website for clinical research the Middle East and North Africa—Widler, whose findings with Roche above informed FERCAP's development of SOPs, comments:

> Because I am a strong believer that we should share tools and best practices, in my opinion there's no need that each institution has their own set of SOPs, templates and other elements of a quality management system but should start collaborating and using shared tools. In fact, a clinical trial is a clinical trial, the fundamentals are the same, GCP is the same for everybody and ethics is the same! Then of course you need to have the flexibility to adapt to the local requirements but there are common basics that we should share and pass from one to the other. (Widler 2012)

In the "exchange" of experiences that the network aims to foster, members also exchange documents; Widler's vision of shared SOPs is being enacted through FERCAP. After a training session in Bangkok that brought together members of many different committees, I spoke with an attendee who had been in conversation with members of a well-respected committee. "They gave us copies of their SOP!" she said excitedly. Juntra joined in, speaking approvingly of the attendees:

> Circulating their own SOP, that's for me the best thing, they share experiences. I saw your SOP and people think, "This could help my committee, we don't have that," and they have to go back and change [their] EC. "Now that's one we'd never thought of, it's a good one."

SOPs have such a central role that in a poignant obituary of one of FERCAP's founding members, the late Indian bioethicist Vasantha Muthuswamy, her colleagues Lalit Kant and Roli Mathur recalled that during her treatment, and "although not in the pink of her health, she continued to guide several universities (like Ashoka) and institutions in drafting their Standard Operating Procedures even between her treatment sessions" (2023b, 24–25). During a Survey, a process I describe in greater detail in the chapter to come, the teams into which the Surveyors split each take sections of the committee's SOPs to examine. Surveyors regularly announce to committees that "you write what you do and you do what you write. Therefore, SOPs should always be an ongoing work rather than a fixed document." On the first day of the Survey in Beijing, for example, the secretary of the committee presented her SOP revision record to the surveyor group:

> Since the Ethics Committee was set up, we have adjusted the SOP four times. The first version was from 2007, October. But when I attended the FERCAP conference in Chiang Mai, I realized some things are not very reasonable, and not very correct. So when I came home, I adjusted the SOP. That was our second version, 2009.10. Then, when I went to Nanjing, I learned a lot, and made a big change to the SOP. That was our third version, 2010.1. Then then I made alterations in preparation for the survey, 2010.03. Each time I edit, it becomes thicker. And now it is very thick, but I say we will do as SOP says, because it will give us more character, and we will be more reasonable as an EC.

Like other committee secretaries I spoke to, this increase in SOPs was seen as a mark of the committee's progress. Writing in the *Bangladesh Journal of Bioethics*, Vimal, Nishanthi, and Kagne wrote that when they started out in 2013, "the SOP booklet had 50 pages and contained 12 SOPs," but after the FERCAP Survey had visited, the "revised SOP is a 283-page document" (Mourouguessine et al. 2022, 55, 58). "We do things right," one committee member said to me proudly, holding her hand protectively over the thick red manila SOP folder, resting on the desk of her committee office.

A Network for Both Centers and Peripheries

SIDCER breaks up the world into regions, allocating FERCAP a regional space in which to operate. How space is done brings some places closer together and keeps others further apart, both in narrative and experience. Toward the end of my first period of fieldwork in 2010, I attended a presentation on the concept of FERCAP to a Chinese ethics review committee in Guangzhou. As a large hospital specializing in cancer research, they were interested in taking part in the Recognition Program. At the time, FERCAP was visiting to promote the benefits, and I listened as Cristina neatly laid out the "natural topography" of ethics in biomedical research:

> The guarantee for a good clinical trial is oversight, but it's hard to do at the regulatory level. For example, China is such a big country there is no way the SFDA will be able to monitor each and every one. But the Ethics Committee is institution based, so it makes it possible to guarantee grassroots level quality in a clinical trial.

The "levels" of this statement seem obvious: a big country, difficulty monitoring activities at the "grassroots" level. Cristina moves from the observation that "China is such a big country" to the Ethics Committee as institution based. The end of her pitch gave an additional role to the committee: "convincing" people of their duty to do good science. Here she reduces the "size" of the object she is dealing with, from the nation to the individual. It is a scale-in-the-making that would be easy to miss, since it so closely resembles how a social scientist might go about "contextualizing" the work of one ethics committee within a national arena: *Of course* the committee is "smaller" than China, or the Food and Drug Administration. One is linked to the "macro," the other to the "micro." Were the framing and description changed, the SFDA might, in other circumstances, be cast as large, powerful. Yet here it is distant, small, made so by Cristina's focus on the physical size of Chinese territory and the suggestion that the committee would be unable monitor "each and every one."

I have introduced this account because "where" is relationalities too, as the empirical philosopher John Law puts it (2008). My fieldnotes are full of moments where location is more relational than Euclidian: April 2010, in Colombo, Sri Lanka, where the decisions of doctors in Tuskegee, Alabama (Rothman 2003), become part of a canon recounted over video-link connections to rooms in Sri Lanka. Taipei, in 2018, in a hospital lecture hall, where the head of the Taiwan Association of IRBs draws on the Royal Free London's controversial relationship with Google's DeepMind and the use of patient data in developing an app. "Euclidianism is simply one version of the doing of location" (Law 2008; Woolgar and Lezaun 2013). These stories become collected, "housed" as the STS scholar Bruno Latour (2005) would observe, in offices, video archives, course materials, and textbooks. This applies equally to the making of ethics centers and peripheries. Casper Bruun Jensen asks us what would happen if "belief in such distribution of the large and the small, according to obvious and commonsense social scales, is suspended" (2007, 837). Correlating the large with importance, he writes, is something "regularly taken as a solution to the problems of sorting perspectives when one moves between contexts" (2007, 837). This scaling effect holds worlds together. It is a key means by which peripherality is produced, as "importance, relevance, size and scale [become] viewed as enacted categories" (Jensen 2007, 837). Let me illustrate from an early part of my fieldwork.

Peradeniya is a university town in central Sri Lanka, with a long-established medical faculty and a now FERCAP-recognized research ethics committee. However, during the spring of 2009, when I visited from my base with the Human Genetics Unit at the University of Colombo, the committee was not recognized, nor was it engaged in FERCAP's activities. Its members explained that distance was the reason why:

> To go to a one-hour meeting, you have to spend four hours on the way there, and four on the way back [in your car]. Colombo is only one hundred kilometers, it shouldn't take that long. But it's a busy road, you get caught in school traffic.

The time required to make the journey grows with the volume of traffic, which results in inconvenience and absences of researchers from other parts of the country. Researchers in Sri Lanka's southern city of Galle were more explicit about how the distance affected their interaction with and understanding of ethics. “It’s easy for people in and around Colombo,” said the researcher Renuka during an interview,

> but for us, Colombo? It’s one whole day, three and a half hours up, three and a half hours down, for a one-hour meeting. So that is how far behind we are, with them briefing us. Not in learning, sharing of information. For example, this Saturday, there’s a workshop on clinical ethics, but none of us are able to attend.

If people don’t travel, the speakers say, then neither does knowledge of research ethics. It gets stuck because of the roads, because of the school traffic. “Three and a half hours” becomes a measure of how far “behind” the geography makes them. In this mapping of knowledge onto distance, and the mapping of distance onto authority, if Colombo was a center, then there were more distant centers, greater than it, referred to often as the “outside.”

But what might that progress look like? Further interviews revealed a reliance on those who traveled internationally. “I learned a lot from Dr. A. She has traveled in the region on the subject,” said Bartholomew, a pathologist on an ethics committee in Galle. “She’s always coming back from Bangkok, saying ‘I was there and they had these documents.’” In this reckoning, through FERCAP’s networking, Galle is further from Colombo than Bangkok.

Networking across Difference

Alongside the refusal of differentiation perceived within projects of regional bioethics, FERCAP’s region-making work is conducted particularly at conferences, where national differences are inevitably highlighted. As I started attending events, I noticed the language coordinators of the network used to describe their efforts. It was “bottom up,” it was “like a family.” Members were described as participating in the making of the network through idioms of food. Instead of just having a meal together, said coordinators, we invite people to “cook” with FERCAP. Extending the metaphor, they said that they refused to tell participants what they would eat, when they would eat, or how they should cook. Another metaphor, that of a house, suggests that involvement in FERCAP is about more than just self-improvement, or improvement for one’s own country:

> If you have your house nice, you cannot just be happy with that. You need to think about what is around it. Are the streets tidy, is there trash? If you are just

> here to talk about yourself, that is not the way, that is not the attitude . . . You need to care about it all, the universe.

Caring here translated to interregional support, the universe made equivalent to the "family region," and took the form of visiting for training, surveys, and a shared distribution of the burdens of capacity building. Cristina would occasionally remind FERCAP volunteers that the network was deliberately developmental, especially in settings where a sense of competition over recognition was taking hold. FERCAP was "trying to help [committees] achieve a level of competence." All those who volunteered as trainers or surveyors knew of huge regional variation *within* the area encompassed by FERCAP. Cristina did too. In conversations that were just between us, told me she saw her role as specifically "articulating the perspective of a developing world country." She was deeply aware of how she could "adjust her language" to serve her purposes:

> Like when I'm in Korea, I say, "You should help. You have a model, you should help other countries in the region." I don't say which ones, but since you have an advanced economy, you should play a leading role in setting up models, developing a better system. I always tell developing countries that there should be no difference in quality of review. It is not an economic issue, not a technology issue. But you do have to modify the way you present.

Cristina's skill in tailoring her perception of a country's role within FERCAP is vital for understanding how she manages the comparisons occurring not between FERCAP, international, and North American standards, but between people from countries within her network. By encouraging "South Korea" to take on a role of leadership, she creates for those delegates a particular role of stewardship and support toward countries that may not yet have the institutional or political pieces in place to push the work of FERCAP amongst their committee members.

Regional hierarchy was invoked when speaking about those who did not participate in FERCAP's activities. A researcher who had been working in Singapore and whom I spoke to at the 2010 Shanghai conference listed Singapore, Hong Kong, Australia, and New Zealand, ticking them off his fingers as "non-participants." He could understand Australia and New Zealand not showing much interest, he said, but the other two? "Well, they are very good," he said, and raising an eyebrow to me, added, "Maybe because they were British colonies, they have no problems for the language." "Too high up," said one ERC member, of Singapore, deploying height as a language of superiority. Japan was termed a "different case" within FERCAP, and to date has one committee recognized by FERCAP's schemes (set against China's eighty-two). Personal friendships had led to individual members being involved in the network—such as the chairperson—but few surveys have taken place. FERCAP members both admired Japan's approach and their involvement with ICH-GCP, and criticized it for being "more bureaucratic than ethical." "I didn't get the impression that they looked into the *essence* of the protocol," one Thai researcher observed, implying that the ethics paperwork was perfect, but not the ethics content: "It's process, not just procedures on paper." Another pointed out that since Japan had national guidelines, an FDA which monitors, "they don't think they need it. They took part in the ICH-GCP, along with the EU, U.S., and Australia, which aimed toward harmonization among those countries."

Over the course of the conversation, I gently probed the notion of a "different case." He initially deflected, suggesting that on my travels I ask why committees in South Korea and Taiwan had sought FERCAP's recognition, since to him, the trials those two countries sought to host were the same. But gradually a sense of hierarchy emerged. "Well, it's partly pride. They can't take being criticized by a lower country. It would be an insult." A Taiwanese man, he had participated as an international surveyor on the FERCAP survey, and said, "That's what happened in South Korea. When we saw speakers from the Philippines, Thailand, the South Korean audience just went out of room. 'Why should we listen to these guys, from countries not as good as ours?'" This brought him round to the point he had been hesitating to make about Japan's lack of participation in FERCAP's activities. "They'd never allow people from South Asia to survey them!" he concluded, slightly exasperated at the anthropologist for forcing him to state the "obvious." "They're Number One! For their self-pride, they couldn't have surveyor[s] from India. U.S. FDA but definitely not other Asia[n] countries. That would be intolerable to them," he said flatly.[4] "The top can improve by U.S. FDA but not by India or Thai."

In this sizing and resizing of countries, just as Cristina is aware that she can talk "up" to countries with funds and well-established research environments, she is also aware that she has the capacity to foreground similarity. This is a technique I saw used elsewhere, particularly during a Survey in Beijing, when a surveyor had remarked with great respect on FERCAP's arrival in the Chinese capital. Aware of tension between China's capital and second city, Shanghai, where FERCAP had already become established, she threw an arm out to her co-surveyors from the Philippines and said:

> We all have our Asian roots, and many of us have Chinese roots . . . Maybe our only difference is our language we speak—if you look at us, we all look the same. We share the same goal and values and would like to protect human subject in research, and do scientific research!

Here, we return to an idea of "Asia" to highlight not only appearance but shared goals. Sleeboom-Faulkner has called the "symbolic metaphor of the 'Asian' family" a "form of grouping [that] has performative value and multiple functions, including regional identity marking, connecting through shared meanings, political positioning and group formation through networking" (2016, 281). If we think about the role of these moments in shaping how FERCAP's regionality is created and held together, social acts of comparison and verbal scalings matter in FERCAP's regional exercise of capacity building. The organizational sociologist Rolland Munro reminds us: "Scale does not exist autonomously as it does with the western conception of levels of wholes, such as the tripartite set of society, institution and individual. To the contrary, it is arguable that changing scale—the effects of 'magnification' or 'diminishment'—is precisely a demonstration of 'capacities'" (Munro 2005, 257).[5] Thinking about how this informs analysis, Casper Bruun Jensen reminds us that cultural imaginaries are important, "not because they *mediate* between lively agencies and fixed structure, but rather because they are part of actors' diverse repertoires for making and breaking relations with others" (Jensen 2021, 126).

Networking for Access

Relations with others include the politics of access, specifically the capacity of different committees to pay to participate in the Conference and Survey activities. For an ethics capacity-building network, particularly one with this grassroots orientation, access—although it is not framed in that language—matters. In the anniversary booklet produced for the tenth year of the network's operation, Cristina presented this as the principle of equity in operation, "shown in [FERCAP] being accessible to both developed and developing countries and in [FERCAP's] socialized costing of programs" (Torres 2011, 50). Taiwan, posed against Cambodia, can pay, "but Cambodia at the moment, TDR supports. Our philosophy is to help them help themselves," commented Juntra during the 2009 Conference. When a surveyor from Taiwan thinks about the funds required to support a Survey team during the course of recognition, he tells me "that kind of money, for Johns Hopkins it's a piece of cake, but for Cambodia? It's so expensive." Thus FERCAP works to subsidize "Cambodia's" participation. As Juntra put it,

> for us, [funding ethics committees is] not a big deal, but for them it is. Delegates from poorer countries have their flights to conference paid by Korea and Taiwan. They ask for money from [pharmaceuticals] because you need sponsors, whether countries or companies. America can't understand that.

In its early years, the network was supported by annual project grant applications to WHO-TDR, and has since become self-sustaining through institutional contributions. It collects institutional fees from recognized committees, which are renewed every three years. In 2009 the conference discussion opened on to how to finance FERCAP in the future, with a flurry of raised hands and whispering in the rows of red-velvet hotel seats. One delegate enthusiastically stood, and suggested FERCAP seek out wealthy donors, who could gain tax exemptions or fame from supporting ethics review:

> Many people want to do something for FERCAP [. . .] We're an international organization, we can change our idea, [get] NGO tax-free donations. Some of our people want to do that because they can create their own dignity. Obama, he [might] put $1000 in FERCAP because he is going to have [the] Peace Prize!

Juntra considered a donation model unsustainable, and returned to the idea of a house to explain her reasoning:

> Do you want to be on the first page of a newspaper, or just want to keep doing [this], sharing same values? This [work] is not only for our country. Our house is really nice, but it's not a good environment for the house. I don't think FERCAP wants millions . . . maybe better to think "OK, we have activities, how can we maintain our activities?"

In the view of its leaders, the organization aims not at profit but at sufficiency. It simply wants to continue doing what it is doing, and do it better. Cristina took countries with "more advanced economies" as examples of this shift in attitude:

> In the beginning, it was different, it was about "my" interest. "I don't want to share." Now, they have a different perspective . . . [T]hey were like that, now they want to host the conference. They want to help those less fortunate to them.

When I asked how this shift had occurred, Cristina was very aware of how the phrasing of her requests affected others. "You adjust the language," she said. "You ask them what they want their role to be." She had suggested to some of the South Korean delegates that perhaps their role was one of leadership, because they were coming from an advanced economy and had resources. "And then they are happy," she said, "they can help others."

What Is a Region?

Regions break up the world. Their boundaries and divisions have histories: Colonial relationships still channel funding, creating patterns of research. They are not stable things. Speaking at the first Global Clinical Trials Forum in November 2023, Tom Nyirenda of the European and Developing Countries Clinical Trials Partnership Cape Town Office presented a diagram of HIV collaborations premised on European schools of tropical medicine, from Antwerp to the London School of Hygiene and Tropical Medicine (LSHTM) and Liverpool in the UK. At that same meeting, one presenter's slides claimed a Western Pacific Region (WPR) versus a South-East Asian Region (SEAR), as well as a category of Southeast and East Asia and Oceania, versus South Asia. By the next presenter's slides, the Asia-Pacific was back. Regions are brought into being strategically.

In this chapter, I have shown how FERCAP's work is region-making, and this is an enactment of definitional power. It belongs to the "ethics package" in Fujimura's sense, where standards and networks both emanating from "outside" an institution—or nation state—can, as we shall see in the chapters to come, be used to mobilize resources and attention toward ethics. At the same time, committees are part of building competitive national research environments, and FERCAP's activities have not always been welcomed—especially when it comes to the proximity between recognition and accreditation. As different capacity building programs set up during the 2010s, different influences flowed through—Memorandums of Understandings, international training programs, U.S. fellowships, WHO-TDR funding programs, philosophers, and bioethicists. It was once suggested to me by a volunteer who had spent time in the United States that "many of them at U.S. NIH were not very happy that FERCAP had developed capacity. They see *themselves* as builders of capacity." At the same time as hospitals in China flocked in the hundreds for FERCAP accreditation, delegates at conferences questioned who FERCAP was to recognize, arguing that their activities were "illegal."[6] But for committee members, the proximity of recognition initiatives and interest from entities outside their own institution can raise the profile of research ethics, redirecting resources and raising reputation. Instrumental use is made of the externality of assessors. As Andrew Kipnis has argued, technologies of governing "often serve some sort of purpose in the management of social relations in a local context," (2008, 286) as researchers have made them do here.

A key question in the coming chapters is why committees and their members have come to participate in what is—and remains—a voluntary process. The reasons are broad. Seen from the perspective of regulators, the "problem" is one of data integrity. But seen from the perspective of scholars who work in the countries where FERCAP operates, ethics committees had become necessary for publishing research. Journals could not fully assess the ethics of research as it was under review, but they could require that it had been through an ethics committee. Growing research environments *needed* ethics committees.[7] FERCAP is already positioned as an organization that seeks, in medical anthropologist Lenore Manderson's words, to "correct the way that knowledge is inequitably distributed worldwide" (TDR Global 2017). A decade after FERCAP's foundation, concern about "foreign" clinical trials continued to drive research in the United States. In 2010, the U.S. Department of Health and Human Services' Office of the Inspector General issued a report entitled "Challenges to FDA's Ability to Monitor and Inspect Foreign Clinical Trials" (Levinson 2010). By that time, it observed, "eighty percent of approved marketing applications for drugs and biologics contained data from foreign clinical trials" (Levinson 2010, ii). However, things had changed, as "with regard to extending its oversight to clinical trials outside the United States, FDA's efforts to ensure data integrity and safety and protection of human subjects must be respectful of the sovereignty of other countries" (Levinson 2010, appendix E). In the years since Cristina expressed her frustration at the absence of national systems, pieces of regulation have been put in place in some countries in the

Asia-Pacific, positioning health bodies, hospitals, and universities as having a role in resourcing—and examining—the practices of their ethics committees. At the time of my fieldwork, the ethics committee community was often seen as being ahead of national programs, but they were well aware of this. At the 2009 Conference, a coordinating trainer based in Thailand laughingly and confidently said during a break,

> Now, ethics committees are more advanced than the regulatory bodies! In the Philippines, they're happy [we run trainings] as they'll learn from us how to inspect! We have to build little by little. Build an ethical review system first. From there, link the system as a whole. FERCAP conference brings in dialogue among stakeholders. That's the aim of FERCAP—to have a research system. Not only ethics committees, that's only part. [The] ethics committee is our entry point.

This statement sets us up for the chapters to come. It prefigures the long hours of reviewing Standard Operating Procedures and observations of committee meetings. It illustrates the vision from the early part of this century, laying out the role of this regional NGO in "creating systems" in their absence, in "building capacity" through relationships, demonstration, and conversation. It resonates with the themes throughout the book, as the region is brought together in a network.

TWO

The Hospitable Audit

Late on a sultry April afternoon in 2010, just over a year after I'd heard Cristina presenting the FERCAP program in Colombo, Sri Lanka, I join a group of researchers and administrators gathered in the medical faculty at a university in Manila, in the Philippines. The ground floor meeting room windows are tightly closed against the roar of traffic outside, and the old metal air conditioner in the corner, painted a medical green, is hard at work. The group has gathered for the closing meeting of a Survey of the medical faculty's ethics review committee, a review in which, over the past four days, I had observed and participated.

Dr. Sam, our Lead Surveyor from Taiwan, stands at the front of the room fiddling with the PowerPoint, about to begin his final presentation. He will be summing up the findings from the Survey's past four days. We, his audience, are both the members of the Survey team—the trainees, local Surveyors, and international Surveyors—as well as the members of the ethics committee that has been under review. His words are to be directed at this last group, who, waiting for the meeting to begin, are shuffling and whispering amongst themselves. There is suspense: A final meeting, where the findings of the survey team are presented, is a delicate social occasion. The standardized sentence—seen on the closing PowerPoint of every Survey—reminds everyone of the combination of help and assessment on offer: "The Reason for the Survey: To assist [insert committee name] in reviewing their practices and appraise their performance against the Strategic Initiative in Developing Capacity in Ethical Review criteria for recognition."

Dr. Sam begins to talk, listing those who have taken part, the trainees in three groups, each under the guidance of the local, foreign, and lead Surveyors. His first fifteen slides identify the research protocols and meeting

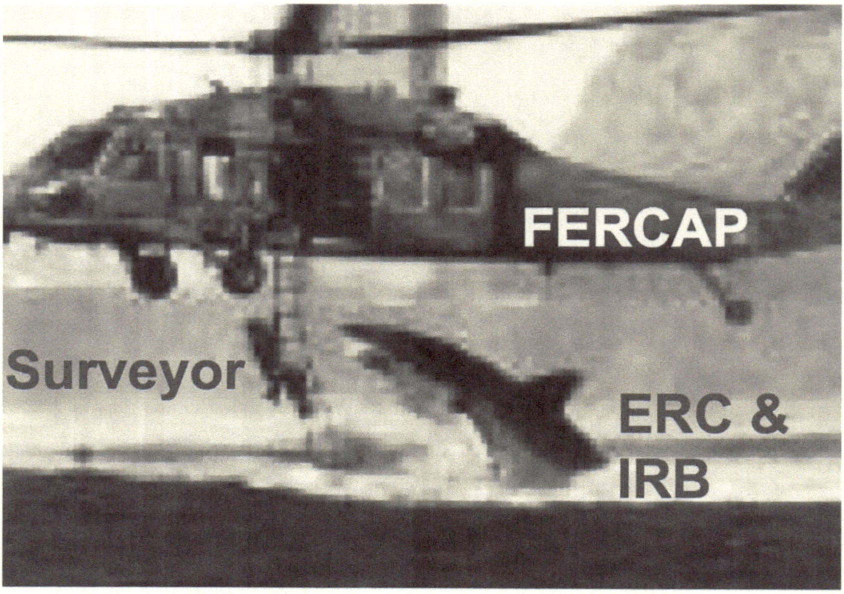

Figure 2.1. Slide Sixteen of Dr. Sam's closing presentation. Source: Author.

minutes that were examined, the Serious Adverse Events reports considered, and the members of the committee who were interviewed.

Slide sixteen (Figure 2.1 above) falls between slides that document the general method of the Survey and its findings. It is a pixelated image of a green camouflage-painted helicopter, flying low over a choppy sea.[1] A rope ladder dangles from its open door. A person clutches the ladder, and to their right, a shark is leaping out of the water, its jaws aimed at the suspended figure. Dr. Sam has typed in labels for the scene: the helicopter, in a large white font, is FERCAP. In red, the person hanging on to the ladder is the Surveyor (him), and the shark the committee that is under assessment, the ERC or IRB. "I stand here, a most vulnerable subject," he comments with humor. The room giggles. Will he, the dangling surveyor, the representative of FERCAP, be eaten by the shark of the committee? Having raised a laugh and dispersed some of the tension, Dr. Sam continues with his presentation of the recommendations for how the committee can improve its practices.

What to make of this moment, and slide sixteen's visual joke? Why is Dr. Sam, esteemed guest and apparent authority, portraying himself as in danger, calling himself a "vulnerable subject"? Standing alone at the front of the room delivering the findings of the Survey, he is clearly worried about how the committee he addresses will respond. Doing criticism well is difficult, especially as an invited guest. Humor can help—a "vulnerable subject" is a category of person that ethics committees have a particular duty to protect in biomedical research, an inside joke that momentarily pulls Dr. Sam under the *protection* of the committee he is assessing.[2] The placement of this slide, between the technicalities and the results, reveals that although during the Survey it is the *committee* that has been under scrutiny, in this moment of feedback, the *surveyor* becomes vulnerable to their reactions.

Doing the Survey is doing regional work through the implementation of the SIDCER Recognition Program. Throughout the year, the network coordinates international and local surveyors in four-day visits of committees, and with participants in their own local Surveys becoming trained to take on the role of international surveyors at a later date. Thus, when people meet, many will have visited or been visited by others. "They're surveyor in one place, surveyee in another," Juntra explained to me, as we stood in the cavernous hallways of the 2010 Shanghai Conference venue. Looking at people greeting one another, she continued: "Instead of competing or being jealous, because of exchanging, people are accountable to one another."

This mutual "accountability" was created by designing a common interest in the quality of the Recognition Program: "The recognized people say we need to keep up with quality—if one of us jeopardizes it . . . so they're looking after themselves. They talk to each other and suggest ways to improve. This model is very good." Despite its large geographic scope, stretching from Sri Lanka and Malaysia to South Korea and Kazakhstan, the model creates a narrative of common investment and the circulation of volunteer assessors, as committees put themselves forward for assessment. It is through this model that FERCAP's work begins to depart from an assessment more familiar to scholars of audit (Shore and Wright 2024). The mechanism of return—of swapped roles—means that those who have held the power to assess in one place become those under assessment in another. At the kernel of the "model" is an investment in the upkeep of standards: If a Surveyor "gives in" to lower standards so as not to offend their hosts, they potentially risk the value of their own committee's standing and achievements.

This chapter considers the four-day Survey as a key technology within the NGO's capacity-building repertoire. It is the main device of assessment through which FERCAP seeks to strengthen the capacity of committees in the region, and the technique through which committee standards are made present. The Survey described above in Manila was one of dozens I attended over the course of my research, the majority in Thailand, the Philippines, and mainland China. The five standards to which committees are held are extensive and cover much of committee life. As such, when they invite the Survey, committees must put their sense of pride in their practices and achievement aside. Dr. Sam's experience at the end of the Manila Survey shows the precarious power of the guest in the face of the potentially volatile vulnerability of the host. To invite the auditor-guests means, as we shall see, to host while surrendering claims to authority.

To understand the Survey as FERCAP conducts it, I bring into dialogue two burgeoning yet largely unconnected fields of literature. The first is social studies of audit, a "distinctly unglamorous" field in its untrusting demands for accountability and transparency, an "idea as much as a concrete technical practice" (Power 1999, xi, 4). The profession of audit carries its own ethics codes, many of which rule out entirely the acceptance either of gifts or hospitality. For example, the "Objectivity Principle," one of four key areas of ethics conduct created by the Global Institute of Internal Auditors, states that auditors shall not "accept anything that may impair or be presumed to impair their professional judgment" (IIA 2018), which, in practice, often rules out dinners, gifts, and tours. All this seems to be the inverse of the second field of literature: hospitality. Hospitable conduct seems premised on gifts, dinners, and generosities of many kinds. Building on earlier academic treatment of hospitality, scholars across disciplines from management to anthropology are again attending to hospitable encounters in an academic renaissance of interest. Anthropologists in particular have demonstrated the breadth of activities that constitute hospitality, from handshakes in space (Battaglia 2012) to Tanzanian "homes" of mosquito experimentation (Kelly 2012), and sought to differentiate hosting from hospitality (Chau 2019). In continuity with this spirit of exploring the character of hospitable conduct, in particular that of the hosts, in this chapter I show how the audit that Dr. Sam is awkwardly summing up above is made to work through techniques of hospitality. While hospitable acts are antithetical to the asocial social relations audit demands, they represent a reinvention of audit through both the network's preference and financial necessity: Audits are expensive affairs. Rather than seeing this as audit done badly, as a failure to maintain the anonymous relations deemed necessary for audit's "objective" evaluation, I explore how, alongside the rule-based ordering practices of the audit, hospitable practices of commensality and ideals of mutual assistance come to the fore.

The critical guests of this chapter—Surveyors—are invited to conduct what I have elsewhere called a "second order audit"—a review of the reviewing practices of ethics committees (Douglas-Jones 2015; see also Power 1994). Volunteer surveyors like Sam travel the region, applying standards and assessment checklists to the work of ethics committees, closely examining their practices, reviewing their archives, interviewing their staff, and reporting back the findings. The Survey's audit traits are immediately recognizable with their emphases on documentation, the need for renewal, personnel selected for their presumed social distance, and objective gaze. Yet the approach taken by FERCAP is distinctive: The language and practices surrounding the Survey are not those of detached outsiders producing an account. Instead, a Survey is full of conviviality and friendship, and it rarely calls itself an audit. The "recognition" on offer is a term that invokes a different register from audit and accreditation, and volunteers share stories more akin to faith-based testimonies as they recount how they came to "see" ethics for the first time.

Reinventing audit plays on what it means to be guest, host, and friend. Each of these terms is well theorized, but thinking of FERCAP's audit as hospitable creates intriguing new intersections that rest upon the need of the participants to manage social relations within formalized settings. I'm interested in the *mutuality* underpinning the way this particular audit is set up. Invitations being the "ambiguous things" (Candea and Da Col 2012, 4) that they are, the auditors are neither absolutely unknown nor divine strangers, as literature in hospitality might know them, but invited friend-assessors. How, then, are the participants in this scheme known to one another? I draw out the fine line these guests must walk between friend and critic by examining how audit's language of "objectivity" is reinforced by the necessity of "strangerness" within a hospitable frame. Surveyors foreground "evidence" as a means of depersonalizing their findings and keeping hospitality's "twin sister hostility" in the shadows (Selwyn 2000, 37) as the results of the Survey are presented to the committee under review. For a committee, the hosting and hospitality work of this audit sits within the broader worlds of which it is a part: those of the international biomedical economy of research projects.

The Auditor Guest

The Survey in Manila was held in a large ground floor room, filled with tables, tall metal framed windows painted green. It looked like it was usually used for teaching, but today it was filled with boxes as the Ethics Committee had brought in their records for us to review. I was filing away research protocols I had reviewed with a local surveyor, Nimuel. Dr. Sam, our lead Surveyor, wandered through the room, reminding us that time was nearly up, adding that we were not "fault finding." Nimuel scowled at this latter remark. "Sometimes that *is* how it feels," he confessed. "You're probably doing the best you can, and here comes a group of people trying to find out something wrong." "Well," I said carefully, "the committees do *invite* the Survey." Acknowledging this, he still shook his head, gesturing at Dr. Sam, who was now hunched over his laptop at the far end of our table:

> I don't understand why [the outcome is] an approval or disapproval, if that's the purpose, to be supportive. Why not make recommendations and then return and see if there's been an improvement? Helping, rather than [acting as a] supreme court?

While Surveyors talk about helping and friendship, mutual and ongoing improvement, at the end an assessment is reached. Every Survey comes with the risk of nonrecognition. Before inviting a team of Surveyors, committees must meet three criteria, today laid out in the newly revised 2020 SIDCER-FERCAP Survey Standard Operating Procedures (Navarro et al. 2020). They must have been in operation for at least a year, have reviewed at least thirty protocols, and have adopted and been working with their own Standard Operating Procedures for at least six months. Before the Survey will visit, the committee must conduct and submit a self-assessment using the SIDCER Assessment Tool. The tool consists of nineteen pages of questions, each tied to a requirement laid out in the "Silver Book" (WHO/TDR 2002) or the Good Clinical Practice guidelines set out by the International Council for Harmonization (ICH-GCP). Sally, an international Surveyor from Taiwan working with Dr. Sam in Manila, described this as a moment where committees could begin to "get outside of themselves." Being within the day-to-day work of a committee, she commented, meant that committee members struggle to "see the things that are not correct." A recognized accounting tool, self-audits aim to ensure an organization is fully prepared for an audit. In this work of defamiliarization, or external interrogation, committees would begin to gain a distance to their own practices.

The next way in which distance is invoked in the Survey process is through the arrival of the Surveyors. "Foreign" or "international" Surveyors lead each Survey, a policy based on their assumed objectivity. Cristina explained the policy to trainees in Manila this way: "We are from [University], so we say, 'We are the best.' Do *other* people think you are the best? It has to be validated. So, people from outside [University] should audit and check the [University] IRB." Cristina's phrasing shows us that an implicit attribute of the foreign surveyor is that they are external to the organization being studied, a (more distant) externality that "checks"; a view that rests on an explicit desire for objectivity,[3] the literal distance that the Surveyor has traveled (from their country) is also taken to offer them the figurative distance, or the "objectivity" so desired for the Survey. Writing about the workings of an Israeli medical committee, Yael Assor has suggested that if we examine "objectivity as a morally desired disposition rather than a static construct," we can begin to see "the process through which subjects aim to assume this disposition" and explore how it is a "subjectively and intersubjectively constituted sedimentation one that operates in light of context-specific interpretations of ideal forms of 'objectivity'" (2021, 115–16). This objectivity has a history (Daston 1992).

While committees invite the Survey, how are they convinced to reveal their inner workings to these outsiders, and how do Surveyors work to achieve the "morally desired disposition" (Assor 2021, 115) of an objective assessment? Building on the ethos built up at the annual Conference, Surveyors announce that they "come as friends," expressing a desire to "learn" from the committee under study. "Learning" from one's hosts is a leveling statement, aimed at reducing the distance from which critique will eventually fall. It is also, tactically, deemed necessary, drawing out the "true committee," rather than a performance put on for outsiders. Take this revealing quote from the opening to a Survey in Bangkok:

> It's like if you're a policeman, I'm not going to tell you my weaknesses. I'm going to try and cover everything up! We are not police! If it's a Surveyor, [the committee] can say, "I don't know how to do this, what do I do?" and FERCAP suggest[s]. It's a different feeling. Though you want to do better, the person who has come has come to evaluate you. You want to show your best, and sweep the bad stuff under the carpet. But with Surveys, it's about quality improvement. Sometimes

> they don't tell you, but because we're like family already, I don't feel so bad if you tell me my child is ugly! The Surveyors come and say, "Your baby is ugly," *but* there's a way to make the baby look nice. Because the Surveyor has a plastic surgeon with them!

In this vivid description the Surveyor is drawing on the "family" metaphor to encourage the revelation of the host committee's "ugliness" to the guests. It is a moment that shows the desire on the part of the speaker for *confession* from the committee, a baring of truths upon which "improvement" is dependent (Scott 2022). It expresses some of the spirit of *kalyanamitra* described by Chitr Sitthi-amorn and Ratana Somrongthong as a philosophy of "intelligent solidarity" (2000, 815) borrowing from Buddhism a concept they translate as "friends helping friends" but that also carries a sense that this person can tell you what you might not want to hear. It recognizes, compassionately, that a committee may wish to conceal its actual practices to retain sovereignty of the home committee (with its "carpet") against the assessing guests. The hosts must therefore be persuaded into a position of vulnerability, revealing their true committee to the authority ("friend") that has come to inspect. The language of family, and of the mutuality of the structure of the Survey, aims to make possible the assessment between friends, and the potential "ugliness of the baby."

However, a danger of the distance in generating objectivity to preserve friendships is that it reduces the knowledge of the "local," of the "complexity of cultural variations, national laws, local medical and research practices and local knowledge" (Karbwang et al. 2001, 3) that the Forum was itself set up to accommodate. Ignorance is the flipside of distance here. Authoritative distance still needed an understanding of the world of the committee, otherwise recommendations for improvement would miss their mark. The responsibility for linking the objectivity of the foreign Surveyor with an understanding of a committee's context falls to the local Surveyor, who serves as an intermediary between the institution being surveyed and the foreign Surveyors. According to the guiding documents of the Survey, these local Surveyors must have "no attachment/affiliation with the EC/IRB being surveyed" (SIDCER-FERCAP 2020). Their primary role is to help provide an overview of the national context and translate committee protocol documents, policies, and Standard Operating Procedures (SOPs) into English from the local language.[4] As Vichai

Chokevivat notes in his summary of the scheme, this work of translation is "time-consuming, as there are a large number of documents" (2019, 1148). This work of translation has the potential to embroil local Surveyors in sometimes highly charged representations of the Surveyors' comments and the committee's responses. Surveyors from other countries, while "objective," are sometimes thought not to not know "enough" about the local context, thereby frustrating committees with requests for "improvements" that would make no national sense. Inappropriate recommendations for "improvements" not only threaten the pride of the host committee, they potentially undermine the authority of the international Surveyors. As we saw in the chapter's opening vignette, the Survey's concluding feedback session is a time of vulnerability for the Lead Surveyors. After watching a number of Surveys in Taiwan, Sally, who had experience both as a local and international Surveyor, told me that she often found that members of the committee under review were "very proud of themselves," making them liable to challenge recommendations. This was particularly the case, she said, if an institute's committee appointment procedures meant that people in very senior positions were asked to sit on the Ethics Committee. "If they think you are criticizing them"—she drew her breath in sharply—"they don't like it at all." She described such people as having "eyes on top of their heads,"[5] indicating with her hands cupped on top of her own head. "So, look," she lamented, bending forward at the waist so her "eyes" pointed at me, "unless they bow, they cannot see."

In the combination of objective distance and the threat of a critical guest, the success of recommendations depends on the interaction between the visiting "foreign" Surveyors and the "local" committee members. The latter must accord the former the right—and authority—to critique, and suggest improvements. Unlike literature on the host's moral authority (Selwyn 2000, 34), hospitality on one's own territory here does not come with a claim to authority. Indeed, the permission to critique is granted largely because it is repeatedly said to be done with the intention to "help," and roles are developed to give those filling them the semblance of an objective position while continuing to allow a narrative of friendship. But the final meeting, talked of as an opportunity for discussion and feedback, also has the potential to develop into dispute if the "recommendations" are not taken well; that is, if critique is taken *as* criticism. As Tom Selwyn notes, "the possibility of rebellion, betrayal, upset and sudden reversals of status, are by definition, always present" (2000, 34). We have begun to better understand Dr. Sam's ambivalence, to sketch out the character of the shark underneath that hovering helicopter. Within straightforward accounts of hospitality, it is the host's moral authority that must be accepted by the guest. In the hospitable audit, however, the guest's authority—to assess—is being challenged by the host. Surveyors must, therefore, draw on further techniques to back them up, should their social authority begin to fail.

Audit's Evidence and Hospitality's Favor

If science has been critiqued for performing as a culture of no culture, then the international implacability of audit longs equally "passionately for a world without loose ends" (Traweek 1992, 162). Even though the sociologist Michael Power's early analyses of audit's rise within post-Thatcherite Britain specifically pointed to its cultural ties to a particular vision of problem solving (this specificity was part of his original expectation that it would be a "passing phase"; see Power 1994, 32) audit practices are today profoundly international, and subject to complex retooling and partial reinterpretation (Shore and Wright 2024). Like other audits around the world, the FERCAP Survey seeks evidence as a foundation upon which critique may rest. "Evidence" is particularly useful for the hospitable audit: As we shall see, it depersonalizes recommendations, creating for the Surveyors the temporary authority that they need in order to speak at the Survey's end.

I became especially interested in how evidence was being thought of during a Survey at a hospital in Beijing. It was FERCAP's first visit to the Chinese capital, with better relationships already established in Shanghai. The feeling was a little tense, a little competitive, as I arrived with the Survey team. The hospital's administrative buildings had tall glass facades, and specially made signposts pointed us to the dark basement meeting rooms, lined with wooden paneling and a highly polished wooden table. Huiying, who had lots of experience with FERCAP Surveys, had taken on the role as the local Surveyor for FERCAP's first visit to Beijing, the corresponding national representative to the international Surveyor's lead. After the welcomes and introductions of the training's first day, she spoke to the gathered volunteers and trainees to explain the process. There were around thirty of us, from different committees, chairs pulled up to the vast conference table. The teams would split up, she said, take photographs of documents, find missing signatures, make diagrams of the committee offices, and lean over the shoulders of secretaries to scrutinize their databases. We were doing all of this, she explained, because in the closing meeting, we needed to present the "evidence." Every recommendation made by the Survey needed a reference: "What protocol number? What page?" Evidence would be collected with the final PowerPoint in mind,[6] details and references hoarded for each end of day summary meeting, and the ultimate feedback to the committee under scrutiny.[7] Huiying's slides explained to her Beijing audience what this work of creating an objective synthesis entailed.

Her first slide depicted how the Survey would reach its conclusions (Figure 2.2), using visual extension of the Chinese proverb "a single tree makes no forest" (独木不成林). Three characters feature: 木 [*mù*], in the smallest font at the back; 林 [*lín*], medium size in the middle; and 森 [*sēn*], the largest at the front. The characters convey leaf, trees, and forest, respectively. Usually, the saying comes as a second part to the phrase "a single thread can not make a cord" (单 丝 不 成 线), conveying the limits of individual capacities in completing large tasks: In other words, everyone must pull together. That day, Huiying explained to the trainees that "the leaves are the detecting method, the forest is the analysis—how we draw conclusions and necessary system thinking." Her second slide (Figure 2.3) was an image of a surprised looking cartoon elephant, surrounded by men in suits, all wearing dark glasses, holding different parts of the elephant and wearing baffled expressions. Around the image, eight large yellow question marks. Huiying warned us that, separated into our teams, none of us could expect to "know" the whole elephant: "Each group is only touching only one part at the end of the day—you [in touching the part you do] don't touch the tail or the head. Try to reconstruct from your observations and reports, what does the EC look like, what are its strengths and weaknesses? How does it do its work?"

Again emphasizing collaboration and working together, Huiying said that Surveyors must be able to describe what the "whole elephant" looked like: "Different people see different things, they see from different parts. We collect everyone's opinion and truth, we put it together, and maybe get truth of whole thing." During the coffee break, I took the handout of the slides to Huiying, asking her to tell me more. The two stories, she told me, were a way of explaining to trainees how the Survey would move from the detail of missing signatures to a final synthesis, a blend both of different (objective) parts to get a whole picture *and* a way of accommodating a range of perspectives to

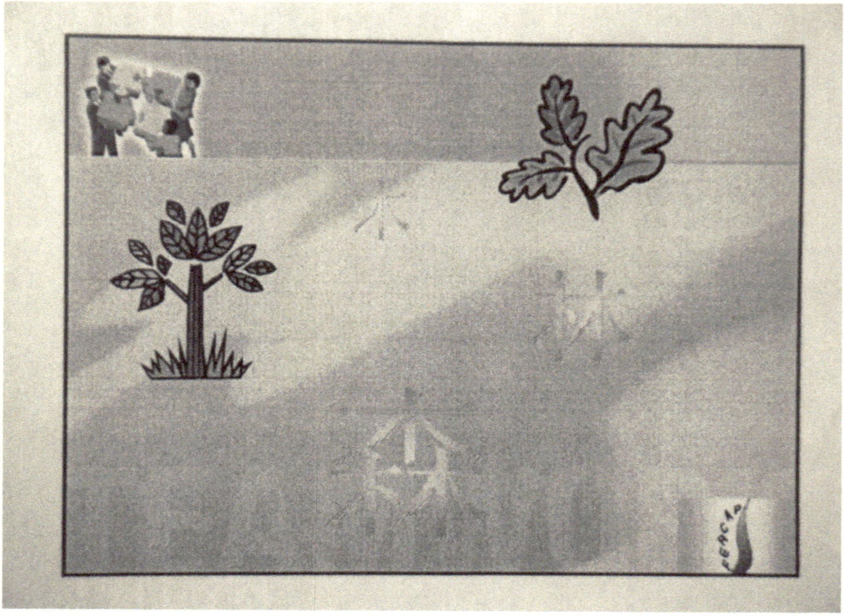

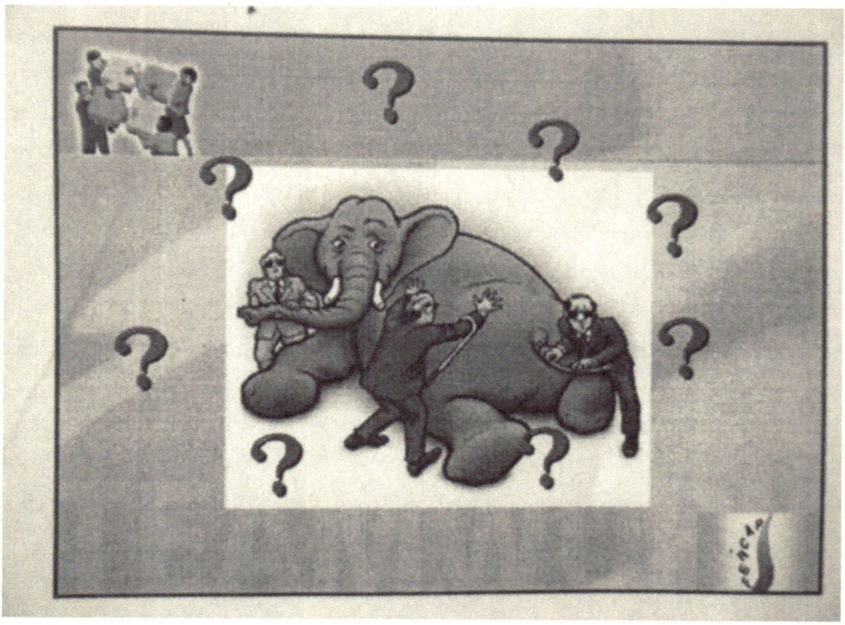

Figures 2.2 and 2.3. Huiying's teamwork slides. Source: Author.

"arrive at a balance." This, for her, was the essence of teamwork: "Everyone may not be completely right, but they may not be completely wrong. Based on teamwork, we can get to the truth," she enthused. Huiying is pulling off a sleight of hand here. The tale of the "Blind Men and the Elephant" is usually told to demonstrate the *futility* of claims to omniscience—nobody has the full picture—not their possibility.[8] Instead, in her telling, the story allows for a "perspective from nowhere" to arise from the "perspective from everywhere," creating objectivity through a strategic renarration. In this version of an auditors' synthesis, the volunteers and trainees will each contribute "perspectives" that "add up" to evidence to be displayed in the form of photographs, diagrams, and protocol numbers.[9]

Evidence is not the only thing to appear in the end of Survey presentations. There are signatures or incomplete files but also photographs of food. At the end of each of these long days poring over documents, Surveyors temporarily let go of their pursuit of an objective account, and committees make time for elaborate courtesy (Herzfeld 2012, S212). After eleven hours around Survey tables in our Beijing hospital basement, for example, taxis arrived and we trudged wearily upstairs to meet them. Squished in the back with the committee's secretarial team, I was driven through the evening traffic out of town, to Beijing's Summer Palace. The complex had closed for the day and was almost deserted—occasional gardeners were sweeping leaves down the Long Gallery as we walked Kunming Lake. Inside the restaurant Tingli Guan,[10] tables were laid for a feast, and the Surveyors and trainees scattered excitedly, taking photos of one another in front of the enormous glowing red gauze lanterns. Unlike the expected ritual expenditures of high finance or corporate life (Ho 2009; Chong 2018), the grand extravagance of this kind of outing, when read within a regular audit framing, would prompt considerable anxiety about, and even undermine, an audit's integrity. Within the calculative frame of a true audit, nothing that cannot be accounted for should be accepted, with newly specific moral boundaries shifting practice toward something more calculative, scientific (Kipnis 2008). Yet the Survey's audit-like calculative behavior has limits because of its extension of "favour, an expression of esteem, of the desire to please [. . .] that is not answerable to coherent reasoning" (Pitt-Rivers 2011, 431). It was not answerability or reasoning that put photographs of delicious food consumed during the Survey into the closing PowerPoint slides, annotated with notes of appreciation and gentle jibes about who had eaten the most. These gifts both of experience and commensality suggest something more akin to grace than calculation, opposed "as the open cheque is to the audited account" (Pitt-Rivers 2011, 431), a suspension within the measures of quality improvement.

Becoming Hosts

The audit-like aspects of the Survey have a particular attractiveness within the international bioeconomies of research. In her analysis of the life sciences in Singapore, a regional hub of activity, Aihwa Ong observes that despite its own "dazzling machinery of genomics and cutting-edge discourse" Singapore is still motivated by a desire to *attract* human and financial capital to its shores (2016, 17; see also Holden and Demeritt 2008). Ethics committees are thought of as integral to this attracting capacity, and when the coordinators of FERCAP present the Survey program of "recognition" to committees, they usually begin by describing the international research arena of global capital to which Ong's interlocutors are oriented.

Surveyors talk about harmonization, compliance, and the pursuit of excellence and quality in research, particularly if researchers in the Asia-Pacific region want to participate in internationally sponsored biomedical research. In this way, ethics review committees come to be trained with a view to their role within a "whole system," which provides a context for their operations. This framing appeals to committees and their members: In becoming hosts to research, they may also gain access to clinical trials, funds, and publications. For Survey participants, *hosting FERCAP's Surveyors is potentially not so far from hosting biomedical clinical trials.* In these scalar movements, analysts of hospitality are at home, as they watch the language and practices of hosting shift from the household to the nation state (Herzfeld 2012, S211; Shryock 2012, S28). So, although the Survey measures, it is also itself a measure: It has the potential to make hosts of these countries, indicating hospitality to outsiders, by outsiders' own standards and measurements. A committee audited and recognized provides assurance that its practices are sound, that they meet "international" standards. Committees are told that they can put their recognized status on their website, and many do. They are also told that it will be of interest to international sponsors who, FERCAP's coordinator states, "like assurance that the Ethics Committee is doing their job."

"Doing their job" is Cristina's shorthand for compliance with international guidelines, an essential factor for sponsors and a measure that a site is hospitable to research: Studies conducted here can be published, and they can also be submitted to U.S. and EU regulatory authorities. To become hospitable in this sense, then, is to do so on someone else's terms. The point has been made forcefully in discussions of bioethics (Farmer 2003; Macklin 2004), but attention to the Survey as a means of participation in "global" research allows us to ask what it means to become, as the literature puts it, a "host country." As Matei Candea and Giovanni Da Col write, "acts of hospitality turn people themselves into things, usable, exploitable assets, indexes of other intentionalities" (2012, S10). This, too, is the potentiality of clinical trials as both bodies and nations seek, in a scalar slip, to play host to experimental international biomedical designs. These "other intentionalities" are discussed in detail across work by anthropologists of global health, whose work analyzes in detail the tensions in becoming hosts to biomedical research funded outside the country where it is conducted (Crane 2010; Brada 2023).

From Dr. Sam's joking ambivalence at the opening of this chapter, I have shown how hospitality infuses the audit-like Survey. Dr. Sam's sixteenth slide shows all too clearly his awareness of the uneasy potential in guesthood. Poised between the ties of friendship and his invited role as the external party whose positionality is necessary for the committee's critical improvement, Dr. Sam embodies the way the hospitable audit compels him to point to his hosts, the source of his own power. Only with their consent can the Survey's findings be accepted and incorporated. Combining the figures of the auditor and the friend subverts the anonymity of auditors, inserting a parallel mode of sociality into the practice of committee review. Invited as guests, Surveyors are hosted by the committee, with both parties bound into a mutual desire for improvement. The language of friendship encourages an openness that audit's severity tends to close: The Surveyors have a plastic surgeon with them!

FERCAP's Survey blends the formalities of both hospitality and audit. This is not a case of doing audit "wrong": The partially unseen, time delayed elements of hospitality (Shryock 2008, 59) are present in its indirect return, whereby each participant visited may become a visitor, where each host may become a guest. I suggest that what Surveyors aim at is not stringently studied informality, not well-managed camaraderie (Herzfeld 2012, S213), but a sense of mutual investment. During audit events, it is hosts who must temporarily surrender their sovereignty and accept the assessment of their guests. Using orchestrated openness, members and Surveyors demonstrate their investment in the mutual upkeep of the Survey's standards. This is precisely the *intended* outcome of the "model"—it creates a self-sustaining system made up of equally invested partners in a dance of reversing places. The hospitality of this paper is not everyday; it is incorporated into formal mechanisms designed to manage relations of proximity, distance, and affect. Following the social lives of hospitality and audit allows us to see them emerging together in peoples' efforts to manage charged relations, the "product and producer of sociopolitical order" (Sneath 2019, 83). Suspended between audit-based ideals of objective, evidenced knowledge and the lengthening friendships of two decades of regional work, the network's Survey is a generative condition productive not only of over two hundred voluntarily audited committees, but also a uniquely self-sustaining system. Even recognized committees remain within the circulation of friendship and critique: Under principles of continuous quality improvement, I am told that "there is no such thing as a perfect ethics committee."

There may be no perfect committee, but there is such a thing as not *yet* good enough for recognition. At the end of a Survey, committees receive a report and must produce an "Action Plan" for the FERCAP Survey team to review. Sometimes a "follow-up site visit," as detailed in the SIDCER-FERCAP Survey SOP-07 (Navarro et al. 2020, 41), will be necessary, as not all committees are recognized in the Conference following their Survey. Some must continue to improve. Talking to one lead Surveyor about their experiences running a Survey for a committee in a country where few committees were yet recognized, he explained that there "was progress." They had found a room, got their SOPs in place, sorted out their membership. But something was still missing: The discussions it was having were simply not "there yet." When I asked what wasn't yet working, the Surveyor explained it was still "just a scientific review" and lacked the qualities needed to be a good *ethics* review. Amidst the administrative and institutional work that the Survey precipitates, at the heart of it is this discussion: Will this committee, and the things they discuss, protect participants in the research proposals that cross their table? The lead Surveyor had already done one follow-up visit and another was scheduled, noting to me that these returns were unpaid time and voluntary work on their part. But until the review itself was good, the committee could not be recognized.

Explored ethnographically, the Survey as a governing device of committee quality is neither entirely hospitality nor audit, but a deliberate and productive ambivalence between them. When Dr. Sam speaks, he summarizes and combines the views of the other Surveyors, his PowerPoint amassing the "evidence" that will be used to support the recommendations. Objectivity emerges as a social strategy, to neutralize the dangerous tensions of critique. While for Assor's committee members, "unemotionality" is regarded as an ethical objective (2021), cultivating an "objective" disposition here draws heavily on bureaucratic tropes of evidence and deflects from the possible insult of judgment as the Survey progresses. But in its foregrounding of evidence and through its mimicry of science, perceived as "good," it leads to Surveyors focusing on that which can be evidenced. This in turn, in a scale shift familiar to the sphere of hospitality, encourages committees to regard evidence for *their own* decisions as essential.

Markets for Audit, Markets for Hosting, Markets for Ethics

It is appealing for research sites who want to create "hospitality" to U.S. funds to be legible on U.S. terms. In 2005, the American accreditor of ethics review committees, the Association for the Accreditation of Human Research Protection Programs, Inc. (AAHRPP), began to visit committees in the Asia-Pacific region. AAHRPP (pronounced "A-Harp") is a U.S.-based not-for-profit accreditation organization founded in 2001 with funds first provided by the Department of Veterans Affairs to the National Committee for Quality Assurance (NCQA) "to develop accreditation standards" (Smith 2008, 68). Like FERCAP, it emerged around the turn of the century, and can be traced to "The Globalization of Clinical Trials" (Rehnquist 2001a). In a letter dated June 29, 2001, responding to "The Globalization of Clinical Trials" report, the nonprofit Public Responsibility in Medicine and Research (PRIM&R), based in Boston, wrote that they had "spent almost three years developing a credible accreditation system for human research protection programs," founding and incorporating AAHRPP.[11]

> While AAHRPP is in its infancy, and it is not yet clear that AAHRPP's voluntary accreditation program will become widely accepted, we do have reason to believe that the community of regulated institutions will embrace a system of

> adopting voluntary performance standards, self-assessment and accreditation site visits by their peers. We agree that an international accreditation program would similarly promote a better worldwide protection for human research participants with uniform standards. This will, however, take time and resources that are not yet available. The goal, though, is a worthy one and should be kept alive and any opportunities to achieve this should be quickly embraced. (Rehnquist 2001b, 35)

The goal has been kept alive. In 2018, its president and CEO Elyse I. Summers noted that "in today's global research environment, where collaboration and multisite studies are the norm, every AAHRPP accreditation has a powerful, positive impact" (BioSpectrum Asia 2019). Operating today from offices in Washington, D.C., AAHRPP's goal is "one standard worldwide" (AAHRPP 2021, 3). The organization has been gradually adding sites beyond the United States: During 2016, they "added [their] first organizations in Africa and South America and increased [their] presence in Asia," welcoming many more to the "AAHRPP family" (Applied Clinical Trials 2016); Osaka University Hospital in Japan (AAHRPP 2022) in 2022, followed by Beijing Hospital of Traditional Chinese Medicine at the Capital Medical University in 2023 (AAHRPP 2023). Some committees visited by AAHRPP were preexisting collaborators of U.S. American universities, while others sought to become so. What could present more of an aspirational goal for committees desirous of association with U.S. colleagues, research groups, and sites than being accredited by a U.S. organization, according to U.S. standards? The idea of hosting research extends the audiences for FERCAP's Recognition Program, but also allows us to see how such markers of recognition begin to create markets for audit and accreditation in ethical review.

The mark of a committee being accredited by AAHRPP is a gold seal, used on websites and documentation. I spoke with Desmond, a Surveyor I worked alongside in Manila and Taipei, about AAHRPP during one of the long Survey lunches. He had recently visited Singapore for a conference, and reported that he once asked colleagues there, "Why are you not active in FERCAP?," to which he received the response "We are a developed country!" Desmond continued to tell me:

> I said so are Taiwan, and Korea . . . but they [Singapore] only like to be seen affiliated with the U.S. That's why they have AAHRPP in Singapore and Hong Kong!

> And now they [AAHRPP] are also entering Korea . . . Some big professor from Korea asked me, "Why [do you] stay with FERCAP, they're not better than us." So they propose to go to AAHRPP. So there may be a competition.

As we talked, Desmond suggested that professional competitiveness in general drove certification: "People will think your IRB is not good enough. So that's the reason why we have to get more and more [certifications]." As an account from the Office of Human Research Protections at the Catholic Medical Center (CMC) in South Korea attests, AAHRPP accreditation can be seen as outranking FERCAP's reviews by virtue of its breadth: "Because FERCAP recognition applies only to IRBs, AAHRPP's accreditation of the whole institution made it much more attractive in influencing sponsors to conduct their trials through CMC" (AAHRPP 2010, 5). The language of accreditation recalls for medical professionals the safety of standardized laboratory practices (Bhosale 2014, 56), and in their "testimonial" of going through an AAHRPP accreditation "journey" in India, clinical research managers Pratibha Pereira and K. L. Bairy show how hospitals working on "global trials" (2012, 81), particularly those regulated by the USFDA, are attracted by U.S. accreditation. They describe extensive preparation at the hospitals prior to the AAHRPP site visit: "Daily training sessions were conducted in order to *internalize the process*" (Pereira and Bairy 2012, 83, emphasis added).

Some of my interviewees worried about the rise of AAHRPP. For a start, the policies held committees to U.S. regulations, specifically "45 CFR 46," known as the Common Rule, or the federal policy that "applies to all research involving human subjects conducted, supported, or otherwise subject to regulation by any Federal department or agency" (OHRP 2009). Then there were the costs of accreditation, which would draw funds away from FERCAP's more distributive financial model by attracting away subscriptions of the more competitive and active research economies. The costs of AAHRPP accreditation for "Non-North American Organizations" sits on a scale, based on the number of active protocols overseen by the IRB. Application fees range from 22,900 USD for committees reviewing between 1 and 100 protocols, to 100,800 USD for committees reviewing more than 7,000 protocols. Once accredited, annual fees sit between 8,760 USD to 30,390 USD for those same size committees (AAHRPP 2024). Noting that the cost is also prohibitive for many U.S. committees, Sarah Babb explains that institutions "relied on the services of private consulting firms to prepare for accreditation, and often purchased new protocol management software," meaning that "institutions that self-selected into the accreditation club tended to be those with high volumes of biomedical research" (2020, 72). In addition to the costs, in my early fieldwork committee members remained skeptical of its regional relevance. While I was participating in a Survey in Taipei, committee member Desmond argued that AAHRPP was simply a "different kind of thing":

> They want to jump into the Asian market. You can't apply a U.S. standard here though. The money is different, the structure, and the mentality are different. FERCAP can operate because it doesn't cost too much, they use rotating volunteers. With AAHRPP, it's "you pay, we send."

In contrast with the careful social strategies described in this chapter, Desmond's perception of AAHRPP's operation relegated it to pure audit.[12] Desmond, after balking at the price tag and volume of work required to undertake an AAHRPP review (which is institution-wide and goes beyond the ethics committee), shook his head at the auditors themselves. "They don't accept anything," he said. Conflict of interest, designed to protect the integrity of the accreditation, meant distance. "They know if they come to Asia they will be treated nicely, so they say no hotel, no meal, only a cup of coffee. Not a banquet, not a souvenir." The anticipated refusal of AAHRPP's auditors to engage socially with committees' desires to host appears as the antithesis of the mutuality that FERCAP has fostered. Auditors, as opposed to Surveyors, will experience "conflict of interest," a condition that a true audit cannot sustain. They would almost certainly have had to refuse a private dinner at Beijing's Summer Palace. What FERCAP's approach to standard-making through mutuality shows is the difference they perceive between their hospitality-based Survey and other recognition programs that generate an "Asian market" of accreditation in the very move of breaking into it.

Reflecting on the early days of FERCAP, founding member Vichai Chokevivat, writes that in the first days of the "Blue Book" (WHO/TDR 2002)—which introduced principles for surveying and evaluating ethics committees—the authors discussed "the concept of auditing" (2019, 1145). Since the "Blue Book" would guide how the SIDCER survey then operated, the language mattered. He continues: "But when it came to the fore at a conference in Washington DC in late 2001, there was a discussion of the meaning and standards of auditing, including assurance and accreditation, and the meeting agreed that the evaluation principle should be used" (2019, 1145). The difference might not seem much, but turning this "evaluation principle" into the Survey program, they have stayed with, as the scholar of hospitality Tom Selwyn puts it, "the rules and principles of hospitality [that] stand at one remove from the principles and procedures of the marketplace" (2000, 35).

Writing from the United States, for Sarah Babb it is clear that the twenty-first century has given the U.S. "IRB field . . . the characteristics of a private industry" (2020, 75). This is in two senses: that committees themselves have become profit-making, "attract[ing] the attention of private equity firms, leading to a wave of mergers and acquisitions" (Babb 2021, 393), and in the growth of accreditation. Committees in this book are rarely profit-making, and Selwyn's contrast with the marketplace shows us the "remove" at which FERCAP's hospitable audit places itself. It offers mutuality shot through with hospitality, recognition rather than accreditation, allowing me to illustrate this distinction in orientations toward standards in ethics committee work more clearly. In his analysis of how the FERCAP/AAHRPP distinction played out in Taiwan, Wen-Hua Kuo observes the tussle over international affiliations, with the Taiwan Association of IRBs (TAIRB) affiliating with FERCAP, and another network, the Human Subject Protection Association (HuSPAT), being set up on the assertion "that service on an IRB was a profession" working with AAHRPP and PRIM&R. As Kuo writes, "backed by international organizations, these institutions identified their positions as genuine instructors and organizers for IBSs" (2018, 12) in a landscape of "lacking proper legal guidance [where] IRBs are actually eager for instructions as to their new role in human research" (Kuo 2018, 11–12).

It was the form of audit that prompted the "defining feature of ethics review as an organizational field since the 1990s: that is, corporatization" (Stark et al. 2021, 274). This chapter speaks to the theme of audit, but with different aims and goals. The FERCAP Survey is neither a response to complex government regulations, nor is what we have seen above fully corporate. In its departures from audit and its collaborative ethos, it remains at a remove from the anonymous relations and objectivity of an external authority given the power to accredit. Yet what FERCAP and AAHRPP share is concern with compliance. While AAHRPP looks to provide organizations with the labor and security that they seek to outsource compliance (Babb 2020), FERCAP is using a version of the same mechanisms as it seeks to equip committees. Scholarship on compliance illuminates the connections further, conceptualizing a "package"—actors, resources, ideas, and networks that can travel along certain vectors of compliance that has served as a "model and object lesson for the rise of a global compliance regime" (Sampson 2021, 111). Read alongside Sarah Babb's account and FERCAP's, Steven Sampson's work on the "compliance package" (2021, 127) points us in the right direction: Instead of the efficiency honed by IRBs of the United States, where "for-profit independent boards vied for clientele by offering speedy turnaround" (Babb 2020, 76), being "recognized" for FERACP's committees has the potential to make international hosts of research sites.

Recognition

When Dr. Sam stood to deliver his feedback from the Survey, the moment referenced the architecture that FERCAP has built—both for economic and political reasons—to make standards travel. It is a sociality that "brings people and things together in a world already full of competing conventions and standards" (Timmermans and Epstein 2010, 84). Dr. Sam's vulnerability is not false, and it is also not entirely his own: He is aware that the reciprocity of Surveyors and Surveyees rests on a relation of that more akin to guest and host than that of auditor and auditee. Using humor to "short-circuit" some of the tension that had arisen in the design, what Andrea Ballestero describes as itself a "short-circuit[ing of] the foundational separation between observers and observed" (2012, 223), he raises a laugh and changes the mood.

When the network gathers at the annual conference, committees are ceremonially recognized. The event takes place on the main stage of that year's conference venue, whether a hotel ballroom or hospital lecture hall. Over the years, the number of recognized committees has varied, not least because recognition—in line with a commitment to continuous improvement—lasts three years before the Surveyors are invited back again. In 2018, the last Conference I attended in person, this meant that committee members from each of the forty-seven committees surveyed that year gathered in Taipei, and in turn climbed on stage to applause to receive their certificate (for renewals) and their trophy (for first recognition). Each year, groups pose for photos that will later end up on institutional websites, joining the other three hundred committees before them who have demonstrated "continuing compliance with" the ICH-GCP guidelines, the Declaration of Helsinki, the Council for

International Organizations of Medical Sciences (CIOMS) guidelines, the World Health Organization (WHO) Operational Guidelines for Committees that Review Biomedical Research, EC/IRB Standard Operating Procedures (SOPs), and Local Regulations and Standards in Ethical Review. These "multiple policy tributaries" (Lea 2024, 6) condense into glass and paper, the certificates and trophies in Figures 2.4 and 2.5 below.

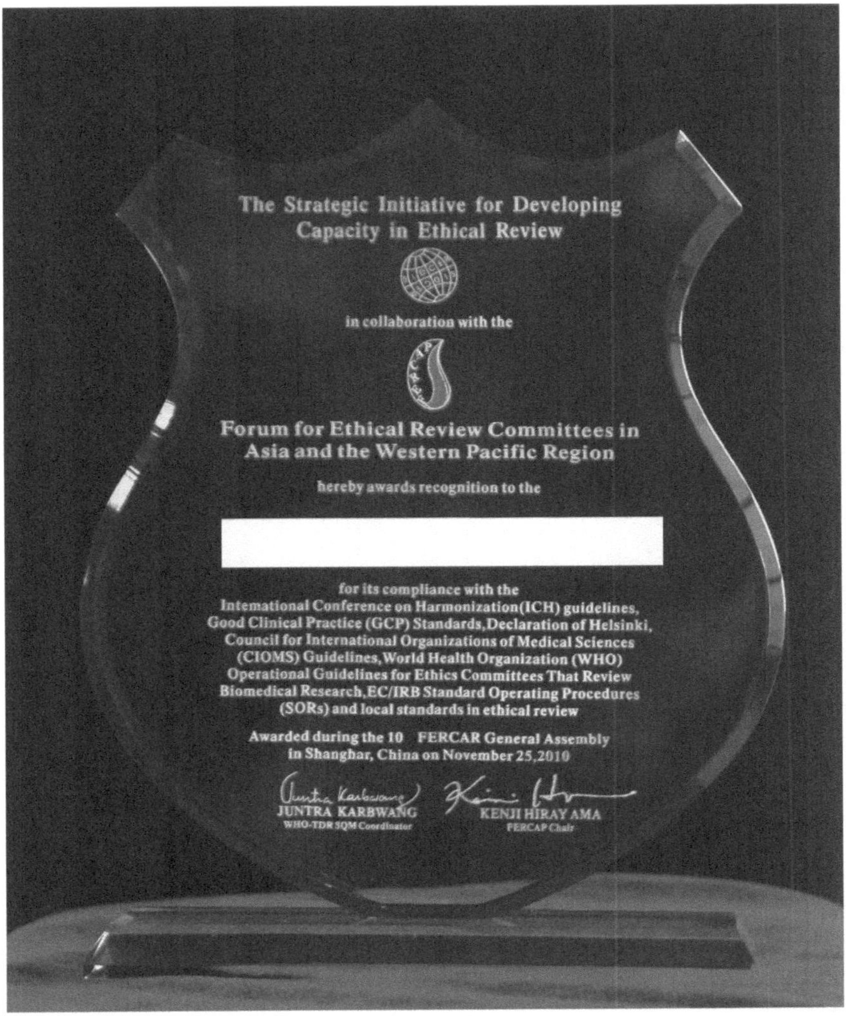

Figures 2.4 and 2.5. The crystal trophy and SIDCER-FERCAP certificate issued to committees on their recognition. The trophy is only issued on first recognition; renewals receive a new certificate with three-year validity. Source: Author.

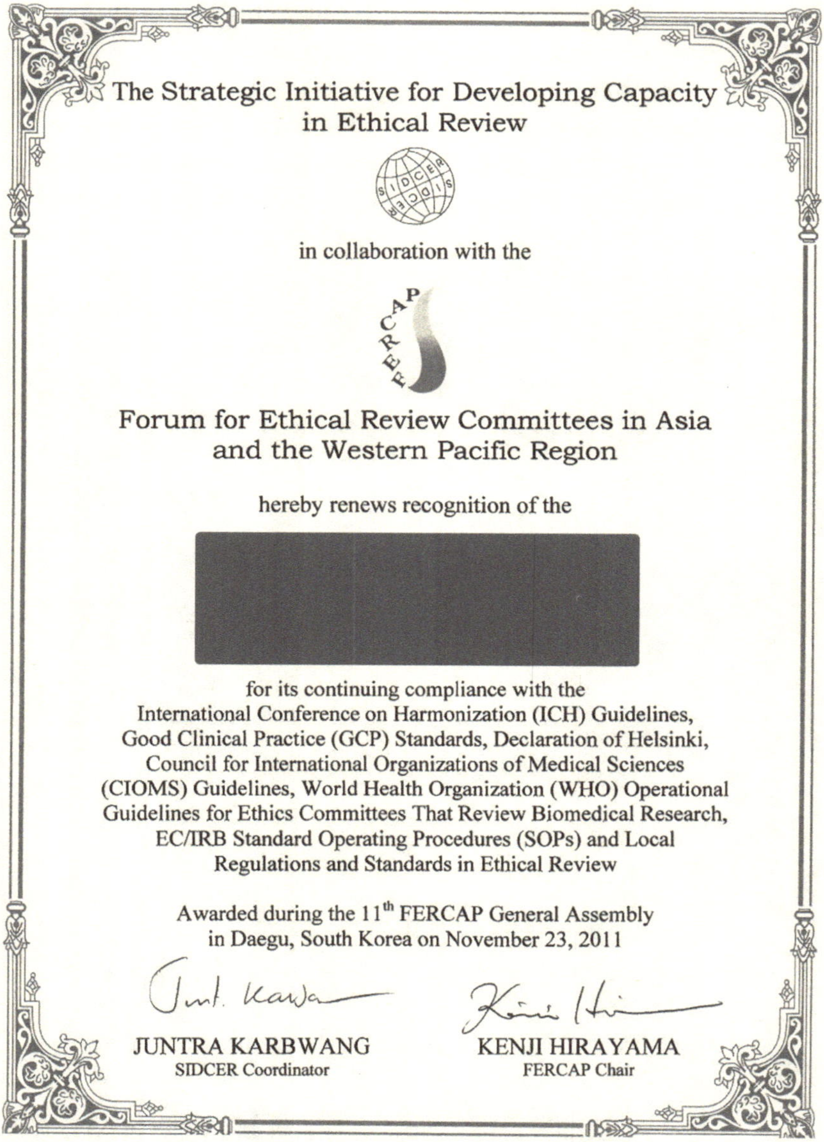
The Strategic Initiative for Developing Capacity in Ethical Review

in collaboration with the

Forum for Ethical Review Committees in Asia and the Western Pacific Region

hereby renews recognition of the

[redacted]

for its continuing compliance with the International Conference on Harmonization (ICH) Guidelines, Good Clinical Practice (GCP) Standards, Declaration of Helsinki, Council for International Organizations of Medical Sciences (CIOMS) Guidelines, World Health Organization (WHO) Operational Guidelines for Ethics Committees That Review Biomedical Research, EC/IRB Standard Operating Procedures (SOPs) and Local Regulations and Standards in Ethical Review

Awarded during the 11th FERCAP General Assembly in Daegu, South Korea on November 23, 2011

JUNTRA KARBWANG
SIDCER Coordinator

KENJI HIRAYAMA
FERCAP Chair

Figures 2.4 and 2.5. Continued

Delegates travel home with these prized material rewards of the Survey and all the work that goes on institutionally and politically to prepare for the visit of a Survey team. In the months following the November conference, official photographs appear across the websites of the region's hospitals and universities, showing committee chairs posing in front of their offices with their certificates, or conducting re-presentation ceremonies with their local deans or department heads. These material artifacts of standard-meeting do institutional work.

Even if Desmond thinks that U.S. standards are difficult to transplant, AAHRPP's activities in the region are growing. In 2019, announcing a further three accredited institutions, the AAHRPP president emphasized not only that accreditation offered assurances "that study partners are protected and research results can be trusted" but also the importance of a "common standard"—indeed, in the words of the reporter, the need for "universal standards is intensifying, in part, because of the trend toward multisite, multi-institutional research," turning AAHRPP accreditation into a "common ground . . . [that] can ease the way for successful collaboration" (BioSpectrum Asia 2019). An AAHRPP audit may not take anything "local" into account, but arguably FERCAP has paved the way for a nongovernmental entity to offer something akin to accreditation, and for that to be seen as a necessary part of not just building but maintaining research ethics. These reflections on the different entities operating in the region also demonstrate the varying interest, ambitions, and expectations of institutions. Hospitality is a frame through which distinct stances toward hosting clinical research can be viewed, and one which illuminates the distinct priorities of committees and ambitions in which they are embedded. A committee that may invite FERCAP may not be within an institution with the funds or will to undergo AAHRPP's extensive full accreditation process. Even as some committees strive to achieve ever more accreditations, others may yet have to secure an office, staff, printers, or their first self-assessment. It is to these material conditions of ethics work that I now turn.

THREE
Committees Immaterial

Ethics is often treated as a discursive enterprise, the stuff of reflection, debate, and quiet meditation. It is thought of as belonging to philosophers or bureaucrats. However, as researchers in the Asia-Pacific region work to set up committees in their universities and hospitals, they quickly discover that establishing ethics review is a material practice, too. Forms must be designed and printed, physical space found for meetings, funds allotted for secretarial staff, and time carved out of schedules for training, reviewing, and meeting. The first ethics committee meeting I saw during my research was being held in the Medical Faculty in Colombo, and I happened upon it entirely by chance. My colleague and I had stopped by the Senior Common Room to fill our water bottles before leaving the department in the afternoon rain. As we crossed the room toward the cooler, to our right, against the tall windows, we saw a wooden table piled high with paperwork, around which a dozen or so people were sitting; I joked quietly, "Looks like an ethics committee." It *was* a joke, because less than two weeks into my fieldwork, I was focused on finding and negotiating access to these committees. I had no reason to imagine I might literally walk in on a meeting. Yet as I stood, filling my bottle, facing away from the table, murmurs of the "benefits to Sri Lanka," and talk of "risk" drifted across the room. "You know, I think it actually is!" whispered my colleague, having turned to face the deliberators at the table: "Here they all are." My colleagues had started their research in Sri Lanka over a year beforehand (Sariola and Simpson 2019) and recognized faces I, too, would soon come to know. I wished I could stay but was unnerved enough to leave: My own ethics application for research on research ethics had been reviewed by that same committee, in the same manner it was now reviewing another protocol just a few meters away.

That the committee meeting was being held in a common room that, while partially restricted by virtue of being "senior," was still open had little meaning for me at the time. In an interview a few weeks later, during a discussion about capacity building, the first hints of a link between the "where" of ethics—its physical institutionalization—and its social robustness began to emerge. My interviewee, Dr. Suraj, was the chair of a department at the same medical faculty. When I met him in his offices, he explained that he been involved in establishing "ethics" at the University of Colombo, and was adamant that unless "local people have capacity to train others, institutions will not develop." He was dismissive, frustrated by visiting lecturers and brief, day-long workshops, which he said did no good. "We need a group of people here, developing knowledge, discussion. Without indigenous institutions as the knowledge base, no subject will live." His experience in establishing psychiatry as a field at Colombo University's Medical School fed into this view. When he began his training in the 1970s, he explained patiently to me, "psychiatry was not a department, it was one person. Now," he said, gesturing out of the open door, "there are six of us. It is a separate subject in the undergraduate curriculum, people can get interested in it." Institutionalization had worked for psychiatry, so he had applied the same techniques with growing research ethics, a process he called "sensitization," by introducing discussion sessions on health equity, research systems, and public health. Over the course of five or six years, he saw that concepts from ethics had become less alien, less exotic, and more relevant to peoples' day-to-day work. Noting to me the absence of guidelines and facilities, Dr. Suraj said he had continued the work of institutionalizing ethics, applying for WHO funding, books, computers, and training programs. "I got us a room," he said proudly. When I asked him why the room was important, he responded a little impatiently, "Otherwise it is person [*sic*], there is not a system. The ERC, I recruited them, but unless we have commitment to the development of ethics . . ." He trailed off.

Leaving the psychiatry offices where we had talked, I stopped by "the room." Pinned to the tall wooden door was a small piece of paper, with a handwritten label reading "Ethics Committee Room." Though the glass was dusty, through it I could see a pair of interconnected spaces. Paint peeled from the walls, and wooden furniture was piled up against one of the tall windows. It was a site of disarray. After the interview, I returned to my visitor's desk in the shared upstairs PhD office of the Human Genetics Unit, an extra space carved out from tall colonial architecture. On my way past the professorial offices, I stopped to ask about the Ethics Committee rooms and was told that progress was slow going, funds were difficult to find. One of the professors suggested that some of the barriers to financing the room were also barriers to the formalization of ethics, but that with dedication it "would happen." It *had* to happen, since having "a room" was a prerequisite for the committee to be surveyed by FERCAP in a few months' time.

These observations and my conversation with Dr. Suraj took place during the first period of my fieldwork in Sri Lanka in mid-2009. By the time I returned, just over six months later, the room had transformed. I had arranged to meet Manisha, one of the secretaries I knew, to hear about how the Survey had gone. I arrived on Kynsey Road opposite the tall white buildings of the Medical Faculty, crossed the parking lot, and headed for the room I remembered. I found Manisha coming into her new office from the committee meeting room beyond, returning to a desk with a computer and brand-new filing cabinets lined up behind. The space had been cleared and freshly painted, a new floor laid. It was filled with new furniture and equipment, chosen with the now-recent Survey in mind. Manisha had just delivered some breaded short eats from the canteen to the meeting participants. As I leaned to peer beyond her into the room, she swiftly moved in front of me. "Confidential meeting," she said.

Spatial Schemes

Over the last two decades, ethics committee advocates in hospitals and universities across the Asia-Pacific region have fought to gain attention, space, resources, and political will from their institutions and colleagues. This chapter is about the implications of space, and what exists in that space. It is also, therefore, about the politics of creating resources to run ethics committees. When FERCAP began implementing the SIDCER Recognition Survey in 2005, committees wishing to invite a surveying group had to meet a few prerequisites, one of which was that their committee had a dedicated office. Suddenly, spaces for ethics took on new meaning. In the Survey's standard on the Structure and Composition of the committee, the SIDCER committee had made the following requirement: "1.4 EC/IRB Office: The EC/IRB should have an office space with necessary equipment and staff for good functioning" (FERCAP, 2024). For many, across institutions and countries, this requirement represented a turning point in persuading their organization to dedicate permanent physical space to ethics committee activities, since equipment, staff, and office space were not always easy to come by. When FERCAP's Survey teams come to visit committees, their assessments consider the facilities the committee has at their disposal and how well the institutions or hospitals are creating a special, professional space upon which the enterprise of a systematized ethics can rest. The inclusion of the room in the standard means that for each setting that FERCAP visits, a version of this room must be duplicated: a space in which certain kinds of operations take place, and in which certain kinds of people are made to convene for ethics to happen.

Space matters. Anthropologists have long paid attention to the relationship between the arrangement of persons in space, their "atmospheres" (Lezaun and Calvillo 2014), and the conceptual work that those spaces are made to do (Humphrey 1974; Mitchell 1988). We can describe rooms as part of the "mundane infrastructure" (Montgomery et al. 2017) of global research and health projects, receding into the background as necessary components that make actual research possible. But as material arrangements, they are often hard-won signs of institutional support.[1] For Dr. Suraj, the room for the ethics committee was a change in the status and permanence of ethics-related activity in the institution. Unlike the people who carried the knowledge of ethics, who could leave, he rooted his hopes for endurance in the physical space. Replete with documentation, secretarial facilities, and a name, the room would remain no matter the passage of temporary "experts" and be sustained through the institutional commitment to literally make space for ethics, in square meters and spreadsheet budgets.

This making of space for ethics has parallels with early contestations over scientific method. Historians of science position the contestation over the public status of science in Robert Boyle's nascent laboratories in seventeenth-century England, with Steven Shapin commenting that "despite various characterizations of science as 'public knowledge' it gets made and evaluated in some of our most private places" (Shapin 1992, 27; see also Shapin and Schaffer 2011). Ethics review is not the scientific method, but committees are regularly asked to assess the scientific methods of proposals under review. The balance is not easy to hold: While the phrase "if it is not scientific, it is not ethical" circulated in my fieldwork, the debate over the role of committees in doing a scientific review remains. The review has become a process through which research proposals must now pass. In the words of SIDCER's Francis Crawley, "Ethics has become both a guardian of and a gateway to research, in the sense that ethical review is one of the doorways that research has to pass through before it can be carried out in a country" (cited in Dickson 2002, 645). As an assessment of proposed work's ethics has been integrated into the making of good science, its materialized practices, too, must spread. Donna Haraway has reminded us that the doing of scientific knowledge has depended on the spread of its materialized practices (1997, 24). This was a question "not of ideas," she writes, "but of the apparatus of production of what would count as knowledge" (Haraway 1997, 24). I find the ethics committee to also operate as an apparatus of production of what will count as knowledge, a technology designed, in Laura Stark's words, to evaluate the kinds of questions that will be asked of the world, "what is knowable" (2012, 5). Through the spread of the committee into regions of the world where the politics and practices of research are not what they are in the sites of committee work's origin, the assumptions and cultural techniques of governance it carries within it become visible. In this chapter, I track those techniques of governance through ethics committee rooms, viewing them as markers of the achievements of long made arguments. Committees may convene and make their decisions outside the remit of FERCAP's assessment, but to call themselves valid assessors of valid knowledge, they must first become assessable. Capacity building in this sense is not critical thinking or principled reasoning, but the marking of space; both claiming "real estate" for ethics in university and hospital premises, and in the political landscape of how questions of ethics come to matter in the administration of research.

Animating the Cause

Despite FERCAP's success in recruiting and galvanizing committed volunteers, during my early years of fieldwork, conference participants often grumbled that their institutions paid little attention to ethical review. Coming together in increasing numbers every year, delegates themselves evidenced the growing interest of ethics review for researchers across the region, but lunchtime conversations and formal presentations revealed anxieties about being taken seriously by managers, bosses, and institutions. At the 2010 conference in Shanghai, Da—a Chinese volunteer working with committees through FERCAP—told me that it had taken a long time to draw the attention of both researchers and institutions. "In the early times," he commented, "most [committee members] said 'We don't have support from the institution, nobody notice[s] we are there.'" Year after year, at conferences and trainings, he heard how investigators dismissed newly formed committees or showed "no respect": "Could you just stamp this letter?" they were asked. It is telling that being asked for a stamp, rather than for deliberation, was insulting to committees who were invested in protecting participants in clinical trials. Committees who engaged with FERCAP's activities were not those at whom the international academic community had leveled critiques of "rubber stamping" (Kass et al. 2007; Lynch and Rosenfeld 2020). The often substantial efforts required by committee members, researchers, and administrators in their own institutions to change the conversation about research ethics—sometimes even to begin it—are not always easy to see. In what follows, I bring these efforts to the fore.

As I spent time with members of the network, I came to appreciate how challenging it was for some researchers to begin conversations about research ethics within their institutions. While numerous informal conversations had implied as much, this insight took its most memorable form as a conference presentation by Hyeon, a delegate from a medical center in the self-proclaimed medical city of Daegu, South Korea. Her animated slide show at the Shanghai Conference outlined the great efforts to which she and her colleague had gone to persuade members of their institution that research ethics mattered. In South Korea, the name IRB, or Institutional Review Board, is used for committees that convene to deliberate the ethics of biomedical research proposals, as it is in the United States. She illustrated their achievements through an animation (Figure 3.1a and 3.1b) she had set to the theme music from *My Neighbor Totoro*, a globally popular Japanese anime. As the presentation played, Hyeon narrated the images on the screen:

> Here is the door [1]. The door is really a difficulty. If you don't overcome this difficulty, I can't work on the IRB. So at that time my friend Sang is coming. Everyone told me she is a very good doctor in Emergency Medicine. She is coming to me. And we are trying together: How to open this door? [2] It's difficult. We have to find the key: The key is the main solution to opening the door, of overcoming difficulty [3]. Now, we find the key, but the door is really, really big. [6] So we don't know how to reach the keyhole. We can't reach. So we have to find a way: What is a good way to reach the key[hole]? We try over and over again [7, 8]. We are cooperating together, but we get a ladder and the key to open the door [10]. We open the door, wow! [11] But when we open the difficulty, another difficulty is in front of us [12]. At that time, nobody is interested in us. Every time we are shouting, they are indifferent. They are just doing their job. They are just in front of their computer [13]. Writing some document [14]. They are

talking among themselves [15]. But we never stop here. We have to overcome. We are shouting "IRB," "IRB" over and over again [16]. At that time we try and speak about the meaning of IRB. Protection! Why [do] we have to do [this]? With our effort they try to understand what IRB is [17, 18, 19]. At first we are just the two, but every persons are [*sic*] getting together and they are shouting together so it [is] impossible to make them understand why human protection subject [*sic*] is so important for developing medical [20]. And what is the right way, and they really understand [21]. I don't think they can understand it fully, but they are trying.

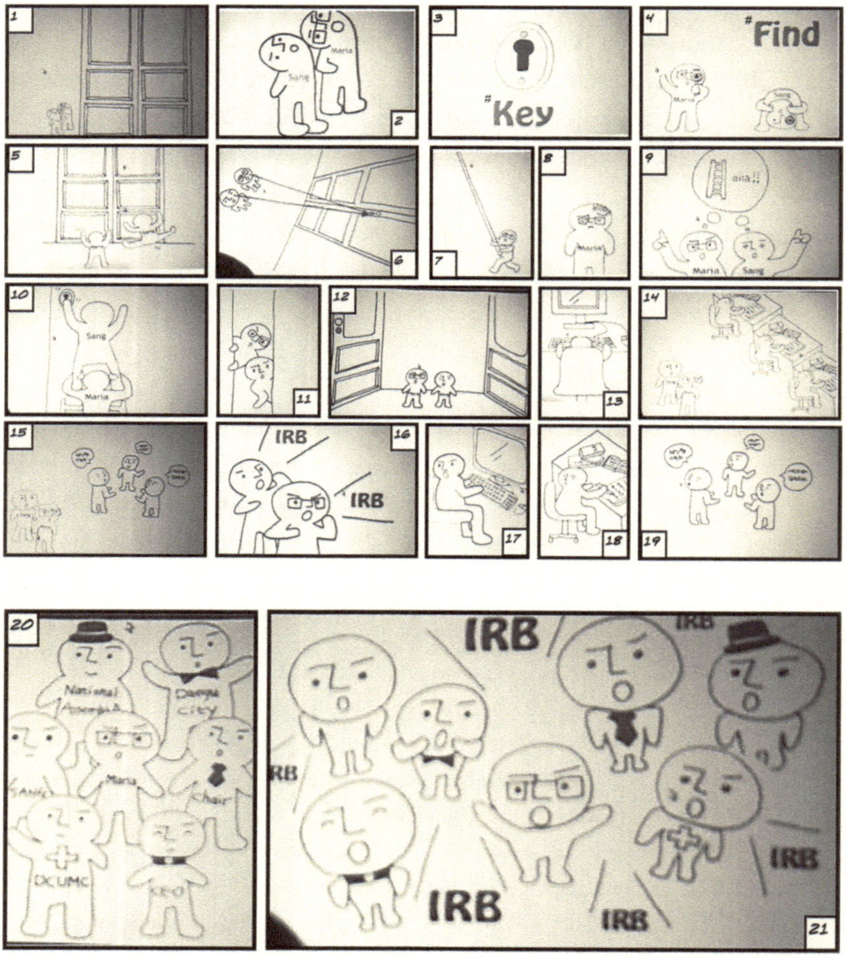

Figures 3.1a and 3.1b. A composite of stills of Hyeon's animated cartoon, compiled by the author.

Hyeon and Sang's story conveyed—with indirect criticism—how, after a long time, they had successfully brought the need for ethical review to the attention of new actors. These new actors—with their clerical neckbands, bow ties, glasses, and top hats—gave authority to the endeavor. Told as an animated adventure, the negotiations and case making were made explicit: a struggle for legitimacy in the face of turned backs and rows of computer-locked workers. Making figurative space for ethics, leading to (for example) funds for trainings, conferences, invited speakers, or committee formation, was not always an easy cause to champion.

Standards for Rooms

During Surveys, a committee's office became a hotly debated topic, since having the room was only a start. The Surveyors were routinely interested in how committee members used a space and its role as a container for ethics committee activity. As I joined the Surveyors on their trips into offices, I often accompanied several of the Survey teams as they examined the room. During a Survey in Manila, I was part of a group that received strict instructions before the tour to "use our eyes." We left the rooms allocated to the Survey and shuffled down the narrow corridor as a group, following the lead Surveyor, who had just done this exercise with another group of trainees an hour ago. It was a little like a tour, but it was not the lead Surveyor who clutched a clipboard, it was us. Pencils in hand, we were to look for accurate archiving, to see if the Declaration of Helsinki, the latest CIOMS publication, and the committee's Standard Operating Procedures were kept to hand on the desk. We were to ask questions of the office staff and see if they had a sense of what they should be doing. Each item in the Survey's standards appeared alongside a checkbox, waiting. The lead Surveyor instructed us to be aware of confidentiality:

> If there's only one office, maybe there is no confidential issue on [the staff]. If there is more than one [staff], who takes care of the lock and the key, who receives documents, who knows the password, who communicates with the PI? In the office, you can take a protocol at random and then you check whether it is complete or not.

Our attention was guided by questions. As we approached the ethics committee office in this Philippine institute, we saw that it was clearly labeled with a sign that hung out into the hall perpendicular to the wall. "Institutional Review Board," it read. We checked off the first box: "Is the location appropriate?" Was there an organogram on the wall? Yes. We were shown the technology: a fax machine, a phone, a shredder, a photocopier, and a printer. The Surveyors photographed these for use as evidence in the summary PowerPoint (Figure 3.2).

The biggest problem on this Survey in Manila was access to the room and the things in it. Let us first deal, as the Surveyors did, with the items within. There are two highly sensitive areas in the office: the filing cabinet and the computer. What is sensitive is not these containers, or their value in themselves (nobody seems too worried about the computer being stolen), but what they contain, namely research protocols and the EC's database of files. In the quiet of our observation, standing squished in the room, a Surveyor asked after the seal of the IRB, the mark of an authentic review stamped on approved documents. The secretary explained she keeps it locked up, in a drawer, and dangled the keys from her keychain. The security of these items is carefully guarded, and in a similar way, the space is, too. I had signed a confidentiality

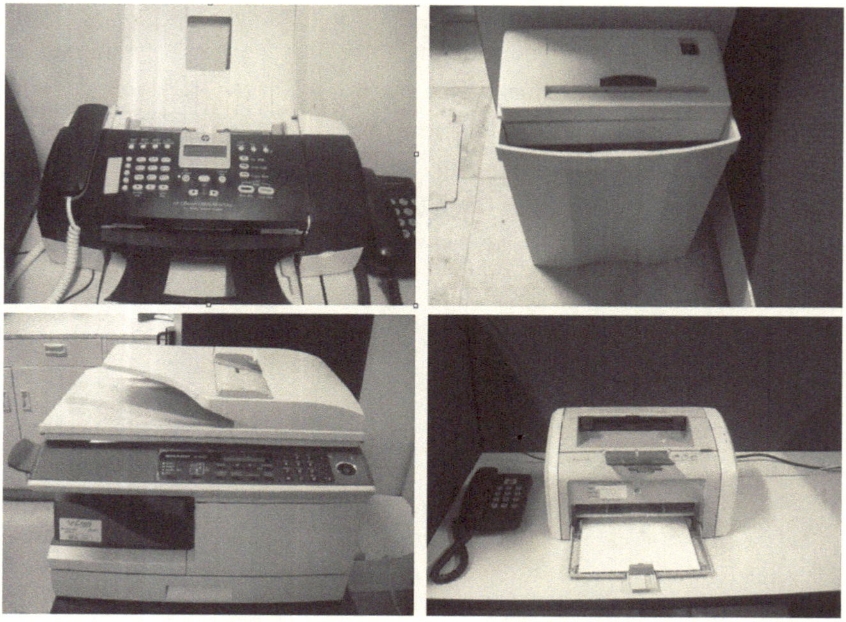

Figure 3.2. Slide from closing PowerPoint, evidencing the presence of the committee's technology. Source: Author.

agreement in order to be inside the room, because according to the secretary taking my signature, we would "see some very confidential things." I asked her whether research proposals were "confidential," and she replied, "Yes!" in a tone that implied "Of course!": "You [an applicant researcher] might be working on something very new or be in competition." Later, discussing this point together, the presence of a shredder in the office corner became a key point on the prepared closing slides: "You must have a shredder," participants were counseled, as they were told not to sell off scrap paper. "Tomorrow you might buy a banana, and the banana wrapper might be an IC form! That is not confidential!" After some discussion, it emerged that while the printed paper with protocols on *was* sold, it was sold in a shredded version to a recycling shop, to help cover operating costs.

In the office, confidentiality arose in new ways. The secretary who had opened the door was asked who else had the keys, and how many people had the password to the computer. She replied that she was the only one, implying that this was good—the room was secure. However, another Surveyor was not so sure: "I'm not happy with just one girl having the keys, what if something happens to her?" As we poked through the cupboards to look at the filing system and worked our way through the checklist, the lead Surveyor shared his thoughts with me: "In Taiwan," he said, "we're crazy for IRB. You have to sign your name if you visit, because that is what they do in the U.S." I asked him why such monitoring of access to the space was needed. "Maybe you'll steal," he said seriously. I pointed out that in most cases, and on the recommendation of the Survey, files are locked in cabinets. "But we need to control people going into the office," he replied, gesturing to the door.

The main door to this Manila office opened onto the corridor. While the room had its own lockable door, it was partitioned off from a larger room with a five-foot wall, in which there was another door. This second door and the partition caused comment from the Surveyors:

> There should be a wall there! This is a confidential space, [it should have] only one door, not two. Someone could jump over the dividing wall, or get through the door from the other side!

The wall became a matter for discussion when the groups came together at the end-of-day summary meeting. One group of Surveyors (I will call them "A") thought the partition ought to be made higher, "because you can reach over." Others ("B") disagreed, arguing that the secretaries of the EC were sharing a photocopier with the office next door, and the door in the partition was convenient for them.

A member of Group A said: "So, she has to go out and round. We should write 'limit the access to IRB office from other staff.'" This was a direction to the person compiling recommendations in a PowerPoint. She in turn paused on the bullet beneath, which, to follow the layout, needed to be filled in with a reason for the recommendation: "If you are a mix of other people you cannot keep confidentiality," the person from Group A continued: "That's why we want a separate building and independent structure." Addressing the typist at the PowerPoint, he instructed her to write: "Partition should be higher." At this point the secretary of the committee being surveyed called out, as she was delivering documents to the usually closed end-of-day meeting. "But we only have one air-con!" she said; "If you make it higher [cool air] won't get through." The possibility of "reaching" over the wall then turned into "jumping," and the familiar secretaries next door became altogether more sinister: "In that office before, researchers actually came in at night and looked for their protocol." Group B protested. They had been shown by the petite female staff in the neighboring office that the partition was far too high for them to reach over. With this, the matter was closed for the evening.

On the second night of the Survey, the partition came up again, because of new findings from Group B. One of Group B's members had spoken to the secretaries, who felt it would be difficult for them to comply with a requirement for a raised partition or a wall. Raising the partition might be possible, they said, on the condition that the new, higher section was *transparent*. The secretaries' spokesperson told the surveying teams this was "because they only have one boss. They need visual access, so the boss can see if they're sleeping!" The Survey team insisted that the entrance to the ERC should be separate, and requested that before the committee received recognition, photographs of this change should be taken. "I will ask for a picture that they made it higher," commented the lead Surveyor. When, on the final day, the lead Surveyor had finished his presentation, including the recommendation that the partition should be raised by *ten inches*, the ethics committee members were given the opportunity to ask questions about the recommendations. One of the secretaries asked why it was recommended that *ten inches* be added to the partition. "Please explain the rationale," she said.

A Surveyor replied:

> It is better to have isolated, secluded space where no other irrelevant people can have access. Now you have two doors but the other side office has access. It depends on the composition of people in the other room. The partition is to restrict access, so there should only be one door. We think it is reasonable to keep the confidentiality of the room. In other IRBs if they share office space, they have to have mechanisms to keep the confidentiality of those people.

The chair then spoke on behalf of the committee:

> Our building is overflowing with people and offices. There is no space for an *exclusive* IRB office. If we had a higher partition, someone can just climb back. We thought putting files under lock and key would suffice. The IRB is competing with other offices for desired space, we're bursting. It's difficult to say it can be done. There is also a leak which has been unresolved for a year.

The Surveyors answered:

> But the recommendation is not asking for *more* space! We know your constraints. The only recommendation is to make it more secure. Make the partition higher and correctly close the door.

I have recounted this disagreement in detail because it speaks to the physical and symbolic segregation of ethics. The Surveyors are not only ensuring that the committee have claimed the space, they also need to ensure it can be made confidential. Surveyors aim to impress on the committee members the confidential nature of the documents an Ethics Committee handles, with careers and perhaps patents on the line. A separate, lockable room was preferable, but where space simply wasn't available other measures were necessary.

The ongoing digitalization of applications and meetings has added new challenges for committees and Surveyors alike. The busiest committees FERCAP works with review one thousand protocols a year, and with ICH-GCP having required the retention of "essential documents" for "at least three years after completion of the trial," limitations on space threatened compliance. When India modified its clinical trial regulations in 2013, for example, Shruti Bhide and colleagues wrote that the five-year archiving minimum had "created a need for space. This has been challenging" (2016, 4). The possibility of holding EC application files digitally has eased some of the need for space, and by 2024, whole tracks of FERCAP's annual Conference were dedicated to presentations on committees' experimentations with different software. As many noted, that meant data security, not just the physical security of a room, has become a new point of collaboration between ethics committees and their institutions. For committees adopting hybrid meetings, Atoy Navarro told me over Zoom, his own home office behind a smart University of the Philippines Manila virtual background, it has become difficult to guarantee that nobody is listening in on the call. "It's not like before, when you could bring your hard copy to the meeting and leave them behind on the table to be shredded afterward!"

The standardization of procedures and practices is well documented (Lampland and Star 2009; Engel and Zeiss 2014; Engel et al. 2014), but these discussions give us another access point: standardization of a space as part of disciplining practice. A reproducible room is a carefully worked out standard, inscribed in the Surveyor's checklists and in the weight of its arguments during the course of the four-day visit. What the "wall" illustrates is the tension inherent to the objective of the Survey: a standardized room that takes in its context. The Surveyors are trying to make a room that can be context independent, while at the same time also trying to take in context dependency.

Materializing Discussion

In an audit-oriented world, evidencing activity is as important as the activity itself. "If it isn't written down, it didn't happen," Surveyors say, emphasizing the importance of documentation to audit and echoing contract research organization (CRO) monitors trained to examine clinical trials. Writing about an international trial taking place in Sri Lanka, Bob Simpson and Salla Sariola note that "things that were not normally documented had to be recorded according to the dictum: 'not documented = not done'" (2012, 568). Following this principle, if any adverse reactions or observations were not recorded in writing, dated, and signed, it would be the same as if they had never happened. As the Survey progresses, FERCAP Surveyors are invited into the spaces of ethics deliberation to observe a committee meeting. For Surveyors, this is a welcome break from sifting through paperwork. For the committee, it is the key moment on which assessment rests. Their paperwork may be excellent, but unless their discussion covers the relevant points, Surveyors cannot be sure that research participants will be protected.

The Survey team are usually given seats around the edges of the room, looking over the shoulders of the committee members (Figure 3.3). Surveyors warn, however, that meeting observation is not standard practice amongst auditors from trial sponsors or the U.S. FDA. If a committee is audited, the minutes will be the only record of meetings, "so it is important that [the minutes] capture what went on," committees are told, so compliance can be assessed. As one Surveyor explained it:

> When they audit, they look at the minutes. Are there missing things there? How did they arrive at decision? So is not just he/she said, it's what you should do. Take notes, mark discussion points. Decisions should be based on discussion points. That is the expectation from the ethics committee. An ethics committee that works without minutes is not GCP compliant.

Meeting minutes materialize discussion, recording and evidencing what happens inside committee rooms. The making of minutes can cause problems

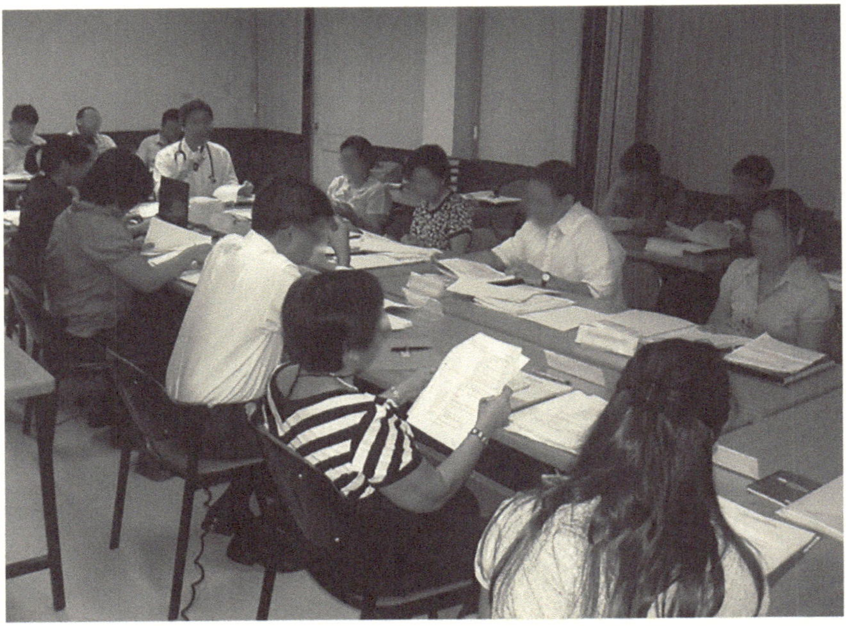

Figure 3.3. Surveyors observing a committee meeting. They are seated at the tables behind. Source: Author.

during a committee's first Survey. "Unlike other areas, where you can look at international guidelines, Helsinki, CIOMS," said a secretary from Manila to me, as she worried about the upcoming meeting, "there is not a guideline for minutes."

During fieldwork, I noticed that some committee meeting minutes were being taken using a laptop, projected onto a screen at the opposite end to the chairperson. This practice was known as "real-time minutes," and FERCAP encouraged it on the dual grounds of efficiency and accuracy. "Everyone will be able to see," said one committee member. "Nowadays," said another, "due to improvements in technology we can do a draft on the spot so members can already see what will be in the minutes. At the end of the discussion, we ask people if we missed anything."[2] Some secretaries worried that they did not have the capacity to type fast enough to "capture" the discussion. In such circumstances, minutes would be typed up using a recording and circulated to the committee members by email, the "old-fashioned way." Accuracy was cast not only in terms of committee members seeing whether their comments had been recorded, but also in terms of ensuring accuracy in discussion by having the themes it would be important to minute already templated. Minutes templates are prepared, waiting to be filled in with discussion: "Then nothing will be forgotten."

FERCAP facilitated the "travel" of this method through trainings.[3] In 2009, during the pre-Conference workshop in Chiang Mai, Thailand, a secretary from the Philippines had created a sample agenda to guide minute making (Figure 3.4). She displayed an anonymized sample document that listed categories such as technical issues, elements of design, ethical issues, assessment of issues, further questions, and required modifications. This was considered easy to generate; "all my staff do it now," she said. It is a way, she noted, "in the future, even if I'm not a member of the IRB anymore, to check what happened."

Meeting minutes can offer what Laura Stark, writing about U.S. American IRBs, calls an "anticipatory perspective" on the study of committee documentation. In her observation, "'board members' sense of how the minutes of their current discussion would be written served as a social resource that they used to manage relationships—between each other and between themselves and researchers" (2011, 252). She suggests that "unwritten minutes [. . .] steered the course of deliberation as it was still under way" (2011, 252). It is clear that committees are aware of the possible future uses to which minutes of meetings

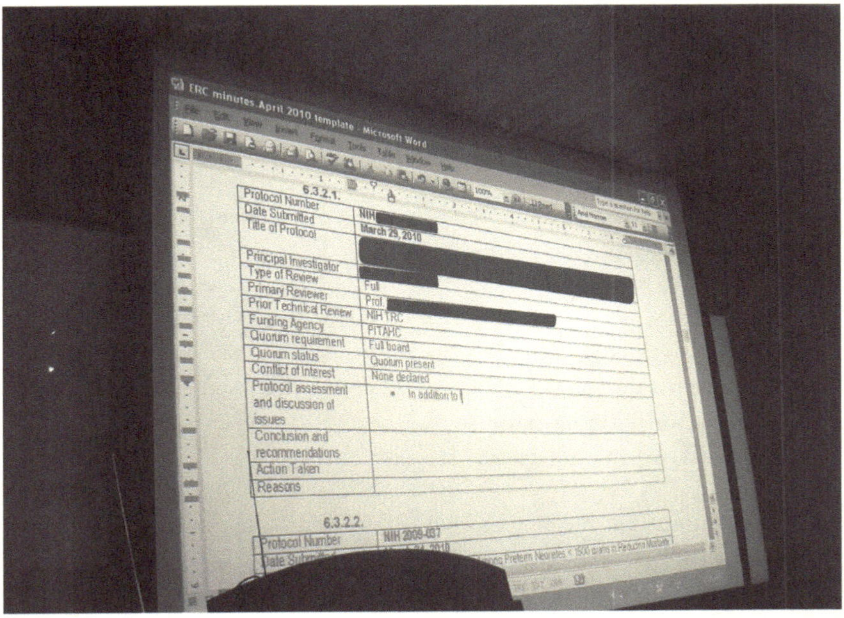

Figure 3.4. A template developed for committee minutes, with dedicated space for the discussion, declaration of conflict of interest, quorum requirements, action taken, and reasons. Source: Author.

may be put, even if the "anticipatory perspective" they exhibit is largely in anticipation of needing to anticipate. But with the creation of real-time minutes, rather than focusing on the deliberations of members and how they put their arguments across, I want to look at those who write the minutes during the meeting.

The creation of minutes is the work of the staff secretary, the network's name for the person employed to administrate the committee. The etymology of the word "secretary," with its roots in secret keeping, is particularly apt for the way Fiona and Karen, secretaries in Manila, the Philippines, describe their work.[4] When I joined the Survey of their committee, Fiona was just handing over to Karen. During our interview, Karen was laughing when she told me how difficult she'd found it to write the minutes. "It was a disaster!" she exclaimed:

> I did not know what to write! I had to keep copying Fi's notes. I had to write it down, so no notes were missing, but I couldn't listen to them speak. I still get so *mesmerized* at how well they speak. At first, I couldn't follow the thoughts.

> At the first meeting, the speakers were speaking, one would say something, one would clarify, another would tell another statement which doesn't correspond to the other, you have to input another line [. . .] I just couldn't delineate as to where to start!

Fiona was sorting paperwork as Karen talked to me, but at this description she looked up and joined in our conversation:

> I was taught by Adelina [a former secretary] how to take notes, and only get those relevant to the protocol. Other comments shouldn't be part of the discussion, so you put them out of mind. So, each issue: What are the recommendations? What are the technical and ethical issues regarding the consent form? I categorize them in my mind during the meeting.

Karen explained that despite her background in biology she found herself ill-prepared for her secretarial role. She learned over time to "organize" her thoughts and take down notes. She struggled most with disagreements committee members had with each other. "Sometimes they have very strong comments on one another, 'I do not agree with your point!' What do you do then?" she asked me. In the "real-time" system, full board discussion is recorded by judiciously editing the speech of the committee members. As I have shown, a decision must be evidenced as resting on a discussion. But both for Karen and many of us who have tried to take minutes, it is difficult to summarize a discussion as it develops. Finding myself in a role like that of Karen and Fiona, trying to transcribe and make sense of unfolding discussion, I also found it difficult to trace by hand discussions as they emerged in ethics committee meetings. Even with the flexibility that pen and paper afford over typed script on a screen; even with the ability to record expressions and gestures, multiply indent, and annotate, it is difficult to say (from my pages of notes) *how* a decision is made, to track moments of persuasion and rebuttal. Fiona took the opportunity of our interview to explain her thoughts not only to me, but also to Karen, her new colleague.

> FIONA: [To be a secretary] a person must know how to organize their thoughts well and be able to multitask and remember. You learn how to divide your mind. Manage your mind and manage your time. You need to have good communication skills and have confidentiality.

RDJ: How do you "have" confidentiality?

FIONA: Like, we put a guard on ourselves—restrain ourselves from commenting, and remain silent, [to prevent] people asking follow-up questions. If in this office, we share. If another office, no, because we signed [a] confidentiality agreement.

KAREN: The other office [staff] do not know what we are doing! They think we prepare for the meeting and we photocopy. They know how to appreciate [our work], that we're always working. They say, "What are you doing, why are you always so home late?" Bosses don't understand when I haven't finished the work. They think it's easy, write a letter, print, send protocols to investigators. It seems easy. But when you're in my place it isn't work that requires intelligence, it requires time.

Fiona's diversion of the conversation toward confidentiality recalls the attention Surveyors paid to this concept in the room. Confidentiality appeared regularly, adhering to persons, times, material objects, and spaces. I signed confidentiality agreements on entering committee rooms in Thailand, the Philippines, and China; filing cabinets were under lock and key "for confidentiality"; computer record systems stayed locked with a password "for confidentiality." A lecture during a pre-Survey training contained the following:

> Reviewers also have rights to confidentiality . . . When [our committee] was new some years ago, the staff didn't know much about confidentiality. So, she gave up the name of the reviewer to the investigator. The reviewer happened to be very, very good reviewer, with many, many comments. Seeming like the protocol will never be approved, of course the investigator wanted to question the reviewer. No! This staff actually gave the name of the reviewer. That's bad, that is not allowed.

I will return to the social dynamics of committee review, particularly in cases were reviewers have "many, many comments," in chapter 5 as "confidentiality" between researcher and reviewer is not the only dynamic of tension in this setting. For now, let us return to the minutes Fiona and Karen are producing. As well as creating a far-future record for possible auditors, the minutes of a meeting serve another purpose: They are the guide from which secretaries proceed. Fiona and Karen are on the receiving end of inquiries from principal investigators, who are often in a hurry to get approval. Reference to "the process" allows Fiona to deflect the blame for delay that PIs might otherwise place on her shoulders, but she finds herself in a mediating position:

> The one who submitted [the protocol] thinks it can be expedited, but the board thinks no. He keeps saying, "Why? Why do I have to go through full board review?" It is a challenge for me, how can I say that board doesn't agree this should be expedited? I refer to chart on the wall to calm them—so we don't have to explain every time they come. "Read our workflow," I say.

In both spoken and written communication with PIs, she finds herself in the middle, compromising, managing emotions. She tells me that she breaks news to investigators gently, rephrasing the words of the reviewers. Seeing my raised eyebrow, she reassures me that the contents don't change, but she rewrites the minutes, softening the "harsh words" voiced in the committee meetings. "Like last week, [in the meeting] someone said, 'This is scientifically unsound,' but we cannot say that [to the investigator]."

I'm interested in the changes that Fiona is describing. "So, what do you put in the letter?" I ask her. "The recommendations from the minutes?"

"Yes," she tells me, "but we edit them. Just to make statements clearer, to make it . . . sound better. Sound softer, so they'll be able to accept the criticism." Studies on ethics committees' authority and legitimacy (O'Reilly et al. 2009; Stark 2012; Clapp et al. 2017) indicate that decision letters are one of the most significant vehicles for a committee's activity, "understood as a solution to the administrative problem that there is a need for a single authoritative ruling on the ethical standing of any application, but there are competing claims as to how that standing should be assessed" (O'Reilly et al. 2009, 258). Karen and Fiona describe tensions between researchers and the committee members in the making of that authoritative ruling. I now turn to the tensions that they must, in the real-time minutes, record: disagreements between committee members as they come toward a decision.

Making Space for Ethics

Paying attention to space allows me to highlight the way the ethics committee—in its physical, enacted form—constitutes a knowledge space. The committee in my opening vignette was, at the time, operating without a room. We could think of the requirements of the space, oft repeated in Surveys—a computer with a database, a fax machine, a printer, a photocopier—as "templates" for, after David Turnbull (2000), the cathedrals of ethics, assembling standardizing, transmitting, and utilizing knowledge. The closing reports of the Survey project images of these pieces of technology as achievements of the space, the space the achievement of the will of the committee. The organization has been convinced.[5] However, I do not want to overemphasize technology. While its presence in the photographed contents of offices is used as a measure in the Survey, to Juntra, good ethical review does not inhere in technology. Any country can "have" good review, in her terms, "developed or not." She explains:

> What I want is [a situation where] everywhere they can analyze ethics issues in their country for public good. [. . .] If you don't have electricity you can still run an EC. If [we're] discussing efficiency, if you have lots of protocols, those technologies can help you work faster. But you can still do it with everything manual. The way how you review [is] still the same, it's based on [the] same principles. You can't follow up as completely as those with technology. It's different from other types of lab. If you don't have technology, you can still function with paper and do it the old-fashioned way. But the Ethics Committee is not a lab, that's why if [they] don't have technology, [they can use] paper, [the] conservative way. They just have to organize the system differently. [. . .] Some EC could be recognized without a computer, as long as they review properly and follow up properly.

The idea is that what constitutes the essentials of good committee work is possible without technology, albeit conducted in a less "efficient" way. Juntra tells me about her work beyond the Asia-Pacific, where she and her colleagues sometimes run trainings in collaboration with other regional networks, such as the Pan-African Bioethics Initiative Network (PABIN). The network was founded in 2001 as part of the SIDCER initiative, and it was revitalized with a workshop at the Armauer Hansen Research Institute in Addis Ababa in 2023. A press release shows Juntra seated centrally, returning to key themes in ethics review (AHRI 2023). By arguing that "quality review is neither an economic nor a technology issue" (Torres 2011, 52), trainers in FERCAP make an argument for inclusion, usually against an implicit scale of degrees of development, within and beyond the Asia-Pacific. While more developed countries were considered capable of financing their own capacity building, developing countries required support. As the FERCAP Research Fellow Atoy Navarro put it,

> The standards are the same, whether developing or developed country . . . We can try to facilitate money for Nepal and Bhutan. Doesn't matter if [the country is] developed or developing, [its quality of review] can be of a par with Western standards.

A functioning office, the capacity to generate reports and minutes. These are a long way from the technologically enabled regimes of compliance U.S. IRBs contend with, as Babb traces the emergence of Natural Language Processing (NLP) in place of "the skilled labor of regulatory interpretation" (2020, 97), technologies borrowed from financial regulation into these bureaucracies of compliance in the "logic of auditability" (2020, 99). But I find it interesting that the committee is, in the quote above, a kind of laboratory: First it is "different from other *types* of lab," and then "it is *not* a lab." I suggest that the lab is present as an idea in these descriptions because the Ethics Committee is a way of thinking, supported by a certain arrangement of space. If we follow the idea of the ethics committee as a laboratory, the enclosed space lends it a robustness, particularly in comparison with spaces where questions are not disciplined (Callon and Rabeharisoa 2008). Through the Survey, FERCAP desires a system in a room that will produce replicable results: In the documents they look for consistency, completeness, and discussion in the meeting. A room can be made and peopled with those who will produce replicable results, within the measures set. The "objectivity" of ethics committee members is sought, demonstrating the "political action in the sphere of attestive visual perception" (Ezrahi 1990, 170) and transferring from the physical to the social world. Sociologist Michèle Lamont's work on the "mechanics" of deliberations shows that "technolog[ies] of evaluation around which evaluative cultures are intertwined [. . .] define and constrain possibilities" (2010, 23). This chapter is evidence both of the material and verbal aspects of her assertion.

The ethics of this chapter have taken the form of walls, locked cupboards, well-phrased letters, Standard Operating Procedures, and organograms. These are what the Council for International Organizations of Medical Sciences calls "resources": "time, training, qualified staff, facilities, clinical and laboratories equipment, hardware and software, communication tools, data protection infrastructure, health databases and biobanks, ethical and legal counselling, etc." (CIOMS Working Group on Good Governance Practice for Research Institutions 2023, 7). This contention that institutional engagement is needed has been adopted into the latest version of the Declaration of Helsinki.

Returning to the emphasis on confidentiality in this chapter, it is perhaps not surprising that an editorial in the *Indian Journal of Medical Ethics* entitled "Ethics in Ethics Committees" (2009) criticized the "silence" on the operation of ethics committees. Frustrated, the medical doctor and consultant Amar Jesani asked:

> Why have EC members not narrated the challenges and dilemmas they have faced, and discussed how to make regulations effective? Would doing so compromise the confidentiality of research and the ethics review process? Unless committed individuals find ways of speaking out on EC functioning, ECs will continue to function as secret societies unaccountable to the public and with poor public credibility. While specific information related to projects and individuals may be confidential, this is not true of the ethics review process itself. (2009, 63)

Confidentiality has, in this chapter, been a material concern. It is a bodily attitude on the part of the secretaries, it is my signature on a form at the door of the committee. It is the shredding of documents before sale of scrap paper, it is the height of a wall. The physical boundaries of the room combine with the attitudes of those who use it to form a combined assemblage: "They don't know what we do," remarks Fiona, speaking of friends in the office next door to her. Jesani's complaint about the silence around committee work and decisions shows that confidentiality must be kept from becoming secrecy. Confidentiality is imbued with virtue in a way that secrecy is not, but ethics committee work is both bureaucratic secrecy and public service, everyman ethics and scientific expertise. Although "bureaucratic administration always tends to be an administration of 'secret sessions': in so far as it can, it hides its knowledge and action from criticism" (Weber 2014, 233), and this is precisely what Jesani queries. As a result, he is asking whether "secret" work on behalf of the public is acceptable, particularly when, Stark reminds us, IRBs "change what is knowable" (Stark 2012, 118).

The secretarial work I have described in this chapter may make committees run, but it remains quite thankless. Writing in the *Asian Bioethics Review*, Salik Ansari, a project coordinator at the Indian mental health network

Sangath, describes member secretaries as, to use Graeme Laurie's paraphrase, "invisible actors behind the machinery of bioethics" (Laurie 2023, 357), arguing that "communication is at the heart of the function of an EC, yet there needs to be more discussion on how assertive or gentle the tone of EC communication should be" (Ansari 2023, 363).

It is these doubts and the labor of these chapters—of surveying committees and getting them ready for the Recognition Program—that are the work of capacity building, both of committees and Surveyors, who return home with newly critical eyes. In the committees visited, Survey requirements intersect with the everyday life of an institution, from space to funding for staff. For the members of committees, the promise of recognition, a form of international attention to the working of the committee, can help make the case for funds and resources for committees to do their work. In recognition that this is still something needed, it is notable that the latest revisions to the Declaration of Helsinki formalize the requirement that a committee have a room, and resources, of its own (Parums 2024).

SECTION 2

Decisions and Models

FOUR

Microcosming Models

The composition of ethics committees—who gets to be at the table—has a complex history and a contested present (Friesen et al. 2023). It matters because a committee's composition not only shapes the kind of review a proposal will receive, but it is also central to its legitimacy, its power to speak. Principles like diversity and representation became embedded in early models of committee-based decision-making, as the ethics committee itself emerged. We might expect to find these principles unsettled in practice, as people move in and out of roles. But they are not settled in theory, either. When I spoke to Atoy Navarro in early 2025, he was just back home in Quezon City after a trip to Bangkok in his now consultant role for FERCAP. The training he had been part of had popped up on my Facebook feed, and as our Zoom connection jumped and glitched, he walked me through the latest updates he had shared with Survey trainees. Flicking through slides on the shared screen, he ticked off the latest updates to guidelines that had an impact on the composition of committees: the 2023 WHO Benchmarking tool; the updated 2024 version of the Declaration of Helsinki; and the new ICH-GCP, released weeks before his workshop.

In this section of the book, I am concerned with the emergence and stabilization of models that committees are expected to work with. "International Guidelines" like those above often make appearances in draft form at conferences, including FERCAP's, and are brought to different fora for consultation. FERCAP members, including Dr. Cristina Torres, are sometimes part of the working groups for their revision. As these guidelines encounter differently resourced settings, the conversation still lurches and falters over *which* standards, and how they should be thought and formulated. Across the three linked chapters of this section (chapters 4, 5, and 6), my interest is in the relationship between these guidelines and the situated, social negotiation of a decision. A committee decision sits in an awkward place between this still new profession of ethics work, and the profession of medicine's long-established and institutionally well embedded authority.

Historians of medicine and its governance have traced the emergence of committees to oversee medical research in different settings. In the United States, these histories offer an analysis of where (public) trust in medicine faltered. Social historian Duncan Wilson examines discourses that emerged after the *New York Times*' 1972 revelation of the Tuskegee study in the U.S. (Wilson 2012). He cites the Yale lawyer Jay Katz, who argued that "fundamental questions needed to be asked about the nature of authority assigned to physicians" (Katz 1972, 606, cited in Wilson 2011, 199). The givenness of self-governance for the medical profession was under scrutiny. In Wilson's summary, "Katz claimed that doctors possessed no unique expertise that justified making them the sole arbiters of medical ethics, and proposed that patients and experimental subjects should be safeguarded through 'more active participation of non-scientists in research decisions'" (Katz et al. 1972, 1, cited in Wilson 2012, 199). Arguments such as this, Wilson argues, led to a profound shift in the locus of governance over biomedical research.[1] Within two years of the Tuskegee revelation, President Nixon established a national commission for the protection of human subjects in research, with the act of establishment stipulating that "no more than five of its eleven members should be doctors or scientists, with the majority drawn from philosophy, law, theology, sociology or the general public" (Wilson 2011, 126). Discussion of the "politicization" of bioethics in the United States ebbs and flows, with some arguing that it is precisely a bioethical role to provide concepts through which to respond to injustice and inequality (ten Have 2022), others concerned that "partisan capture" risks the field's "independence and credibility" (Lawrence 2025). Yet in defending the U.S. President's Council on Bioethics (PBCE) from accusations of politicization, Leon Kass, its former chair, stated that:

> The Council has been "in microcosm, and in the best sense of the term, a *political* body," because of the way it has sought to incorporate diverse perspectives, avoid expert jargon, and engage the public. (Kass, cited in Brown 2009, 43)

The history of committees as models for decision-making matters because it is tied to their legitimacy. While they may have received training in North American bioethics controversies, or even participated in training programs in the United States, members of committees in this book do not necessarily share North American ideals of public engagement or accountability. The histories of medicine as a profession may trade in concepts of expertise and authority, but how such authorities are handled and managed in the face of scandal has not necessarily given rise to new accountabilities for the medical profession. So, the ethnographic question motivating this chapter, and the section overall, is: What happens when the worlds carried by the committee, described in Kass's and Katz's work, are brought to bear on distinct contexts? What a committee is assumed to be—and how it becomes situated in local bureaucracies—varies enormously across the settings where FERCAP works. While FERCAP's Standard Operating Procedures can be uniformly applied and committees assessed according to shared criteria, the model itself, with its incorporation of "diverse perspectives" or capacity to "engage the public," play out in radically distinct ways outside of the bureaucratic settings and civic epistemologies. Legitimate decisions through a committee in Kass's account may not resemble those challenged as the committee form arrives in countries where imaginings of "society" as something to be fully represented do not result in expectations of agreement or unity.

In the World Health Organization's "Research Ethics Committees: Basic Concepts for Capacity-Building," the authors argue that "in ethics, the process by which a decision is made is as important as the outcome. For a decision to be ethically legitimate, it must be made in an open and inclusive process that takes into account the views of all stakeholders" (2009, 22). The role given to each member forms part of the justification of the committee, each role with its own history. The idea of the ideal committee runs through trainings on ethics work, focusing particularly on the ideal composition. Members of FERCAP participate in and react to the making of new standards, and they query the purpose of standard-making along the way. The conversation among practitioners is live, and I develop this into an analysis of what I term "microcosming work" done through committees and their members. My suggestion is that the interaction between their "lay" role and the ideal of the committee reveals the agonistic epistemics at work in the relations between the kinds of expertise they are thought to bring to the collective decision. But first let us turn to some of the language games of making models in the first place: the verbal politics of how such ideals get into international guidelines and regulations.

Represent, Reflect, Have Knowledge Of

When standards are being written or updated, they go on tour, and acknowledgments to those who responded around the world appear in prefaces. During fieldwork, I realized that FERCAP had become part of the consulting networks for the World Health Organization, having made itself into a useful site where diverse representatives from a range of countries in the Asia-Pacific would gather. So, as I sat in the Grand Hall of the Hotel Equatorial Shanghai and listened to the draft of the new WHO *Standards and Operational Guidance for Ethics Review of Health-Related Research with Human Participants*, I knew I was watching a struggle over how standards for committee composition would be shaped.

It is November in 2010, and Carl Coleman, a former advisor on bioethics and the law to the World Health Organization, is presenting the latest version of what the network knows as the "Silver Book" to the gathered FERCAP conference. Standing at the Hotel Equatorial's red velveteen podium, he opens his slides. The room, chatty, quietens down. Laptops are brought out, glowing in the dark of the ballroom. Coleman is here to share what a large working group has been doing, and he wants to give the room some context for the draft. "Let me preface this," he says, "by saying the standards are all phrased in the same way: phrased as describing a state of affairs that would be a good state of affairs, the way things should be. There's no verb in there, such as 'should' or 'must' or 'encouraged.'" In the large plenum hall, conference-goers look to the screen and to their programs: Coleman has the first after-lunch slot, so we are all quietly heavy with food and our bodies are sluggish in the air-conditioned space. "It's simply saying," he continues, "that in an ideal world, this is what happens. [. . .] They're describing the situation as it should be. The question in evaluating any given system is whether in fact this description is being satisfied."

A document that intends to bring something into being through description is idealistic in its normativity. The new *Standards and Operational Guidelines* document is a means, as the anthropologist of documents Annelise Riles would say, that points to an end beyond itself (2001, 93). The endpoint of these documents was, however, contested. By forcing a description of the ideal, and bringing it to the Forum for discussion, Carl was holding open the gap between the ideal and what people sitting there considered realistic. The feasibility discussion went back and forth, committee members raising concerns.

At the height of the exchange, a delegate from the Philippines put it best: "I feel the standards are supposed to be aspired toward. Not the standards conforming to what is reality but reality being improved to conform with standards." Supporting the "unrealistic" standards meant giving them reality-bending powers, pushing that reality to meet the description of the world put forward in a document—a document with an end beyond itself.

This work of improving reality is an everyday task for committee members who campaign and lobby their home institutions. Carl's challenge lay in creating a standard about moving from the system to the entity that is establishing the REC, which could be a national or subnational entity; it could be an institutional entity. The REC is defined as follows (he reads from the screen):

> The appointing official ensures that the REC has a multidisciplinary and multisectorial membership, that its composition includes both genders, that it reflects the social and cultural diversities of the communities from which research participants are most likely to be drawn, and that it includes individuals with backgrounds relevant to the areas of research that the committee is likely to review. Committee members recognize the limits of their knowledge and seek external input where necessary, particularly in relation to research that involves participants whose life experiences may differ significantly from those of the committee members.

Carl formally summarizes the standard as being about "a diverse representation on the committee and it goes into a little bit of detail about what diversity means." He stops, then looks out to the crowd and asks for questions. In the discussion that follows, definitional work is being done. Committee members gathered here in Shanghai are challenging what work standard-making could or might do in their settings. What they contest are the imaginaries of representation and resource put forward in this draft. It is not just a contestation of feasibility—though it is that, too. It is a contestation over logics of representation embedded within the draft.

The first hand in the air is Vasantha Muthuswamy's, at that time the senior deputy director general of the Indian Council of Medical Research.[2] "Of course," she begins,

> [the standard] only talks about backgrounds relevant to areas of research the committee is likely to review. It's not always possible. That's why you need consultants, experts who are attendant to the committee to do the expert views.

The session chair points out that this is addressed in the next sentence, that committee members "recognize their limitations," but the chair thinks it's important that the standard notes that "individuals have backgrounds relevant to the areas of research," even if this is not always going to be possible. Carl agrees, and takes up the point:

> *Ideally* you would have representation from all the areas of expertise. In reality, that may be a standard that is going to be difficult to meet in a lot of cases because the committee just doesn't have a lot of options to draw from. That's where the next sentence about limits of knowledge would come in.

Vasantha worries that by making "representation from all areas of expertise" mandatory, it becomes impossible for committees, particularly those in developing world settings, to achieve the standard.[3] There is a pause. People shuffle and the tension rises. Cristina responds, interrupting the silence: "I think I'd still emphasize that an EC should have the expertise to review the types of research it reviews," she says:

> If it has no expertise, it should not review it, no? I like this guideline because it emphasizes that this EC should have expertise, otherwise what's your business accepting that protocol? And you seek external input where necessary. That's the consultant.

At this point, an invited speaker from the U.S. raises a hand. The chair motions for him to speak. "This is only a suggestion," he begins, conscious of his accent and his positioning. "Not imposing?" jokes the chair. "Just a suggestion," he repeats:

> When it says that the appointing official will ensure that [the committee] reflects the social and cultural diversity of the committees, you imply that you must have representation from that participating population you are doing research in. Perhaps it should say that they ensure that they have *knowledge* about social and cultural diversity. Not every REC has an HIV infected person on their board, nor do they have poor people, or others from these vulnerable populations that we'll do work with. So, it may want to say that rather than ensuring the committee *reflect* the diversity, that the committee have the *knowledge* of that diverse population.

The invited speaker has enlarged the problem—which started in the possible limitations of medical expertise in developing countries—to the *kind*s of knowledge that are sufficient, who might possess them, and how both people and knowledge should be made present on a committee. "How can we get those people from that community?" asks one audience member. "I think it's about having the relevant knowledge," continues another: "I think it should say, 'The committee should have the relevant knowledge,' rather than the committee itself *reflecting* those . . ." We reach a point where this change is being contemplated and Carl speaks again:

> There were a lot of people saying that there wasn't enough in the existing "Silver Book" to emphasize that this isn't a committee that is looking *at* the community and making decisions for it but that it is a committee *of* the community. At first it said something like "*represents*" and then there was some concern that that was a little ambiguous and what does it mean to represent a community? So *reflects* was seen as a little bit . . . But *knowledge of* is almost expressly saying that it's people who are not [of that community], it's someone from the outside who *knows of.*

Li Ling, a delegate from the host city of Shanghai, suggests "emphasis on the cultural or community consideration of the committee composition," worried that unless this is specified, it will be ignored. Cristina replies to her,

> It's about the layperson not a community representative. [The standard] says that members whose primary background is not in science or research should be appointed in sufficient numbers to ensure that they feel comfortable voicing their views. And that was intended to emphasize that you shouldn't just have a token member that is the community or a lay member, but there really should be a critical enough group.

The shift from sufficient breadth of scientific expertise to "social and cultural" issues provokes the invocation of three distinct terms: reflects, represents, and "has knowledge of," each carrying its own connotations.

Why do these words and terms matter? While Dr. Muthuswamy's concern with the scientific whole can be readily supplied with "experts" and "external consultants," the breadth of "the social" is less easily satisfied. The discussion shows disagreement both about the qualities of persons who embody the social, and about how they are to be brought in. North American literature on the topic is clear: While no committee can represent all elements of the community where research will be conducted, the REC must be capable of assessing the impact of the research on the community and determining whether the research is relevant in the local setting (Rivera and Borasky 2009, 50). However, Li Ling's intervention allows Cristina to reframe the problem of representation as one of the committee's expertise. This in turn becomes a question of quantity: "You shouldn't just have a token member that is the community or a lay member, but there really should be a *critical enough group,"* Cristina says. Researchers try to ameliorate such intimidation when conducting research. Consider these notes from a discussion at a workshop in Canada in 2005, following presentations on community consent in the "Promotion of Equitable Research Practices":

> One way to achieve informed community consent is through community REBs. Then it will not simply be a traditional band or tribal leader consent—one person who decided for the group—but a more balanced consent. It is an epistemological question: are we individuals first or members of groups? The answer seems to be neither, and this is the problem. (Dubois-Flynn 2006, 63)

Anthropologists are likely to recognize this "epistemological question" of the tussle between individuals and communities, refracted through the issue of consent. When confronted with community consent, the certainty of the researchers (and of their "ethics") in the primacy of the individual evaporates. Informed consent is the ground upon which this tension becomes most evident and has garnered a large share of academic attention (Sankar 2004; Molyneux et al. 2005; Reubi 2012; Hoeyer and Hogle 2014). Within the concept of "society" the individuality of its members is constructed as primary; individuals first, their relationships second (Strathern 1996a, 62). What the apparent problem of "applying" principles of individual informed consent to others reveals (again) is that—as anthropologists have long known—*the individual is a particular way of thinking about the person* (Corrigan 2003). In the closing of her contribution to the 1989 Manchester General Debates in Anthropology, Marilyn Strathern puts the consequences of this foregrounding strongly: "The unfortunate outcome of conceiving of society itself as an entity has actually been to make relationships seem secondary and not primary to human existence" (Strathern 1996a, 55). When the individual whose consent must be sought is not found, indeed the concept itself is not found to hold, researchers look for groups. Groups then require representatives, and the problem recurs.[4]

When I interviewed Carl nine months after the consultation in Shanghai, he clarified that the draft at the time read "reflects,"[5] for what he called "practical" reasons:

> Will you be able to find people who truly represent? "Having knowledge of" might mean anyone who has read a book. The reflect is more in-between. "Represent"—you'd need to find someone who could speak on behalf of the entire group. "Reflect," you could be a part of the group, or it means you're somehow part of it, it's not necessary for you to stand for everyone, you're not necessarily typical. But "Reflect" also goes some way to preventing a total stranger . . . So we had to try and find a word . . . Everyone will interpret [it] in a different way, not everyone will read it this way. For people who wanted the word "Represent" it helps them, and so in a way it serves both sides. It doesn't say that they do . . . [it] comes on a little weaker.

Carl's later analysis reveals assessments about the adequacy and type of "knowledge" desired from persons on an ethics committee. It also makes a careful distinction between types of learning. Book learning seems too little—the person could be a "total stranger." Representing seems too much of a demand, indeed, perhaps impossible. Sometimes, for Euro-Americans, "simply 'knowing' about other perspectives may [. . .] be regarded as a respectable end in itself," writes Strathern (2022, 252). But the discussion around the revisions of the "Silver Book" suggests that this is not one of those cases. In discovering the inadequacy of "having knowledge," we are led to ask for what purpose it is inadequate, and what is instead required. What is desired is no longer the characteristic of *knowing* something, but of *being* something: being "of" or "from" that community, being a patient with a disease that is under discussion. The "ideal" standards describe not only a broad range of persons in whom scientific expertise resides, but also types of people. Though the standard was ultimately published using the term "reflect" (WHO 2011), the first "guidance" point for Standard Two states that: "Members include individuals with scientific expertise [. . .] and lay people whose primary role is to share their insights about the communities from which participants are likely to be drawn" (WHO 2011, 8).

A Tale of Two Microcosms?

These conference contestations in Shanghai show that it is not easy to agree on what should be inscribed in international, aspirational standards. Does one convene a committee that, in Carl's words, "isn't a committee that is looking at the community and making decisions for it but that it is a committee *of* the community"? Does one emphasize the equality of participants, aiming for a conversation in which everyone is of equal standing? Or does one emphasize the need for scientific expertise, in the knowledge that unless research is scientific, it is not ethical?

In what follows, I build the argument that within these models for committee membership is a process of imagination that imagines this thing called society in microcosm. "Microcosm," from the Greek *mikros kosmos*, little world, is used to describe something "encapsulating in miniature the characteristic qualities or features of something much larger" (Oxford American Dictionary), of imagining one thing miniaturized inside another. Conceptualized as a process, it becomes microcosming. For me, it is an analytical means of drawing attention to *their* sets of strategies, in the way Michel Callon and Bruno Latour intend the term "macro-structuring" (1981), marking how ideas of macro and the micro *were part of the artifact under study*. Calling it "microcosming" allows me to point to the replication, scaling, and movement of shrinking that happens. How can you bring "society" into conversation with a person? The presence on the committee of a particular version of "society" is perceived as a miniature, drawn from a "larger" imagined externality.

In the sections that follow, I argue that there are two different types of microcosming going on in FERCAP's engagement with committees. The first concerns the *committee* itself as a microcosm, a move of representationalism. The second involves an image of "society" contained within a *person*, who comes then to represent "society" on the committee. My analysis follows through two different techniques of making microcosms, both of which seek to materialize "society" in the face-to-face environment of a committee meeting.

The Committee as Microcosm

When a committee is imagined as a microcosm there is—implied—a macrocosm from which that microcosm is drawn. When bioethicists look for "public opinion," "representative" committees are convened, or specified sections of "society" consulted. Here, the ethics *committee* needs to sufficiently make whole a fragmented outside whose diversity needs to be "represented." When representatives are found and arranged onto a committee, it can be thought that in the single voice of this committee's decision, "science" and "society" speak together.

But making society speak through the committee in this way is not always as straightforward as imagined. Indeed, Marilyn Strathern advises us to be wary of analysis that "hypothecates *society* as a partner [. . .] An abstract notion of 'society' [. . .] is pre-emptive. It demands demonstration rather than investigation" (2005, 476). The coherence of "society" depends, arguably, on denied incommensurabilities within a given totality, and the committee's ambiguous faithfulness to this totality leads to hesitation. At a 2009 FERCAP preconference training in Chiang Mai, Thailand, discussants noted how the committee was "*supposed* to be a microcosm of society where people have different backgrounds and trainings." Imagining society as something that can be shrunk to the size of a committee has another effect: that of democratization through miniaturization. Throughout her work, Cristina argues that ethics should not be a specialist activity, that it should be the kind of conversation that everyone on the committee can follow. In this genre of the committee the different backgrounds of members are valued, a "cross section" is sought.

The idea that "everyone" can follow the discussion prefigures the comparison with juries I will discuss in chapter 5. While the jury is a great deal older than the ethics committee, they hold in common a Euro-American tradition of *equal civic participation*, which comes forward in declarative moments. In 2007, for example, the UK barrister Helena Kennedy represented Shuja Mahmood, a man accused of involvement in a plot to cause explosions in London using ammonium nitrate fertilizer. The BBC reported her closing speech to the jury: "Because you are drawn from the public at large you represent something more—you signify law is not left to lawyers or judges; it is not some specialist preoccupation" (BBC 2007). Kennedy's concern that "law is not left to lawyers or judges" repeats a distinction made in ethics: Committees are told that while their professions are important, the committee's work is ultimately "not about your profession." Both juries and ethics committees must deal with hierarchies of expertise, types of people and knowledge, and yet sometimes, both insist on the value of nonspecialism.

It seems as though both Cristina and Kennedy are arguing for the same principle: that both the law and research ethics should be accessible to "everyone." Put another way, it matters that they are decisions that could be understood by all. Through their principles of composition, both the committee and jury contain the essential fiction that "society" can be made to speak. What differs is who it is that makes up "society" in each of these groups. It was because a jury was supposed to be a "cross section" that when, in early 2002 in the UK, Louis Blom-Cooper QC "argued that defendants should have the right to be tried by a panel of experts instead of a jury" (BBC 2002a), there was a rapid response from civil rights groups and barristers (Home Office 2002). Blom-Cooper had claimed that "the question of evaluating evidence in the courtroom is a professional job, it's not for amateurs" (BBC 2002a). During the response to this suggestion, the Bar Council framed this as a matter of public trust: "The public trusts the jury system, the government needs to show it trusts the public" (BBC 2002b; *The Observer* July 14, 2002). Public trust and confidence are precisely what Coleman (2003, 1185) and Koski both desire for science, and ethics committees are posed as a route to it. I suggest that as states borrow from science techniques of knowledge for their legitimacy (Ezrahi 1990), the technique of transparency is beginning to be applied to ethics review committees.

The reason usually given for the "closed" nature of an ethics committee meeting is that of confidentiality, and the risk of proprietary protocols and drugs-in-development being disclosed. However, pursuing the jury analogy, Coleman argues that confidentiality concerns "should not be used as a shield to limit the public's ability to participate in and oversee the decision-making process" (Coleman 2003, 1186). As much as the committee *is* "society" in microcosm, "publics" must also be able to inspect this microcosm in operation. Indeed, he goes as far as to claim that "both IRB deliberations and their written opinions should be open to the public" (Coleman 2003, 1186). In the U.S., committees *are* federally mandated (Stark 2012, 157), and like Coleman, Laura Stark speculates on the closedness of IRB meetings (2012, 35–37). She writes that "many questions raised about declarative bodies as a tool of government have gone unanswered precisely because administrative bodies work outside of public view" (2012, 37) and argues that

> decision makers are persuaded by different forms of evidence for administrative choices made behind closed doors than in decisions made publicly, with doors flung open, TV cameras rolling, and full transcripts available. (2012, 38)

In the widely read account Shapin and Schaffer offer of early experimental science, Hobbes and Boyle famously disagreed over what counted as public witnessing. Donna Haraway writes that "Boyle's 'open laboratory' and its offspring evolved as a most peculiar 'public space' with elaborate constraints on who legitimately occupies it. 'What in fact resulted was, so to speak, a public space with restricted access' (Shapin and Schaffer 1985, 336)" (1997, 25). That questions are starting to be raised about the closedness of ethical review is significant when one remembers Stark's succinct summary: They can change what can be known in their review and revision of protocols.

So how is a legitimate *macrocosm* chosen? It is a question suited to empirical study. Stark's work on committees as "declarative bodies" concerns itself with the way they are "empowered by governments to make decisions without consulting citizens" (2011, 233). Working with FERCAP, I have not found it to be the case that "citizens," "the public," or "society" are invoked or thought of as needing to be consulted; nor have I found that the committee is a device that, through its decisions, is used to make science "accountable to society," to use language familiar in Europe and North America.

In Singapore, Kerry Holden and David Demeritt expressed concern that the focus they encountered on "the international marketability of research results" and the "highest international standards" (2008, 81) drew from a macrocosm which was, for Singapore, mislocated and mismatched. As they write,

> the bioethical model being put into practice in Singapore anticipates a certain state-society relationship in which the populace is invested with a series of rights, both individual and participatory, such that it can give active asset to new and novel forms of science and technology. (2008, 82)

When Holden's interviewee, who worked for Singapore's national ethics committee, pointed out the absence of "autonomy," replacing it instead with "respect for the individual," Holden and Demeritt were—at their own confession—"flummoxed": What, they asked, was ethics without its "guiding principle" of autonomy? (2008, 82). They argue the "the mapping of ICH guidelines onto Singaporean society defies the very logic of those guidelines," that it was not about the meaning of "autonomy" for committees or the Singaporean state: "As long as the consent forms are signed and the paper trail is clear, there should be no qualms about what it all means" (Holden and Demeritt 2008, 82).

Laypersons as Microcosms

But what is the meaning already in the making of the paper trail and the social relations *it* makes? In comparing an ethics committee with a jury, I found that in neither judgment nor discussion are all perspectives equally valid, even if they "should" be. This is also what Stark finds in the United States:

> Is everyone equally an expert in IRB meetings? In theory, the answer is yes. In practice, however, the answer is no. [. . .] Cordoned off from traditional avenues of public oversight, declarative bodies have been imagined as democratic by virtue of their design. Each member is expert in his field; each member is equally valuable. (2012, 38)

The authority of most of the committees I worked with did not come from an imagined ability to represent the considered opinion of a population. "Society" is present, nominally, but through a second microcosming, through laypersons. Instead of regarding committee itself as a microcosm, this second version considers "society" to be present in a single person, who then comes to "represent" the everyday person, a person whose expertise is precisely their inexpertness, their normality, everyman-ness. This specific kind of person is a "layperson," a well-established figure in Euro-American discourses of public engagement with science. Looking back at his 1995 text on AIDS activists, the text which introduced the term to the literature, sociologist Steve Epstein suggested that in the mid-1990s he "placed no great weight on the term, and [he] was vague and inconsistent in reflecting on its provenance and meaning" (2023, 81). Today, the idea is enmeshed in a "semantic web, one that concerns various forms of knowledge seen as alternative, subordinated or contrarian that stand (explicitly or implicitly) in contrast to forms of knowledge deemed official, standard, universal or authoritative" (Epstein 2023, 81–82). Recognizable renditions of laypersons are distinguished by their medical ignorance, and standing in contrast to the medical members of the committee, they assist in *creating* the latter as experts (Michael 1996; Strathern 2004). Alessandro Maranta et al. suggest we look to laypersons for their "*action* in the knowledge production which ascribes epistemic and functional competences to lay persons" (2003, 154, emphasis added). This action plays an important role in both types of microcosming that I argue result in ways of doing ethics committee work.

Stopping to think about this more carefully, in the way that Carl and the FERCAP conference did, means that underlying principles embedded in the form of the committee, the model that creates legitimacy for a decision-making that is itself ethical, begin to emerge. Writing about the United States, Stark's suggestion that "declarative bodies have been imagined as democratic by virtue of their design" becomes an idea with a particular history, a specificity possible due to the North American representationalism present in research ethics. Similarly, in his study of the "epistemological commitments underlying American conceptions of individualism, politics and public action," the political theorist Yaron Ezrahi notes "the idea that the life of every individual is in some respects a microcosm of the life of the community" (1990, 201). This imaginary of society/community-in-the-person allows commentators to turn away from the imaginary of "segments" of society being represented on the committee to a person "in whom" society/community is contained.

In my earlier discussion of Carl's struggles around the terms "reflect," "represent," and "have knowledge of" above, we begin to discern that *who one is* and *how one knows something* both matter. The detail of the slippage in discussion shows two outsides: the professional realm of medicine, which seeks representation through expert knowledge, and the remainder, imagined as society, with its cultural and "lay" specificities. Making standards that describe a committee sufficient to both of these is, as the representative from the Indian Medical Council, Dr. Muthuswamy, noted above, practically impossible. While FERCAP works to "educate" committees on the role of the layperson and tries to measure the impact of their approach in terms of whether or not the layperson speaks, this cannot be an indicator. The layperson needs to be "heard," and this is difficult to measure. We have seen that both "laypersons" and scientists or experts need to "learn." Thus I would suggest that the capacity FERCAP builds is a matter of seeing problems as they are framed by the makeup of the committee.

So, this second form of microcosming, which takes the layperson as the microcosm of societal interests, has a "type" of committee associated with it. By condensing "societal" concern into the layperson, the remainder of the committee is made up of scientific experts, shifting committee discussions closer to the scientific soundness of research. The tension between ethics review and scientific soundness of research has been noted before, most clearly in follow-up discussions to the Nuffield report on the ethics of research in developing world settings. Published as a follow-up document, Nuffield reported that while participants in the discussions contributing to the report agreed that "both the scientific quality, and the ethical issues raised by the proposed research should be reviewed," (Nuffield Council on Bioethics 2005, 48), the meeting could not agree on how this should be achieved. No minutes are available, but one can imagine the conversation resembling the situation faced by Carl in Shanghai: What resources exist to make sure both reviews happen? As the document notes, in Kenya, "a scientific committee usually reviews the scientific protocol before it is submitted to an ethics committee [. . .] in a much smaller country such as Fiji, there are not currently enough suitably qualified experts to make it possible to create two separate committees" (Nuffield Council on Bioethics 2005, 48). In a formulation very similar to Carl's Shanghai ambitions, the discussion group concluded that "*ideally*, and where feasible, it was suggested that these [scientific and ethics] review processes should be separated" (Nuffield Council on Bioethics 2005, 48, emphasis added).

During my time with FERCAP, trainers repeatedly argued that if research is not scientifically sound, it is not ethical; that *no risk* to participants can be justified if the results will not be scientifically valuable. During the two decades of FERCAP's work, ethics committee trainers have had to acknowledge that in some countries where they work, hospital or institutional ethics committees may be the only point through which international applications for research pass. *As such, the scientific members and their expert knowledge come first*, upholding the maxim that unscientific research is always unethical. The priority of this version of the ethics committee, in which the social is microcosmed into a single layperson, is to oversee *good science*: that is, create publishable papers, monitor research coming into a country from overseas. Ethics committees' attention to matters considered scientific can frustrate, no matter where the review takes place: "Clinical researchers are exhausted by the demands of ethics committees that seem more concerned with the science (which they cannot necessarily judge) and editorial control of patient information sheets than with ethics" (Warlow 2004, 241). How and where the distinction between science and ethics is made is an ethnographic question. Juntra is thinking of this part of the committee's role when she expresses concern about the lack of doctoral qualifications in some countries where trials are to be held, or when Chatura, a committee member in Sri Lanka, tells me that they spend most of their time discussing methodology, criticizing proposals:

> When you think about it, [research ethics is] a highly technical subject. You can't just walk off the street and be a good ethics committee member. Just because they are clergy or a teacher, doesn't mean they can come. I don't agree with taking one of each kind and saying everyone is represented [. . .] Some methodologies are unethical because if research is not scientific then it is unethical to subject people to risk.

Historians of science Shapin and Schaffer note that "democratic ideals and the exigencies of professional expertise form an unstable compound" (2011, 336). I suggest that this unstable compound is present in globally circulating models for how ethics committees are assembled. As FERCAP works to "bring perspectives together" on an ethics committee, following semi-tacit principles of equal contribution and common discussion, it also *re-creates the separateness of those views*. Shapin and Schaffer's witnesses of science acted as "transparent spokesmen [. . .] whose only visible trait was their limpid modesty, they inhabited the culture of no-culture. Everybody else was left in the domain of culture and society," writes feminist critic Donna Haraway (1997, 25). The separateness resurfaces in Chatura's comments on the technicalities of research ethics. However, when committees review ethics they are *also* witnesses of science (Nuffield Council on Bioethics 2005, 48) when their decisions not only *rely* on the scientific expertise of members but are also *about* the science. Those moments give double meaning to the making of "good science."

Perspective Machines

In this chapter, the committee emerges as a means of controlling the formation of perspectives. This control is bound by the limits of time, particularly in the Asia-Pacific region where committees are made up of academics and physicians, volunteering time. The committee is limited by those chosen to be on it, those who sit in the room. As a form it gains its legitimacy from having multiple views present, but in acting as a committee it must arrive at a decision: a committee decision. The "one voice" with which the ethics committee speaks takes a single body, sometimes the chairman, sometimes the stamp of "The IRB" (Stark 2011, 235). This both lends authority to the image of combined and considered views and conceals the identity of those who have swayed the opinion in the meeting. In this "corporate" sense, the committee members are less themselves and more the features of many.

The capacity being built is not just to do with histories of ethics or even modes of thinking, but with the inseparability of those modes of thinking from the form of the committee. What emerges is sometimes imagined—as the experienced Sri Lankan microbiology researcher Wedika put it—as a dialogue between those who speak for everyday people, and those who, through their training in medicine, have "lost" that way of thinking. In its purpose and modeling, the committee simultaneously assumes that viewpoints are comparable and works toward ensuring that they are. The possibility of misunderstandings at the committee table is expected, indeed desired. Misunderstanding and discussion contribute to debate, considered as a necessary component (measured in FERCAP's Survey) of what an ethics committee is. But that the misunderstandings might not be the *same* misunderstandings is not something that can be entertained or desired.[6]

Many scholars remark on the Western origins of bioethics, and the problems that this causes. At the turn of the century, Zulfiqar Ahmed Bhutta, a pediatrician based in Toronto, cited in his article a fellow Toronto-based colleague, Abdallah Daar, as stating "so long as all the ethicists are in the North and the South is just the recipient of ethical principles, nothing will change!" (Bhutta 2002, 118). Contemporary voices continue to call for "epistemic justice for a global bioethics," problematizing how expertise is constructed and valued, and critiquing the way "the field silences the epistemologies and experiences of the very populations on whom global health ethics are inscribed" (Pratt and de Vries 2023, 333). Discussing the latest revision of the Declaration of Helsinki with Atoy following his training workshop, the themes of this chapter—still discussed—came to the surface. He flicked through his slides to find the one he wanted, a summary of the Declaration's latest changes. This was something he was happy about, he said, as a social scientist. Now, the Declaration "calls for participant and community access to research results" (Bierer 2025, 18) as well as "meaningful engagement with research study participants before, during and after the study has been undertaken" (Parums 2024, e947428-2).

What this will—or could—mean for committees remains to be seen. In its current form, its ideals of operation owe a great deal to Euro-American ways of thought about what people and their relations are, and they also replicate the tensions that constituted anthropological analysis for a large part of the twentieth century: the micro and the macro, society and the individual, local and global. There is and remains an implicit distinction that treats the *form* of the ethics committee as separate from the "western" origins of ethics *content*; as though it were in some way neutral, as though it could host any kind of discussion. Viewpoints were always comparable. What is this space, in which all must be equal, but some are afraid to speak? As Shapin asks, "What relations obtain between the authority of knowledge and the character of knowers?" (2008, xvii). But who sits on the committee matters deeply to the decisions that are made. In explaining the difference that FERCAP training was oriented at, Cristina referenced a workshop where a case had come up about "the Malarone study in Indonesia, you know it? Well their analysis was very . . . academic." How so? I had asked. She responded:

> Well they were focusing on fair subject selection, and thought it was bad because the study would exclude locals, but not migrants. And you ask why, well it was because the area is malaria endemic! The migrants would be clinically naive! They don't know what they are talking about. In things like this, you have to consult experts, that is what I do, defer to experts, and not give an academic opinion without really knowing the realities of sites where trials go on. But that is the job of the ethics committee, to be familiar with local conditions. They [bioethicists] cannot make conclusions, it's not how their training works. But an ethics committee, it is supposed to decide.

It is this doing of knowledge, an ethics as embodied and enacted, where the stakes for the committee as a form lie. It is the aspiration of creating groups of people where an understanding of the connection between a study's exclusion criteria and local geographies of malaria that would render the study meaningful. But it also organizes and creates the conditions of a decision, which, as we will now see, is the task that a committee must do together.

FIVE
Dynamics of Decision

Decision-making in ethics review is political work. It is also work that committees *must* do—postponing decisions is unpopular, and tales of delay and inefficiencies haunt bureaucratic ethics. "You cannot be deadlocked," FERCAP Surveyors tell committees sternly. But as scholars of social decision-making have argued, a decision is a textured and interpersonal form of action. It is not always easy to trace how it has been made, what contributed to it, or at what moment a group of people settled. These characteristics make it a challenging, if ethnographically observable, form of "social knowledge" (Camic et al. 2011). It is also a live discussion at the intersection of bioethics and practice, with ongoing debates about consistency of decisions (Friesen et al. 2019). I had been interested in committee decision-making since the start of my research, curious about how people arrived at decisions as a group, how they handled disagreements and disputes. How was this thing, an ethics committee decision, formed? What constituted expertise and the "group"? How did committees feel out sufficiency of information, how were principles put into decision-making action, and upon what resources did people draw to make their case? Fortunately, this topic that drew my interest was also high on the FERCAP agenda.

As we have seen, standards for committee formation and practice can be sources of aspirational authority. Standard Operating Procedures promise a "right" way to conduct the review. Vasantha Muthuswamy, FERCAP's founding secretary, wrote in her capacity as the president of FERCI (the Forum of Ethics Review Committees of India) that one kind of reasoning, "risk-benefit analysis is the main responsibility of ethics committees," but noted that "how this is being done is anybody's guess, and the capability of the members of doing such an analysis is a debatable issue" (2013, 10). For sponsors, discussion is an unknown. Writing in FERCAP's tenth anniversary booklet, Lisa

Hamadian and Allan K. Johansen, both experienced clinical auditors, write that the observation of a full board meeting, as undertaken during the Survey, "is carried out to evaluate group dynamics, the management of COI, and the actual adherence to written SOPS—Are the EC's decision-making procedures in line with their SOPs? Do they follow the 'write what you do and do what you write?'" (2011, 20).

While committees can be encouraged to ensure they consider various aspects of a research proposal there is another dimension of a committee that Standard Operating Procedures cannot template: its interpersonal life. Dealing with the personal within the official is problematic. Committee members struggle when the principal investigator of a proposal under review is one's boss, when a reviewer is also a colleague, or when those sitting around the table with them, deciding, are their superiors. With its historic roots in a merger of cultures of expertise and ideals of public participation in the oversight of science, the ethics committee is *in principle* a community of equals sitting around a table. Yet this ideal inevitably intersects, through its embeddedness in institutions, places, and cultures of medicine, with institutional and national politics of seniority, prestige, and friendship.

In this chapter, I show how committee members put the form of the committee to work when they decide. Drawing on the differently designated roles of members to manage ambiguity, chairpersons steer conversations that veer between deference and open hostility, negotiation and compromise. Close empirical attention to discussion and dialogue is difficult. Given the competitive nature of scientific research proposals, few committees are open to observation. Through the repeated observations of the Survey, and as a trainee auditor within the Forum's Recognition Program, I gained admission to the otherwise closed spaces where this work took place. I was able to be present during discussions and deliberations, listening for and exploring the delicate question of how decisions arise, how they are communicated, and how they orchestrate the authoritative speech of the committee. There are, however, two limitations to this access. First, committees are on display to the wider Recognition Program: There are stakes to their deliberations on Survey days, and they take care to ensure they demonstrate the kind of committee meeting the SIDCER standards require. Second, given the network's commitment to supporting committee work in the languages in which it takes place, international guests at these observations worked with translators, usually trainees participating in the Survey, as local support. While they were often extremely knowledgeable about the processes of the committee and had the vocabulary of review, the the form of translation—whispers and notes on paper—did not always convey the full nuance of debate, neither to me nor to Surveyors. At times, committee members would switch language during discussion, moving rapidly between topics and speakers. As a result, my analysis examines what is at stake in the politics of representation embedded within ethics committees, focusing in particular on the problem of how a committee member takes a "perspective" on a protocol. By putting decision-making at the center of my analysis, I tune in to the way trainers and committee members reason through the problems of perspective and presence. The visibility of disagreement in the vote and the invisibility of personal ties both create difficulty for committee members, leading to moments of training or contestation where expected behavior is made explicit. Through these, I explore how people find ways to make criticisms, and the dangers in carrying out the task that committees must undertake: decision-making.

Bodies and Decisions

In its most simple description, the committee is a group of people physically sitting around a table. But then what? At a training on Good Clinical Practice (GCP) at Thammasat University, just outside Bangkok, Juntra, Cristina, and I were discussing decisions in ethics review committee meetings. As trainers, they were trying to convey to committee members that it was important that they not only draw on their expertise, but also bear in mind the patient, protocol, and contribution of the research to society. From this breadth, Juntra's first concern was to avoid discussions that led to position-taking:

> In a debate, if you adopt a position, you take that and see if you win or lose at the end. You won't compromise your position. But it's not about winning or losing, that's not a good attitude for an Ethics Committee.

Cristina agreed:

> It's not who you are, [if you take a position] you won't be moved, so it's not what you really think. Real life is about decisions, not hypothetical unreal stories. In an ethics committee, everyone should think: "How could we come up with a decision appropriate for that study that will be the best for people taking part?" The minute you take positions, you try to protect them. All you have is that position.

> If, instead, all of you have one position, how to contribute to the protocol—if you have *that* position, you can have your eyes open for another's view.

Her reference to hypothetical unreal stories is a gentle jab at bioethics cases. Juntra, who was sitting opposite me, pointed to the water bottle on the table between us. "I can't see the other side of your bottle," she said. "Our job is to ask 'how can we describe the whole bottle?'" Cristina nodded, saying:

> Huiying has a nice picture of this. There are three blind men and they are all holding different parts of the elephant. There's this elephant and you touch different things, one has the tail one has the foot. And you say the elephant looks like this, but you only have a part. But together, they'll be able to describe what the elephant looks like.

We saw Huiying's slide in chapter 2, during the training of Surveyors in Beijing. In this retelling, the table is part of making the committee meeting recognizably a committee meeting. As a regulator based in Geneva noted, committee work "can't be two people in a corridor, but a meeting around a table." Juntra intends the bottle between us as the applicant's protocol, forcing the bottle into view not only from the literal perspectives of those around a table at an ethics committee meeting, but also their figurative perspectives. That she and I can literally see different sides of the bottle is equated with the different (figurative) "perspectives" that the members on the committee will bring to the discussion: They may have clinical experience, they may have knowledge of the law. When Juntra uses the bottle she is calling on a literal example of perspectives to illuminate a figurative perspective. In an ideal discussion, we describe the whole bottle—the whole protocol—and what it looks like seen from all sides. The imagined objective of Cristina and Juntra's committee view on the protocol is one that finds resonance with "a kind of cubist presentation in which every side of the object is presented simultaneously to us in a single—though 'general'—perspective" (Willerslev and Holbraad 2007, 334): the decision of the ethics review committee.

It is when figurative *perspectives* turn into *positions* that Cristina becomes critical: "The minute you take positions, you try to protect them." When, during a mock review at a training in the Philippines, the trainer announced that "in [an] ethics committee, you can change your mind as you discuss," the statement was greeted with applause. "It is not like a debate, where you stand by what you believe, no matter what," she said. What Cristina is recommending instead is the holding of a "common position": that of improving the protocol. Using the water bottle as she does, Juntra is using figurative language to get around what Rane Willerslev and Martin Holbraad see as the stumbling block to a "view from everywhere": that "we can never actually see things in their totality, simply because seeing in its nature is embodied and therefore perspectival" (2007, 334). But why would the embodied nature of ethics committee decision-making matter?

When a trainee asked Cristina, "Isn't it the point of having a diverse composition, to get diverse points of view?" during a Survey in the Philippines, she responded with the importance of decision-making: "When there's a difference in opinion, you arrive [at a decision] by voting [. . .] You cannot be deadlocked. The Ethics Committee is about decision-making." Opinions voiced in committee rooms become notes, become letters that change protocols. Anthropologists have long observed how the arrangement (and disciplining) of bodies in physical space betrays ideologies at work (Mitchell 1988, 78–79). When Hannah Brown and her co-authors summarize ethnographic attention to the meeting format, they describe a space "for the alignment and negotiation of distinct perspectives," spaces that are "constituted through the contextual interplay of similarity and difference. While multiplicity (e.g., people, perspectives, knowledge) is often their point of departure, singularity (e.g., in the form of objective agreement) is often their achieved outcome" (2017, 14). Even though Juntra is locating the perspective in the body, her figurative location of perspective is in the minds of the attendees, differently trained, each with different knowledge. In an ethics committee, perspectives are thought to be brought in and made present by the bodies of the room. They, too, are the materiality of ethics. What it makes visible relative to those sitting around the table is how perspective becomes tethered to identity. An ethics committee is not, for example, arranged with a circle around the chairperson, nor could it take the form of stage and seats: The idea is not that the chairperson is superior in wisdom or knowledge to those who accompany her. This in turn demonstrates the concern of the form with democratic reasoning. Yet as we have seen above, members of ethics committees are persons often chosen for their seniority. How do we reconcile these things?

In the opening section of this book, I brought forward the narrative anxiety of a "global clinical trial system" that may not be able to hold all its parts together—that it may fragment. Greg Koski's image of the finely woven silk cloth in chapter 1 provided an image for this fragile complexity. When attendees are prompted to imagine how this global system works, and their place within it, capacity is being built. Imagining is the skill. The same can be said to occur here, on the ethics committee itself. The parts of the committee—chair, secretary, laypersons, reviewers, and experts—learn how reviewing works. This observation allows me to return my attention to what that "form" of the ethics committee allows. As Marilyn Strathern puts it, "the idea of there being numerous perspectives and viewpoints 'on' phenomena implies that one could ideally formulate some kind of summation of all possible views, or at least a framework or perhaps a generative model for the production of the perspectives themselves" ([1991] 2004, 108).

Operating as a theory, the committee links identity, representation, and perspective, with the objective of producing a balanced view. But such a balance is itself fragile because of the potential for the proliferation of perspectives arising from "a constant sense that any one approach is only ever partial, that phenomena could be infinitely multiplied" (Strathern [1991] 2004, xiv). Too many perspectives, or too much representation, could lead to deadlock for research: It could be impermissible for any number of reasons. Cristina's recommendation of a common position acts as a limit to redescription, a way of bringing to rest "expandable narratives" (Strathern 1996b, 522). When she responds to a question about diverse composition and diverse viewpoints by emphasizing the importance of making decisions, Cristina is pointing to one method of delimitation. The limit of time is another and, as I illustrate below, the mapping of the figurative "perspective" onto the body a third.[1]

The One and the Many

A committee as a device assembles many views and combines them in decision-making. This makes it a device of Euro-American pluralism, "ontologically grounded in one world and many viewpoints" (Strathern 2011, 92), what Bruno Latour terms mononaturalism (2004). To do the work it needs to, the committee must be both a composite of many perspectives (representative) and a single voice (authoritative). Thus, having collected these potentially infinite—but practically and politically delimited—points of view, the next move is a shift between the singular and the collective. We have seen why it is socially advantageous for the anonymity of the reviewer—their point of view—to be concealed within the eventual decision of the "full board." Committee members are told: "In full board discussion your opinion can change, the final decision is a board decision, not an individual one." This combination into single-ness allows it to speak "as though" it were "one."

This "many as one" is a technique with considerable history within English political thought, and its implications have attracted anthropological study. In his long-term reflections on "the cultural epistemology that enables knowledge to become an enabler itself" (Corsín Jiménez 2013), taking up Hobbes's theory of representational personification as a political innovation that "brought about a political transubstantiation: the Many became the One, which contained, but also transcended, the Many" (2010, 3), Alberto Corsín Jiménez draws on the historian Noel Malcolm's observation that this "transubstantiation" resulted in "a curious structure of argument that requires two different ways of seeing the relation between the individual and the state to be entertained at one and the same time" (Malcolm 2004, 228, cited in Corsín Jiménez 2010, 3). There is a version of representational politics at work, and I suggest a version of this "structure of argument" is repeated when an ethics committee must be both one who stands outside to assess ethics and made up of many points of view. For the committee to "work," it must be seen twice: As Simon Schaffer writes of representation in politics and pictures, "you have to see each member of the group in its own right. At the same time, you have to see the group itself as a singular thing" (2005, 196).

Differences in viewpoint are no longer visible in the "one voice" (Stark 2012, 164) of the committee, and yet their input remains necessary for the decision's eventual "legitimacy." Being a "one" that becomes part of the "many" requires a certain capacity to detach oneself from one's argument (and context). The following interviews with Sri Lankan committee members Colin, a lawyer, and Wedika, a microbiology scientist, show their perceptions of how the different identities on the committee inform its discussion. Telling me about his fellow committee members, Colin said:

> They're from different backgrounds, it's a good composition of people, diverse backgrounds and those who have done well for themselves. They're not reliant on others for work, they're not worried about what other people think, so it makes for healthy discussion. At the moment, the committee is looking at guidelines for stem cell research. It's an old argument, what should be prohibited and what restricted, and at our last meeting, there was a lot of give and take, looking at the moral and religious issues to have a fairly objective discussion.

"Objective?" I asked.

> Well, people left their beliefs at the door. I don't think people's personal beliefs should have anything to do with what is being discussed at the table. [We are] not there to pass religious judgments. It is a question of what is lawful, and what can be done. The point is that members of ethics committees are not of any particular faith, unless they need to be for the purpose of representation.

What is Colin saying here? He is emphasizing the independence of the committee members, separating them from financial ties that might sway them. But he is also emphasizing a capacity for objectivity. How can one leave "personal beliefs" at the door, and yet be present for the "purpose of representation"? Colin is placing a positive valuation on the diverse "backgrounds" of the members, but finding one *part* of that "background" problematic.

Wedika, the microbiology researcher who sat on a committee in southern Sri Lanka, told me that his committee was "more confident" if it comprised several different disciplines. When we spoke, they had just added a statistician to their ranks, and he said that they found she was able to comment on the mathematical appropriateness of the sample size of a protocol, relative to its scientific aims. Using this as an example, he argued that a variety of perspectives would ultimately be good for trial participants. But Wedika's desire for variety had limits. While a statistician was an unambiguous positive, and a lawyer was also considered to be important, clergy posed a problem. "They are important too," Wedika said hesitantly, clearly struggling:

> But it's difficult to have *lots* of people coming—you lose control. Which religion are we going to choose? If all, then we have to give equal [weight] to all: Buddhists, Christians, Islam. They have their own areas they are very concerned about. If all three are there, I find, I feel some research projects might not go through, which should not be the case.

As Wedika saw it, *these* additional perspectives would clog research possibilities. Were the ideal of equal representation according to census figures or demographics actually enacted in the Sri Lankan town where he worked, he thought a great deal of research would stop:

> They may go on minor details, say, "In our culture, our religion, this should not be asked or questioned or investigated." Research will all end at that point [. . .]

> If a monk would sit in our committee, none of the animal research would be possible. They bring in teaching of Buddha, nothing will proceed—though we have thought of having [them on the committee].

He did foresee some possibilities for including such perspectives, albeit in a rather contradictory fashion:

> If we have such people, they need to be educated enough in ethics, so the religious thing doesn't apply to the proposal itself . . . Until we can have a panel of educated clergy, better not to have [them].

Embarrassment was another difficulty in including non-medics: "Even with the lawyer, it's difficult. It is not possible to invite them and then not accept that person's opinion, because it's embarrassing to then disregard it." At the same time, he worried about "losing the social part" of research: by concentrating on one issue, "we medics have blinded ourselves to other things."

These two interviews give a sketch of what a non-medical person who sits on an ethics committee in Sri Lanka is thought to be. The comments depart from the expert/layperson dichotomy of Euro-American studies of science, in which the literature on democratic of participatory decision-making shows roundtables, open fora, and consensus events are "intended to involve the lay public in decisions" (Flear 2009; Weingart 2017, 140). Shedding my *personal* religion, I come to stand in for a generic social concept of religion, one that is put "outside" the committee (which has concerns for "all" of society), and is channeled into the committee through me. Am I then an individual as "an internal constellation of plural elements," as conceptualized for example with conflict of interest, or a "life" "merographically conceived as belonging to many external systems" (Strathern 1992, 167)? The Sri Lankan material I have discussed here shows both versions in use. People are brought on to ethics committees on the basis of a "merographic image of the individual person as a part of diverse systems of domains beyond him or her" (Strathern 1992, 167)—but some of these domains are cut off. What the committee as a form effectively creates, I argue, is a space in which all perspectives are *notionally* present, but the relative value of these perspectives is contextually predefined, pre-weighted. Some matter more than others.

Voting and Consensus: Decisions and the Visibility of Opinion

Guidelines exist on how committees should make their decisions. In World Health Organization documents current at the time of my fieldwork, committee members are told that

> most committees make decisions through a process of consensus. This means that, instead of taking a vote and following the decision of the majority, they strive to make decisions that most people in the committee feel comfortable accepting. (World Health Organization 2009, 22)

However, the majority of committees I met with tended not to explicitly aim for consensus, even though it was acknowledged as the ideal. Anxieties circulated during a training session outside Bangkok: "We have to have consensus," fretted a newly appointed chairperson, "but what if the group is not at consensus?" Cristina, who was running the session, responded:

> That's the problem with consensus, if you do not vote [. . .] Consensus means you cannot vote. In Thailand, they table the protocol![2] Consensus means everybody agrees, or at least there's only one who disagrees, but how do you know?

The question asker persists: "Isn't it the point of having a diverse composition, to get diverse points of view? What if both points of view are valid?" Cristina nods, but challenges back:

> But how do you make a decision? You *have* to arrive at a decision. That's a problem. When there's a difference in opinion, you arrive by voting. There should be something in the SOP that gives you a way out. You cannot be deadlocked. An EC is about decision-making. Sometimes it's like this: The chair sits there, the EC members are fighting and they finish then the chair says, "Approve!" But what did you approve? It has to be very clear, otherwise we cite that as a weakness. Decision-making is very important to us as Surveyors. The reviewer has no authority to make a suggestion [to the researcher]. It's the full board. This is my problem in [Country X]: you give feedback and then they quarrel with the investigator. The investigator finds out you're the one. [. . .] In full board your opinion can change, *the final decision is a board decision, not an individual one.* (emphasis added)

The difference revealed in this exchange between a consensus opinion and a board decision is subtle, but important. Consensus, the term used conversationally in my fieldwork, meant both the discussion and the decision: It was a process that contained a result. Discussion and voting, on the other hand, could be separated. In Cristina's example, the board members are "fighting," and then the chair says "approve." She is using this as an illustration of poor behavior, since no link can be discerned between the discussion and the decision. In Stark's detailed research into how decisions are made on IRBs in the U.S., she writes that rather than consensus being the formal requirement and voting being the norm, voting is the formal requirement and consensus-making is the habit: "Group members act *as if* they should each agree on a shared judgement that they all can get behind" (2011, 236). Her observations brilliantly show how people persuade one another and how a committee comes to arrive at recommendations. What I want to look at here is how American models of open discussion and a consensus vote (see also Guston 2006) are not easily adopted.

A change in staff at a hospital in Taiwan had prompted the decision to send an administrative secretary for training in Olympia, Washington, at Western Institutional Review Board (WIRB). Edith, the committee's long-serving secretary, was chosen, and she spent six months there as part of the International Fellows Program of the Middleton Foundation for Ethical Studies (MFES 2013). The international fellowship programs FERCAP has facilitated have gone under different names over the years, beginning initially with the WIRB Fellowship Program (2002–2009) after Dr. Angela Bowen, then CEO of WIRB, met Juntra at a SIDCER meeting in Brussels in 2001. In Juntra's words, "many who attended that meeting were skeptical about the chances for SIDCER to succeed, being such an ambitious project with such an enormous vision. During the meeting Dr. Bowen sat quietly at the back, observing. At the end of the meeting, she said to me: 'What can I do to help you move this idea forward?'" (Karbwang Laothavorn 2016). The ensuing friendship led to jointly established fellowship programs, one of which Edith had benefited from. In our discussion, two years after her return, Edith focused not on her time in America but on the changes that she had implemented once back in Taiwan: "When I came back I just follow[ed] this way [they taught me] and have something to make the IRB more strong." Not all the changes Edith had tried to implement had been successful, however. In hopes of effecting greater efficiency, Edith tried to get her committee to change their manner of making decisions. She had watched and participated in committee meetings at WIRB during her training and seen "the rule": "[They] say 'OK, did anyone have different opinion, or don't agree. If [you] agree [with the proposed decision], say aye, and raise [your] hand.' When I came back," she said, "I tried to use this, but," she shrugged and shook her head. It hadn't worked. "This way," she paused, "maybe not good."

"Why not?" I asked her.

"If a board member sees every other board member raise [their] hand, maybe they just follow." She had spoken to her colleagues at other Taiwanese committees and considered introducing the voting paper that they used. "They just write, agree/disagree. But I think this spends more time, you have to give the paper, calculate, collect." Stuck between her desire for efficient processes and a concern with "following," she brightly told me that she had introduced "computer voting." I hardly needed to ask Edith whether it worked better. "We don't know who voted for which one!" she said, with a big smile:

> We just only have the number. 1 for agree, 2 for disagree. So, they press, we don't know [which] they press. Then maybe they have their own decision, not affected by other members. Another [good thing] is that it's very quick—I just press enter, see how many agree.

Decisions cast in the language of efficiency take in a variety of points and are the moment at which interpretation ceases. I decided to ask Edith why raising a hand might be okay in WIRB, but not in her hospital. Her answer was considered, but she rested it initially on the idea of "cultural difference." "Because I think the culture is different," she said, telling me that if she saw me raise my hand against a protocol, she might do the same: "I don't want to become the different person."

For Edith and her committee, the moment of decision itself was a moment of uncomfortable interpretation that needed a solution. The invisible vote provided it. While all could vote equally under the invisible voting system however, opinions given in discussion could not be disassociated from the speaker. Her ingenious voting system creates the space for a difference between points of view that is assumed to exist, and permits the expression of it by removing the social visibility that would otherwise—she claims—hamper its expression. The ability to conceal a single person's vote is also useful when one wants (or needs) to see the outcome of the vote as the decision of a committee: The decision retrospectively creates that which decided as single, rather than multiple. As Cristina emphasized in the training earlier, a final decision is a board decision. Similarly, when the lecturer slipped from the reviewer of an article for publication to a review of a protocol in an IRB meeting, he was at pains to remind his listeners of the following:

> When your EC reviews, it is your committee that is reviewing, it is not just one or two people reviewing. *The board speaks as one.* So it is only the name of the chair of the IRB, not everyone, in that communication [to the PI]. It is a mistake to inform investigators or authors that "Dr. so-and-so reviewed and found your article questionable because of the following." Okay?

During an interview with Chandeep, a Sri Lankan committee member, I found he wanted to make the point explicitly: "An ethics committee is not an *individual*, it's a *committee*." Procedure, he thought, would help a committee *be* a committee:

> You realize that there are many factors making committees not work as committees? There is this thing called groupthink. People fall into line, perhaps because of who said something, say I say "blah blah blah" and because it's *me* who said it, or because a certain individual told that, people aren't going to critique. I don't think that's *real* decision mode. Dynamics should be set in such a manner that all get the chance to speak [. . .] [and] ethics committees should have an operating procedure to make decisions on consensus basis.

Chandeep's description of a committee as a procedure reveals his assumptions about what a "real" decision should look like. When he described to me the perils[3] of "consensus" he revealed concern with *who* makes a point and how that affects decision-making: "With groupthink, if there is a catchy personality, then the rest of the ideas [fall away] . . . The role of a chair is to ensure there is good participation so there is proper consultative decision-making."

His reference to groupthink reveals his education in an American bioethics tradition. William H. Whyte coined "groupthink" at a time when American tensions between individuality and "the dark forces of conformity and collectivism" (Shapin 2008, 120) were at their height. Bureaucracies were regarded as a threat for those like Whyte, who sought "to protect the creative scientific spirit that resided in the unique, autonomous, and free-acting individual" (Shapin 2008, 119). Whyte's anxiety was with "rationalized conformity—an open, articulate philosophy which holds that group values are not only expedient but right and good as well" (Whyte 1952). As Freeman Champney summarizes: "Tentativeness and humility are needed in group processes, not only because a group can be unanimously wrong but because the unreconstructed individual (however much he may sand up the group bearings) has a vital role to play in the total picture" (1952, 384).

This "unreconstructed individual" is Whyte's "layman, the what-the-hell sort of character who carries his center of gravity on the inside of him" (Champney 1952, 383). This particular reading of the layman puts an era-driven positive spin on the individual point of view in a group setting.[4] In her work, Laura Stark uses transcripts of EC meetings to demonstrate how opinions are evaluated; how people persuade others, or fail to. Her concern is to demonstrate how, in the creation of "the social actor known as 'the IRB,' documents liberate individual evaluators to make what they consider to be extreme judgements" (2011, 235). She draws on a committee meeting she observed where Kevin, a junior researcher serving on the IRB, found fault with the protocol of a more senior researcher he knew. Citing his professional experience, he persuaded fellow members that a change really should be requested, but he was reluctant to allow the board to act upon it, however, since he would be "dead meat" on campus. The senior researcher, he thought, would know it was he who had recommended the change. It was not calling upon his "duty" to protect human subjects that swayed him to permit the change, but the fact that he would not be identified in the meeting minutes. To Stark, "the fact that individual opinions can be presented as the view of 'the IRB' erases personal accountability" (2011, 235), creating a situation in which documents enable the "impression that there is no *one* to hold accountable" (2012, 71).

Where Chandeep wants a board decision to be made through a consensus in which "all get the chance to speak," he observed that sometimes committee members (particularly laypersons) felt slighted if their thoughts could not shift the tenor of conversation in a consensus-oriented discussion: "Why end up with consensus? Why is my comment more or less valuable than someone else's? Sometimes [my comments are] not taken well, not appreciated. I feel [my comment] is supposed to be out there, otherwise, why [should we] still get a diverse composition? Get doctors and that's it."

Yet discussion is "part" of what makes a committee a committee, according to the measures FERCAP has set down in the Survey. When I visited a committee meeting in Taipei, my host took pains to translate the conversation and point out to me the kind of concerns that the various members were raising.

A lawyer had asked questions about the validity of the informed consent form; a layperson had queried terminology. "Our discussion," he said proudly, "is as good as America." However, as Edith discovered, applying standards, largely American, did not always go smoothly.

Conflict of Interest

Decision-making can stumble not only on recognizing the importance of others' views, but also on "conflict of interest" (COI). As I attended trainings and Surveys throughout my months of fieldwork, conflict of interest came to take different forms. At times, it seemed like a structural consideration for committees and their Surveyors. In a dim corridor in a hospital in Guangzhou with a team of Surveyors, checklists in hand, for example, it was a question of titles and labels. "This is the EC?" asked the lead Surveyor, sharply. The local Surveyors nodded. "But it's called Science Research Admin!" In my analysis of the Survey in chapter 2, I showed how physical space for committees mattered, as the lead Surveyor immediately observed, "You cannot have science and ethics together, there has to be a marked division." But the need for a division was as much about establishing importance as it was about establishing independence: In an interview, Atoy told me that this was something some committees continued to struggle with because of where their support comes from institutionally. When a committee is "under" a research office, for example, a member of the research office that has facilitated or even funded the research may sit on the committee. Space, names, and committee membership can all risk the independence of a committee's decision.

During my participation in a Survey in Manila, Cecilia, who was the chair of a number of national health boards, had accepted the role of providing a national overview on the first day of the Survey. Explaining to the international Surveyors and gathered trainees some of the challenges of conducting ethical review in her country, she classed conflict of interests as an "obstacle to quality in ethical review," lamenting that

> in the Philippines [w]e do not understand or easily recognize conflicts of interest. One time, we had a member in the National Ethics Committee, a very respected researcher who was also a head of a health institution. He said, "I think our health institution should be exempted from ethics review because we've been doing research for so long." I said, "OK bye!" So, it's not very clear yet

> what this is all about. Since we do not recognize conflicts of interest, we do not manage [them].

Cecilia chose this moment to highlight that both researchers and institutions needed to adapt to the changes brought about by GCP and research ethics: Neither experience nor seniority provided exemption from external evaluation. Therefore, as internationally sponsored research increased in the Philippines, so did attendance at trainings on international standards. Later that day, I joined a lecture at the Manila College of Medicine, where some forty or fifty GCP course attendees had gathered for a presentation on conflict of interest by Dr. Rodriguez, a professor of legal medicine and ethics at the School of Law. His lecture echoed the concern that conflict of interest was something "difficult to see." He acknowledged that the *potential* in conflict of interest made people anxious. In the same way as "confidentiality" flipped from being a concept committees *sought to ensure for participants in the trials that they reviewed* to being *something the committee itself must demonstrate*, conflict of interest is a topic committees examine in the protocols review *and* one that affects them directly. Although committees are tasked to consider the former concern, Canadian commentator Trudo Lemmens (2006, 32) pointed out that COI has a vast reach. The assessment would include the clinical trial agreement between researchers and sponsors, the budgets of trials (particularly the incentives for the recruitment of subjects and any payments to them), publication agreements, the scientific validity of the trial, access to data, and the publications that result. "Should RECs be expected to do all of this work," Lemmens asks, "indeed, are they capable?" (Lemmens 2006, 32). In his view, they "cannot take sole responsibility for unraveling the complex relationship between scientists and the companies that sponsor them" (Lemmens 2006, 32).

The knowledge that brought committee members to their "expert" role on the IRB was also the knowledge that made the exercise of this role problematic: If they knew the field of cancer, say, it was also likely that they knew who worked on cancer in their institute. Even with anonymized protocols, reviewers would probably be able to deduce whose protocol was under review. Rodriguez described this social proximity as "bias":

> There is always this tendency of bias, when you talk about a committee who are all *barkadas*[5] of the one conducting the research. You know our culture,

> Philippinos. Our *barkadas*, as medical students we are a close group, close friends there who went through thick and thin all throughout. "Hey, this is a proposal from Dr. so and so. And I'm the one reviewing it?" So there is always this potential.

Rodriguez reminded his trainees that they will often know the applicants: "We are faculty, same institute. It is a problem as much as you *like* them, as if you *dislike* them. You still feel something toward them." He also reminded investigators who sat on committees that they may know how to do clinical trials, "but when you sit in the EC you wear a different hat because you are supposed to institute that check and balance. You're supposed to present an alternative perspective, not the perspective of an investigator."

Those with experience of the clinical research environment were often considered useful people to have on ethics committees, so the appointment did not prevent them from conducting research. However, Rodriguez pointed out that "practically everything you do now you see a sponsor, a multinational corporation funding the researchers." He warned committee members to be careful:

> In the U.S., all members make a declaration about their investment. They think anything over $10,000, in WIRB,[6] if they do Pfizer protocols. Those with stocks in Pfizer have to leave the room. That's how they look at COI [. . .] In the U.S., it was said that the $10,000 is a minuscule, a negligible amount. But here in the Philippines $10,000 U.S. dollars is really something.

Translating from dollars to Philippine pesos was an attempt to evaluate the amount of money that would cause an "undue influence." Things got more complicated, however, as money, he told us, was the "only tangible thing in the array of secondary interests. It's always easy to address it because money is there, you see it." Other things were less visible and required different forms and degrees of self-awareness.

Secondary Interests

"We think of COI in terms of your perception," counseled Rodriguez. "You are an ethical individual," he says, projecting the inner thoughts of his audience in the room, "and therefore you cannot do anything wrong. But that's not the definition of COI. COI means that you are ethical [and] at the same time you recognize you have a different role and a different interest." Recognizing these different roles and interests meant being aware of "secondary" interests—and with this, we entered the realm of the intangible. "We cannot come up with a researcher without conflict of interest," Rodriguez told us. "Life desires to have fame. How do we measure that desire?" Secondary interests applied as much to ethics review committee members as to those who conducted research, but as I observed above, often these persons were one and the same. While those who sat on ethics committees tended to have an interest in research, *interests*, as Rodriguez put it, were something different:

> Problems occur when secondary interests dominate, unduly influence, distort, or corrupt the integrity of a physician's judgement in relation to patient health. Fortune, fame, and family threaten the integrity of the professional judgement.[7]

So how are these "interests" to coincide, to come into "conflict"? The extension of "interest" reveals for anthropologists the starting assumptions on which COI disclosures are based. Anthropologist Chris Gregory, in revisiting anthropological readings of economist Adam Smith, finds them selective, focusing only on greed and rational self-interest: *The Theory of Moral Sentiments*, he argues, is more subtle (Gregory 2011). Smith scholars such as Charles Griswold (2006) and Pratap Bhanu Mehta (2006) would agree. Consider the passages of Smith selected by Griswold, writing on the imagination and its relation to self-interest:

> Moral self-consciousness requires that I "divide myself, as it were, in two persons" (III.I.6). The idealized judge is still a spectator—the stand-in for "the public." [. . .] The "natural misrepresentations of self-love can be corrected only by the eye of this impartial spectator" (III.3.4 cf III5.5). (2006, 37–38)

Based on these excerpts, Griswold argues that "the theatrical relation is thus internalized; we become our own public," concluding that "our understanding and moral assessment not just of others, but of ourselves as well, depend on an exercise of the imagination" (2006, 38). Through contrast with other ways of thinking about persons, we can see the contrivance of imagination at work in the concept of conflict of interest. As Strathern remarks, "the center is where the twentieth century Western imagination puts the self, the personality, the ego. For the 'person' in this latter-day Western view is an agent, a subject, the author of thought and action, and thus 'at the center' of relationships" ([1988]

2001, 269). What COI makes explicit is the tension inherent in this model of the individual subject, modeling how people belong "to a matrix of radiating relations" (Strathern [1991] 2004, 68) and creating a context in which relations that might otherwise be considered ordinary become suspect. During the lecture, participants were encouraged to "think about" what conflicts of interest they might have, as Rodriguez assured them that "half the problem is solved if the presence [of interests and their possible conflicts] is recognized." A conflict exists, he cautions, whether or not decisions are shown to be affected. "Conflict implies only the *potential* for bias or wrongdoing. And the basic step that you must consider is *failure to disclose is wrong*." Having listed various potential conflicts of interest—with conflict itself understood as "potential for bias or wrongdoing"—disclosure was introduced as the next step. "Disclosure is the cornerstone of the conflict of interest guidelines and regulations," Rodriguez announced:

> You can keep it to yourself, but you will be taking a risk because once its discovered or if a third party disclose it, then you are in deep trouble. [. . .] You simply cannot hide one or two and disclose the rest because eventually it will be discovered. That is a requirement that you alone can perform [. . .] So you might as well start by disclosing it.

The revelation of conflicts of interest, Rodriguez counseled, required "discipline," as there was "no other way for others to know" if one was harboring a conflict of interest around the table at the committee meeting. It would also, he implied, be difficult for those who knew to point to someone. "It's a cultural thing, if we say 'You have a conflict of interest, get out,' there will be hurt feelings." This sort of discipline, the revelation of internally held knowledge of relationships external to the committee, meant committee members were told they could not "be silent," but had to "manage" their conflicts "preemptively." The "perceived relationship between inner and outer worlds" (Strathern 1992, 184) provides a model of human thought, and action lends itself well to a consideration of "interest" in the phrase "conflict of interest." Interests are not visible attributes; they must be declared, moved from internal worlds to external. The focus for conflict of interest has moved, too, replacing an examination of relationships between committee members with an examination of one's relationship to oneself (thought of as containing or composed of relations), by finding a position from which this can be viewed. I return to the work of Griswold above, as he traces Smith's comparison, or conflation, of moral and visual judgment:

> Smith [. . .] compares the process by which we learn to exercise balanced *moral* judgment to that by which we learn to make correct *visual* judgments. He has Berkeley's *New Theory of Vision* in mind, a book of which he thought very highly. The basic idea is that just as I cannot gauge the correct proportions of objects of different sizes and at varying distances, except by "transporting myself, at least in fancy, to a different station, from whence I can survey both at nearly equal distances," so too I cannot accurately evaluate the magnitude of my passions in comparison with another's except by viewing them "neither from our own place nor yet from his, neither with our own eyes nor yet with his, but from the place and with the eyes of a third person, who has no particular connexion with either and who judges with impartiality between us" (III.3.3). (2006, 38; emphasis added)

The creation of this third person, a position in moral terms equivalent to a physical or proportional space, resonates with the creation of objectivity in chapter 2's Survey through the "distance" of foreign Surveyors, and recalls the moralization of objectivity in the historical work of Lorraine Daston and Peter Galison (1992, 81). Rodriguez is asking members to problematize concealment and revelation, which for the duration of the meeting is a moral act that only the individual member is capable of performing. He is asking committee members to think of people as already related, with their relationships, and thus their potential conflicts, "built-in."

In the Philippine ethnography above, COI may not only jeopardize the desired "objectivity" of a researcher, but it can also cast doubt upon the research enterprise itself. Members' relationships outside the committee come to be constitutive of the trustworthiness of the committee as a unit. When a person discloses a COI, they will usually stand and leave the room. The recognition and management of COI can be evidenced by minuting that bodily action. Cecilia and Dr. Rodriguez both indicate that conflict of interest has the potential to inhere in any of the relations of which a person is made up. It can reside in their internal attributes (their ambition) and their relationships (through kin or money) which, during the committee meeting, are seen to be carried in the body of the (in)dividual committee member.[8] As Rodriguez says, it is not that some of the *people* to whom one might be connected might be bad. Rather, it is that the *connections themselves, unrevealed* might cause difficulties. The distinction, as drawn by the lecturer, was that the crime is not to have conflicts of interest, but rather to not declare them. Thus it becomes the responsibility of each member to scan their relations. This is the nature of their "disciplining."

The Decision

The ethics committee, as a group of people sitting around a table in a room, both relies on and denies the relations those persons bring to that room. The dynamics of decision-making are embodied, yet what I have brought forward is how committee members aim to move different parts of that which informs a decision in and out of sight. A decision arrived at through invisibly expressed views is preferable to Edith and her colleagues than a situation in which the "individual" disagreement of a member might be socially damaging outside the committee room. Decision arises not only from dialogue and the discussion of a particular case. It also arises from these techniques through which the committee can continue to exist as a committee, persisting in time, as a learned disposition of its constitutive members. Considering conflict of interest training as a site of cultural transmission requires considerable reflexivity about how persons and their relations are perceived from outside—both outside the committee and outside the institution. Dealing with the personal that attaches to the official is problematic, as many working in institutional settings will recognize. A PI is one's boss, a reviewer is also a colleague, those sitting around the table with you, deciding, are senior to you. By routing these concerns through bodies, and through the room itself, we are required to acknowledge the permeabilities and the inevitable sociality of the decisions that take place in this room.

In choosing to emphasize the decision, trainings in FERCAP are also setting themselves apart from bioethics training and the implicit luxury of philosophical questions without answers. The fact of a decision as the site of an intervention on practice is, for Cristina, a divergence from the games of "suppose" I recounted in chapter 1. If the decision is the core, then the questions of documentation, voting, and consensus, even the marshaling of the most appropriate perspectives, become practical matters that can be written into SOPs and offered to committees to work with. But the sociality of the committee does not go away, as it makes its decisions in institutional settings. It is to the risk of collegial judgment that a decision carries that I now turn.

SECTION 3
Future Capacities

SIX
Ethics and the Law

Across the universities, hospitals, and research institutes I visited, I listened to account after account of the network's successful interventions. Being involved with a regional network had brought legitimacy for ethics champions in institutions. But in more private spaces, FERCAP trainers would express their frustrations and doubts about the progress they were making in capacity building. "We *have* to change perceptions of what it means to be involved with ethics," they said to one another. Although trainings were happening, it wasn't clear that "knowledge" was being taken on board: "People still tend not to *say* when they don't understand," trainers lamented, "they don't admit to not knowing the difference between the Declaration of Helsinki and the Belmont Report and Good Clinical Practice." Sometimes, trainers reminded one another of small changes they had started to see in the universities they visited. Perhaps some researchers had started to drop by the ethics committee office to ask questions. Perhaps there was more engagement in training sessions, a greater circulation of the desire to "do research better." Indicative of this gradual change in attitude, at one lunch I attended, Rosa, the chair of a committee, commented that the "culture" at her research institute had changed. "Researchers now take responsibility, they say 'I should be trained on this.' Before, it felt like we, the ethics committee, were a jury—to give a sentence."

This reference to a prior state where the committee was "like a jury" resonated with something I had heard earlier in my research. Six months before, I had been in Sri Lanka interviewing Harsha, a layperson on a Colombo ethics committee. We had been sitting in plush executive chairs at the long, black boardroom table of her employer's office, waiting for her secretary to bring us tea. As it arrived, I asked about her experiences on the ethics committee: "So, what's it like?" I asked open-endedly. "Well," she began,

> It's like a jury. Sometimes, the common man's view is taken up, and the questions that are asked by us three [laypeople] they are *so* non-medical. Sometimes, they give them ideas, they discuss while we're completely clueless, they go into detail for us. Sometimes, our responses give them an idea of how the common man might react. For example, if there was organ donation or something, the questions we ask—for example, how explicit is it, is it usefully explained? What is its history? Has there been testing on normal patients? The cross section of members is useful, as in a jury. I wonder, sometimes, whether we're just there to add acceptability to the ethics committee.

Though the emphasis and reasoning are different, the common comparison both women make is that an ethics committee is "like a jury." Rosa's concern is with judgment and the relationship between the committee and its applicants; Harsha's with the relationships within it, how different people deal with information: weighing it, making decisions, knowing why those decisions were made. My concern in this chapter develops this section's theme of how people experience committee membership, in particular the *consequences* of their key task of decision-making.

Although FERCAP has not primarily been agitating for legal change or especially engaged with government initiatives, I use the comparison of the ethics committee with the jury made by Rosa and Harsha to extend work by legal scholars who disagree on the purpose and nature of ethics committees. My interest is in the limits of ethics as a form of soft law. It speaks to the quietly expressed desire for law and what people feel it would bring. The analysis tracks between the idea of the jury and questions of judgment, arriving at salient disagreements on whether the law is an appropriate vehicle for changes in ethical review.

Are Ethics Committees Like Juries?

Are ethics committees like juries, or should they be? The first exchange that drew my attention to this question started when Carl Coleman, whom we met in chapter 4 presenting the new WHO *Standards and Operational Guidance for*

Ethics Review of Health-Related Research with Human Participants, published an article called "Rationalizing Risk Assessment in Human Subject Research" (2003). In response, his colleague and friend Lars Noah wrote "Deputizing Institutional Review Boards to Police (Audit?) Biomedical Research" (2004). Coleman's riposte "Why Have IRBs at All?" (2004) concludes the exchange. Racing across the pages of law journals, this academic disagreement splits open a dichotomy central to FERCAP's concern with the role of the committee for ethics. In brief, Coleman (2003) draws strong parallels between IRBs and juries, and suggests training committee members in legal reasoning and the use of written opinions. Objecting, Noah likens the IRB to a peer review system, arguing that IRBs should instead focus their efforts on "inculcat[ing] a commitment to ethical behavior" (2004, 291). Coleman considers this wholly "inadequate," stating that "this sort of vague directive to 'do good and avoid evil' is so devoid of content that it provides no useful guidance for those genuinely concerned with protecting human subjects from unjustifiable risks" (2004, 301).

Seventeen years later, in 2021, David Resnik, a bioethicist at the U.S. National Institute of Environmental Health Sciences reopened this discussion with a desire to "stimulate interest in descriptive, empirical investigations of IRB decision-making" (2021, 18). Lamenting the absence of "standards of evidence" in U.S. federal regulations, Resnik considered different *types* of evidence IRBs might use (legal, scientific, medical), suggesting that "an IRB should require that evidence be more than clear and convincing as a condition for approval" (2021, 18). Again, a conversation emerged across the literature. Responding, Elise Smith and Emily Anderson called his suggestions "justifiable," with the potential to bring "much needed rigor and transparency to the system," but argued that while the suggestion "seems to incorporate a small change with respect to a standard, in application it *would actually require a novel system*" (2022, 55, emphasis added). What is of interest to me in these disagreements are the differing approaches to the research ethics committee as a tool of governance, and their unresolved character. To what extent should committees be "like juries," and how close are they to the law? One way of answering this question is to consider how the idea that an ethics committee is "like a jury" fits a certain kind of imaginary. In 2021, socio-legal scholar Mark Flear and bioethicist Richard Ashcroft put forward the first "law-led interdisciplinary accounts of imaginaries," aiming to explore how "imaginaries underpin law's engagement with biomedical technologies and science" (Flear and Ashcroft 2021, 1). Expanding on conceptualizations of imaginaries across disciplines, they argue that "imaginaries have an important role to play in mediating the boundaries of responsibility and accountability": for my purposes, the sense of how a decision *should* be taken. To understand the emphasis on the *process* that emerges in this chapter, we need to consider the sense of suspicion that sits as the tacit backdrop to Coleman's 2004 intervention.

The World of the IRB

"Americans," writes Coleman, are "deeply suspicious of medical research" (2003, 2). Fear of being experimented upon, the deaths of healthy research participants, and the revelations of "deep and pervasive problems" in "systems" (Coleman 2003, 2) all lead Coleman to ask how public trust in biomedical research can possibly be restored. His article suggests the reform of IRBs. His premise is that in the U.S., "IRBs are engaged in a process of *legal* decision-making, insofar as they interpret specific regulatory requirements pursuant to authority that has been delegated to them by administrative agencies" (2003, 4). Hence his comparison with the deliberation of juries. Ethics committees, he says, share with juries

> a reliance on general, impressionistic judgments unsupported by specific reasons; the absence of any obligation to explain or justify decisions; a focus on individual cases rather than general principles or rules; and the potential for inconsistent determinations in similar situations. Juries are also justified by the same values of localism and community input that underlie the current system of IRB review. (2003, 16–17)

The thrust of his argument is toward the reform of how decisions by ethics committees are made, with a particular focus on risk assessments. Using the similarities of form that he detects, Coleman outlines decision-making methods used in law, such as the use of written opinions and reasoning by analogy. He considers how IRBs could take up some of these "strategies," and in doing so, he makes explicit the parallels he sees between healthcare and legal judicial systems. When calls came for local capacity building, particularly from the European Union, it was felt that a review that was otherwise competent in Geneva would still be either inadequate or worse, inappropriate in some way, if it were done for research that would be conducted elsewhere. "Juries," writes Coleman,

> are justified by the same appeal to local values and attitudes that underlies the IRB system. The most common justification for jury decision-making is the jury's ability to "bring the common wisdom of the community to bear on the resolution of the private dispute" and "to legitimize that solution in the eyes of that community" (Brodin 1990, 15). These justifications mirror the emphasis on localism in the system of IRB review. (2003, 1154–55)

He points out that familiarity with "the actual conditions surrounding the conduct of research," is thought to give local committees an advantage over regional or national review. His reference points are from the United States, and, drawing on the National Bioethics Advisory Commission's 2001 report, he cites the former director of the U.S. Office for Protection from Research Risks (OPRR) who writes that

> it is local review by individuals who are in the best position to know the research at the site, the resources at the institution, the capabilities and the reputations of the investigators and staff, the prevailing attitudes and ethics of the community and most importantly, the likely subject population. (Ellis 1994, 31–32, cited in NBAC 2001, 119)

With the development of multi-centered trials, however, "local" review often leads to many committees reviewing the same protocol, and changes demanded by one can have knock-on effects for others.

Noah's response to Coleman's original article makes evident that they share a common concern in the operation of IRBs: "consistency and transparency" (Noah 2004, 269). What they disagree on is how to go about ensuring these principles are adhered to. Where Coleman has advanced an argument that plays to the strengths of his legal background, Noah insists that the parallel to juries is problematic, and that improvement can come from methods that "do not necessitate mimicking the judiciary" (2004, 269). In an earlier article, Noah expresses the concern that

> IRBs may become preoccupied with reviewing the niceties of the consent form and perhaps less concerned about their separate obligation to make independent risk-benefit assessments about the research protocol, confident that

> potential subjects can "vote with their feet" so long as the consent form contains all of the necessary information. (2002, 384)

In his view, the comparison with juries is unsustainable, as he does not think IRBs "resemble juries except in the most superficial of ways" (Noah 2004, 271). He offers an alternative comparison, suggesting that what IRBs "much more closely (and appropriately) resemble" is "peer review mechanisms utilized by the scientific community" (2004, 268). He sets himself wholly against the "recasting" of IRBs as "adjudicatory bodies" (2004, 26), a move which he says "may appeal to those with training in the law, but the scientists and physicians who staff IRBs will predictably—and I think appropriately—recoil at any such suggestion" (2004, 274). He suggests instead that "IRBs may do the most good by helping to educate researchers at an institution about the basics of federal law, as well as working to *inculcate a commitment to ethical behavior*," with a

> flawless protocol crafted with extensive collegial input by an IRB following guidance from institutions around the country and accompanied by a thorough written opinion mean[ing] *nothing if the researcher has not "bought into" the process*. (2004, 292, emphasis added)

Coleman and Noah are talking specifically about U.S. American IRBs, asking how best to reach their common goal of "human subject protection." They sketch their answers between the poles of law-like enforcement and the encouragement of responsibility, each having sought to pull ethical review in their own direction. Their debate offers us at least four versions of the committee/jury comparison laid out already: that a committee is like a jury because it judges; a committee is like a jury because it deliberates and evaluates information; a committee is like a jury because of its localism; and a committee is like a jury because it performs a delegated legal role. I arrange the following sections around the implication of these four versions. When, around the lunch table in Bangkok, Juntra said that committee work felt like jury work, she wanted to change that perception. Pursuing the comparison she made may help us find out why.

Politicians Don't Need a Protocol

In 2006, the American press reported that Japan was embarking on "an experiment with democracy," with a plan to reestablish juries within three years. From 1928 to 1943, Japan had operated an "American-style" legal system, but a wartime lack of men (and it was only men who could serve as jurors) made the system impossible to sustain. In 2006 the new *saiban-in* ("lay judge") system promised consequences for the citizenry of neighboring countries such as China, Taiwan, and Thailand, all of whom were said to be "calling for greater involvement of citizens in their legal systems" (Precht 2006; see also Kage 2017). The international attention attracted by Japan's "experiment" included a seminar held by Cornell Law School,[1] where the pros and cons of the new system were aired. "Japanese people pay more respect to authority than to the individual and are afraid of being isolated by the majority," Kiichi Nishino, a former judge now at Niigata University, was reported to have claimed; "unless a juror is bold enough to disagree with the legal professionals, then this system is meaningless" (Parry 2009). Professor of Law and Public Health Jeffery A. Fagan speculated that was "a difficulty of human nature to argue with someone of a higher status." These concerns seemed to be borne out in the comments of the first jurors on their experience: "I don't like the idea of judging other people," said Mr. Number Two, his and his co-jurors' code names designed to allay fears of retribution.

Looking back at the reintroduction of juries in Japan makes us aware that at no point in the IRB/jury comparison in the American legal debate does status, hierarchy, or even discomfort in making an ethics assessment arise. Yet these are issues of high and explicit concern for both Japanese and American commentators on the Japanese take-up of *juries*. As discussed, members of institutional ethics committees will often know the applicants personally, as colleagues. As Edith strove to find a way to comply with her American WIRB training, she ended up introducing an electronic voting scheme that ensured each person's vote was concealed. We have also seen some of the tactics used by Surveyors to soften the impacts of criticisms, with people creating a distance so that the Surveyor could be considered "objective," avoiding the potential referencing or inflection of personal relationships through the fiction of a corporate person.[2] All these tactics also neutralize potentially hostile or fractious tensions associated with the problem of assessing a proposal, and they make evident how the assessment is *also* one of the principal investigator applying to conduct the research. In the stories that follow, I focus on the *education* of the principal investigator as a strategy, a committee's external means of dealing with the problem that (their) judgment causes.

The principal investigator (PI) of my research notes is a multifaceted character, cast sometimes as an enemy, sometimes as a friend. In trainings, PIs are often presented as criminal, such as those at Tuskegee (Reverby 2013). Where trainings localize bioethics stories, the "Hwang scandal" in South Korea (Kim 2008) and He Jiankui, whose gene editing "experiment" was announced at the Second International Summit on Human Genome Editing in Hong Kong to international distress (Wahlberg et al. 2021), often come to the fore. While well known, these types of PIs were rarely thought to be present in the institutions at which committees were working. Rather, they described their PIs as, at worst, thoughtless or "cold," trained to "think scientifically." They may not wholly "understand" why ethics is important. Describing "PI" figures as they appear to their committee in Bhopal, India, Salik Ansari tells us that "PIs may want to get ethics approval as soon as possible. Deadlines and incredible collaborations all lie ahead, and they do not want to miss it. Someone once said in a lighter way that for many of our PIs, the EC seems to be the only barrier to getting a Nobel prize!" (2023, 361). Impertinence may be a sign of disrespect, with the feeling that "important persons" might be capable of swaying the "objective" judgment of the committee if permitted to put their case in person, not in writing.

We were halfway through a Survey in Shanghai, China, when a disagreement arose between Surveyors and committee members on a "new practice" that the committee had introduced, ostensibly to smooth relations between the PI and the committee. Cristina, Juntra, and the team of local Surveyors were sitting in the rooms designated for the Survey, around two long trestle tables draped with velveteen red tablecloths and covered in baskets of lychees and water bottles. Everyone was struggling to remain focused—we had spent the morning interviewing committee members—but we had a slide template to begin filling out. The laptop on the table was connected to a projector, displaying Criteria 3 of the Survey, "Completeness of Review Process." We were discussing something the committee being surveyed considered a "major innovation": They invited the PI to present their protocol to the committee during the meeting. During interviews, one of the committee members had explained: "We have an interaction with them and we've received a positive reaction to that." Questions that arose for the committee could be resolved there and then. Having seen a quality management–inspired emphasis in FERCAP, I expected the Surveyors to approve of the apparently efficient innovation.[3] But they did not, and were preparing to list it in the slides as a problem. "The documents should speak for themselves. It's not speaking for itself, then it should be revised":

> JUNTRA: Decisions are based not on what you hear but what you read. Sometimes, you're affected by the person presenting. In China, we always hear "famous famous." You're not looking at how famous he is, it's the document he made. It affects your objectivity. He is famous, I'm not famous . . . Prepare questions first, don't rely on what you hear. The only reason to do all this [have the PI present] would be that the documents not clear enough for people to make [a] decision. We should encourage people to do more documentation, 'cos that's what it *is*—that'll be there forever. Sometimes you don't capture what the person says, but it's in the documents. You may say many things, just to convince me. You listen to Obama and he convince[s] you. Doesn't mean it's going to happen.
>
> CRISTINA: Sometimes their way of speaking influences you.

The room goes quiet because the local Surveyors are surprised at the strength of this rejection. How could something seemingly so efficient *not* be adding to the completeness of the review process? The local Surveyor tentatively suggests that the secretary "can document what the PI says at the meeting, though?" Juntra's response is quick:

> But *you're* documenting. It's second hand. You ask [on] paper to say "we don't understand," it's all documented. That'll teach them. [It'll be] a learning experience for [the] investigator to do next time. Make it very clear. I've seen conflicts arise when not very professional—it becomes personal. That's why [we] need objectivity—clarify what [you are] going to do. Lots of people who have skill to speak—politicians . . .
>
> LOCAL SURVEYOR: Politicians don't need a protocol!

The room erupts into laughter at this idea and its sense of license. As we adjust the slides, the Survey prioritizes documentation over presentation. The Surveyors are concerned about persuasion, about charisma, and about the arts of the "politician." These worries speak to longstanding discussions in the study of research ethics committees, particularly what Adam Hedgecoe (after Anthony Giddens, after Erving Goffman) calls the "facework" of presenting one's character (2012), arguing that when committee members *do* present, this often reshapes how the written materials are viewed. Written material here both provides "crucial insight not just into what researchers *say* they are going to do but what they are *actually* going to do" and ensures that the committee is making decisions it can provide future evidence for. It is ensuring it is auditable. In the discussion about the jury in Japan, what was at stake was the possibility of a juror disagreeing with legal professionals. Here, the Surveyors are concerned that committee members will be swayed by the presentation styles of the researchers, persuaded to allow research to go ahead. In her overview of the crystallization of the current review system, Laura Stark confirms the perception of researchers as "contaminants, rather than aids, to sound moral evaluation" (2007, 784) amongst the ethics committees she studied in the U.S.[4] The other side of this concern is FERCAP's focus on documentation as a technique of "objectivity."[5] In Shanghai, the Survey turned the PI's absence into an opportunity for education, making the distrust in the PI's tactics of persuasion a (solveable) matter of ignorance, in which good intentions could be preserved. In the presentations later, in over-air-conditioned rooms around large, polished tables, against calligraphic wall hangings, the point about the "politician" in the PI resurfaced. It was not settled anywhere in my fieldwork: A Taiwanese doctor who had been working on an ethics committee for more than five years put it:

> I think all PIs have to be educated and because they . . . Everyone *wants* to do the right thing, they don't intend to do harm to patients. The problem is they don't know *how* to do that, so we have to educate. That's why I teach young investigators [. . .] Older men—my age, nearly retired, sixty—you think that is not necessary, sometimes we take it for granted.

Education, then, is seen as part of the preemptive apparatus of the committee. The role of a jury, as the new Japanese jurors learned, is that of assessing the evidence presented and reaching a verdict. But in an ethics committee, the assessment is preemptive; as Hedgecoe astutely puts it, "at the core of the REC process are decisions about whether researchers who are applying for approval can be trusted to do what they say they will do" (2020, 10). It is thus *possibility* that motivates the review. "Education" is the action of the committee's forward-looking temporality. The comparison between juries and committees highlights how an ethics committee tries to ensure ethical, moral action through intervention *before* the events that are assumed to hold potential for harm have occurred. Ethics review is anticipatory, preventative. Its own potential lies in its scrutiny of the detail, its knowledge of the relevant size of samples or the necessary frequency of blood draws, its knowledge of the intended participants. Its potential as an activity both anticipates and is generated by the potential in research.

For research ethics committees, it can seem that oversight duties grow, but their ability to enforce change is limited. As one Surveyor put it somewhat helplessly, "an IRB doesn't have police power, but it has to ensure things are right." While I have, earlier in this section, emphasized the necessity of decision-making, I would now like to foreground how the *finality* of decisions can be eroded. When the committee limits the validity of its approval, it grants itself the license of maintaining connection with that investigator, who must return to be "re-approved," a practice known as continuing review. However, this changes the relationship between committees and researcher, introducing new questions of resources and monitoring.

The difficulty of performing continuing review arises in the languid break following lectures at a workshop in Bangkok. We have spilled out from the lecture hall into the canteen, which is open to the warm afternoon air, a counter with sweet tea in plastic cups and fruit has been set up for the participants. As we talk about the arrival of the rain and enjoy the fresh air after hours inside, we also talk about how far the senior researcher from a committee in the north of Thailand has traveled. What has he learned that was new to him? I ask. "Many breaches!" he says, speaking of the cases we have just heard. "I can't tell whether it is just because they don't *know*, or if they intended [the breach]." "How might you tell?" I ask. The committee member explains that he has found that researchers get defensive, and while the door of the committee is always open should issues arise during research, and PIs *can* come, few do.

> Every week we see lots of projects come. But we don't have the time to go and check up on them. We will not shock them [hitting motion]. We'll try to help! Well, very carefully. Go see them, "Hi, how is research going?" Little by little, approach the point, "I heard someone went to IRB . . ."

The hope is that through education, PIs will come to "see" ethics for what those who take part in committees see it as, a necessary protection of research participants: "human subjects." A member of an ethics committee in Taiwan spent an afternoon telling me about disputes between his committee and PIs. If staff and PIs "don't have the same understanding and knowledge, then there is fight between the IRB and investigator," he told me. "We want them to *know*, to think it is very important." His approach was to cast the problem as one of imbalances in knowledge, ameliorated through education: *reason* will prevail. Asked for his opinion on a dispute that had arisen in a local committee, he had informed his colleague of the following:

> Ethical review by IRB is kind of business based on "reasonable" judgment. Therefore, I will not say which side of decision is right or wrong. But I think all can be discussed based on this reasonable person standard. I guess the IRB's decision is always of good intention, and sometimes might be a little bit exaggerated. The only effective solution for such dispute is continuing mutual learning between PI and IRB.

The education agenda therefore is directed toward a future in which judgment is hardly necessary, both the IRB and the PI have the same attitude and objectives, and the situation is marked not by tensions or disagreements about delayed research, but by mutual understanding. We know, however, that this is not the case at present.

The Continuous Committee

Harsha, the Sri Lankan layperson whose comments opened this chapter, had been a member of her committee for a little over a year. Unlike a jury, convened to assess a single case and subsequently disbanded, an ethics committee member is appointed for terms often of lengthy duration. In their debate, Coleman and Noah both acknowledge as a significant point of difference between a jury and an IRB that the latter are "continuous bodies whose members decide multiple issues over an extended period" (Coleman 2003, 1155). The comparison of the standing ethics committee with the transience of the jury allows me to highlight some of the particularities of continuity, and to relate the anxieties of committee members I spent time with, for whom maintaining continued relations in their immediate setting was experienced as both a primary concern and a silencing constraint. Peter, a Taiwanese researcher with whom I had conducted Surveys and trainings in Beijing and Bangkok over the course of several months, spent some time explaining to me the dynamics of his ethics review committee meeting and the strains on its long-term members. We had worked side by side on several Surveys by this point, and he had become frank with me about the experiences he had had over ten years of working in ethical review. He told me that the struggle in his committee, he reflected, was always in "the boardroom," finding ways to reduce conflict between physicians and IRB members. Disagreement led to lengthy meetings and "conflict" in in the boardroom, yet he maintained that it was important for each member to air their "different thinking." But as he had taken on a mentoring role for new committee members, he had begun to see their precarity in a way that he hadn't seen for himself. "Committee members needed to be aware of the decisions the board took not only for the sake of patients, but also for themselves," he said seriously. "One day, if you disapprove something, maybe next time, 'Okay, no time for you!' Someday they get promotion, they say, 'Okay, IRB, you have too much budget,' and maybe they will cut you down." The "they" of Peter's sentence is the researcher, who stands to lose time and possibly funds if their research is delayed or "disapproved." Peter did not think these problems were contained to his own country. "In Asia," he generalized,

> people's relationships last from position to position, especially in older life. If there is someone you disapprove, if you kill the approval with your opinion, maybe they'll say, "I'll get revenge on you." Your operation can affect the project of the IRB.

Choosing to raise an issue that derails the wrong research project, Peter implies, could lead to disaster for ethics review itself. He had, in discussions with other FERCAP members, found that they too struggled with these same issues. Citing "The Dr. Hwang scandal" in South Korea,[6] he speculated that if committee members were under social pressures to produce success, "they might not check everything, approve something, and disgrace themselves." However, he reflected on recent developments designed to "protect" the committee members. "If there are twenty-one people on a committee, who disapproves, nobody knows." Electronic voting allowed committee members to disagree, but not be targeted for their disagreement, he said:

> Even in records of meeting[s], it doesn't show who speaks. Before we had names in the minutes, now we use member A, B, C. With the subject protected, [we] also try to protect our members.

But some committee members feel that their opinion, and their assertion of it, is a virtue. When I interviewed Camilla, a Taiwanese former IRB member, in an office off a hospital corridor during her lunch break, she told me that she had just returned from a nearby hospital, having just given a talk on Genetic Ethics. "I went to threaten them!" she said, laughing. She wanted to make her audience more aware of questions of privacy and the relevant regulation. "I can't tell how much they change," she told me, "but gradually they change their thinking of ethics":

> Medical doctors, they think of research; [the] patient, who cares? A lot of MDs, their mind is set on research but not really ethics. They might not think of it at all, before someone convinces them. [The] medical doctor way—"I treat you," their thinking is different. [. . .] Sometimes it is hard to change their attitude or thinking. Sometimes they still argue. It's a long-time process to educate these people. Even in a committee you find doctors still doing things very unethically—after all the education, I am always shocked that you still see these kinds of people around, still.

I asked her to elaborate on "these kinds of people." She shrugged, and told me she herself had been one of them: "When initiating research we'd do unethical things, for consent—ignore things we were supposed to do. Just say, 'Hey, give me my proof—my IRB approval letter.' [Then] forget everything about ethical things." Her criticism is aimed at researchers, but she extends it to the committee—suggesting that under pressure, committees bend to the expectations and demands of their colleagues:

> The hierarchy system is very strong and people are afraid to lose their job. Committee is a nice way to do this, 'cos we have backup from each other. We can speak out. [We are] not afraid to have a "big mouth."

She was quiet, reflecting on what she'd said about speaking out for a moment, then seemed to change her mind. Her account of the committee as a form of challenging authority through group discussion dissipated as she went on to reveal that it was *her* enactment of this ideal of speaking out that led to her becoming an *ex*-IRB member. "Well, I was kicked out!" she exclaimed, with a wry smile.

> They want smoothly run, obedient ones. [For me] it's about whether, at the right time, are you willing to speak up for something. Especially for ethics. You're

> *supposed* to speak up. That's our principle. It's the right thing to do, for myself and participants. You set your mind on the ethical thing and you do it. Not different to becom[ing] a martyr. I'm martyr of the IRB! Honesty, integrity, things you believe in. That's our problem [in Taiwan]. IRB independence.

There are details of a case that she does not reveal, but the point is made. Not everyone is equal, nor is everyone able to speak in the same way.

On the Problem of Relations

While most interviewees told me they felt confident to voice their views and comfortable speaking their concerns in committee meetings, Vinaya—a Sri Lankan ethics committee member—openly told me that she thought people were afraid to criticize their superiors. "They're afraid for their careers," she said, "even if they think something, it is better for them to stay quiet." I had arrived in the Sri Lankan hill town of Peradeniya to speak with her, and in our interview in her campus office, Vinaya told me that she served on a committee that had recently been reconstituted. "New faces" were brought in because the older group had been, in her words, "dysfunctional." The Peradeniya committee had been established in the early 1980s as a joint research and ethics committee, "until a separate ethics committee was established in 2003" (Dissanayake et al. 2009, 111, cited in Sariola and Simpson 2019, 37). Vinaya explained that the committee primarily handled research proposals of the university's own faculty, and that the committee meetings had been poorly attended due to the posts being packed with many "senior persons." They simply did not have time to come to the meetings. Describing her own workload, she told me that a minority, herself included, had been doing most of the work of reading through the proposals, thinking about them and checking them. "It takes time," she said, "very few senior people can prepare." As we talked, she explained that her medical research career had taken her to the U.S. for a few years, and she used this experience to illustrate how her perception of authority and questioning had changed as a result. In the United States, she gradually found that her colleagues did not find asking questions derogatory, and they did not think it would, in her words, "hurt." Vinaya had appreciated this; she found it "a good way" to interact and learn, but at the same time, she had been uneasy with the sense there was little respect for the experience of older people. Returning home to Sri Lanka, she reflected, she had found that even "asking questions may hurt the person, and the person being questioned regards it as something not good because you're questioning your teacher or your elder." A solution to the problem of question-asking, she thought, was blinding the review, so that the reviewers did not know the name of the person whose research was being reviewed. "I may be more free, then, to give my view," she said. What that view would contribute, however, she didn't quite know. In the end, on her committee, the chairperson and the dean took the overall decision, "because everyone can't take the decision, we can give our views, but in the end, they take the decision." She expressed doubt about whether the decisions being taken were "correct":

> This is how we do it: We look at whose research it is. So-and-so has been doing it for so long, their influence, they've done so much for the country, they're faculty. At the same time someone is trying to start, they may be harsher on the evaluation of that research. That has big reputation behind it, this doesn't. Animosities, maybe, or at the same time, friendship. There are large, bloated egos in research.

While Vinaya longed for the freedom that "blind review" would give *her*, it is very clear that ethics committee work is embedded in existing social relations, often to the frustration of committee members. This was foreseen by the 2000 gathering of the Global Forum on Bioethics in Research, with Bebe Loff, Karen Hofman, and Vasantha Muthuswamy noting that "serious ethical debate could be problematic in cultural milieu lacking a tradition of egalitarianism or in an environment in which challenging authority is unusual" (Loff et al. 2001, 63). However, I often found that this equation was turned around, with ethics being used to *manage* existing social relations. A depersonalized approach—to employ standards that must be complied with—was considered an advantage, particularly when ethics review was being newly introduced to faculties. Malika, a social scientist at the Open University in Sri Lanka, had encouraged the establishment of a committee in the humanities. When I interviewed her and her advisor, who had founded the committee, he explained that they had run a

> step by step introduction of it, we made it known to everyone. In a sense, no proposal can deviate from the established mechanisms, it has to abide by the mechanism. There won't be any different treatment because you're my friend, or you're my enemy.

Relations—friends, enemies—find themselves circumvented through an appeal to "established mechanisms" and the manipulation of the externality of rules. Malika told me that she often contacted the researcher applicant in advance:

> I contact the person if the application form is not well written, I get some things clear. Some people process the application in a hurry if they want to make the deadline. Some don't understand certain aspects of the ethical approval form. So, in that sense, giving a call and getting[7] is very effective.

She did find that PIs could be "defensive," concerned about being penalized or delayed, and most were "afraid of being rejected by the committee." What Camilla's and Vinaya's comments about committees with "high up" or "senior" figures in the chairperson's role indicates is that this person may well play an important role in sustaining existing hierarchies within a committee setting. Discussions over who is chosen for the chairperson are revealing. As one Thai FERCAP conference delegate, with considerable experience volunteering as a Surveyor for the network, said:

> I'm impressed when I go surveying in China, and I see that the president is the chair of an ethics committee. They get a lot of support! I go back home and I ask my director to be chair. But you have to balance that. What are the risk[s] and what are the benefit[s]?[8]

Having high-status members of research institutes and universities serve on ethics committees causes debate amongst FERCAP members. Some worry that having presidents on committees means the jobs of committee members are at risk if they do not perform well, or if they disagree too much. Others argue that if the head of the institution is the chair of the committee, there is nobody to whom they can bring a complaint. This overt concern with the consequences and intricacies of seniority is part of a wider trend. Where literature originating in the U.S. and Canada notes that committees sometimes struggle with authority, it is often the case here that those who are appointed to the ethics committee are chosen *precisely* for their seniority, and hence, authority. While there were, no doubt, many stories of conflict and professional tension that I did not hear, the discussions above show that amidst the document-oriented work and attention to the "clerical side" of bureaucracy, it would not do to leave "no space for the study of affect"

(Navaro-Yashin 2007, 83). These moments show that how the ethics process feels to committee members—and researchers—matters.

Ethics and the Fixity of Law

By comparing the ethics committee and the jury, I have brought forward the complexity of relationality within committee work, when brought out of policy documents and into institutional settings. Places and their history matter, different contentions arise in rightness of how much is known (and by whom). I now move away from that direct contrast, turning to the wider issues in the apparent poles of Coleman and Noah's debate: the tension in the concept of ethics between compliance and aspiration, between external regulation and an exhortation to "do good." Their debate frames ethics review committees and juries as comparable on the basis that they are both instruments of the law. Indeed, as Stark reminds us, in the United States, the ethics committee *is* empowered to make legally binding recommendations (2012). This is not the case for many of FERCAP's committees. Despite FERCAP's aversion to the "red tape" of working with governments, many nonetheless held aspirations for their countries to implement a legal framework. At the same time, however, many also did not feel that "law" would be a suitable vehicle for change.

Throughout my fieldwork, committee members sifted through documents produced in the wider research ecosystem: the standards in the Survey, national regulations, World Health Organization's Blue and Silver booklets, ICH-GCP, the Declaration of Helsinki. In 2010, the hope was that WHO standards could be adopted by countries involved in FERCAP as the basis for their own national laws, offering, as the WHO discussant put it, the same "the minimum floor of ethical principles" fixed everywhere. Even at moments of "saming" work such as this, researchers point out that their countries don't have legislative frameworks, or their FDAs don't function in a particularly "regulatory manner." Understanding the different legislative and regulatory systems in which these standards aim to operate causes confusion. As the delegates try to fix the "levels" on which things can be done part of the challenge is that countries do not organize their governments in the same ways. Are those who issue regulation authorized through legislation? If regulatory is less than legislative, is it sufficient? What counts as regulatory? If legislators speak of the "duty of medical colleges to regulate," does that make them into regulators? Delegates are worried that the inclusion of language about legislation will exclude them. Carl is polite, but agrees: "Guidelines are good and guidelines should exist but guidelines in themselves wouldn't meet the standard of a legal framework." The Sri Lankan delegate points out that in his country, legislation can only be made by government, which affects who the "relevant national authority" being addressed is.

> So, if we are to use this document as part of lobbying, to get governments to get laws enacted, then you must say "national governments should ensure." It needs to address the government as the responsible authority in enacting the law. And I think that's what is going to strengthen our hand if we are to go to government and say, "Look, WHO is saying that you must do this." So I think we mustn't undermine that because yes, the Forum of Ethics [Review] Committees in Sri Lanka [FERCSL] [. . .] have guidelines, but those have no *legal* authority and that is the reason why we have a lot of problems of enactment.

Indian delegates agree, arguing for regulations over guidelines, feeling the latter are "not mandatory so if people do not follow them you cannot take [give] punishment." During FERCAP Conferences, then, legislation is usually formulated as an absence, where countries *with* legislation list it amongst their achievements, marking routes of progress on PowerPoints. The relationship of ethics to the law is in part a question of what the law is taken to be. During an interview with Lakmini, a Colombo University lawyer who also served on a medical ethics review committee, she reminded me that the law was often regarded as something static. "Here, it is archaic," she said, "not amended in years. What happens is society outstrips the law, and the law becomes redundant." While it might be useful to have legal backup for the committee's work, she thought it would ultimately cause problems. The courts, she said, were slow and weighted.[9] "Law," she said, "strives to divorce itself from ethics and morality," citing the debate in the UK over the limits of criminal law between Lord Patrick Devlin and Professor H.L.A. Hart during the 1950s following the proposal of the Wolfenden Committee to decriminalize homosexuality.[10]

> This raised huge issues for us, the divorce from religion—[the idea that the] secular should regulate morality and ethics with it. That's the fear: When you fix law with morality, there's the danger of having it be stagnant.

An interview with Dr. Chatura, a neuroscientist committee member in Colombo, I heard repeated the sentiment that ethics ought not be set into law, but his reasoning was that *ethics*, not "society," changes. "As far as the law is concerned," he said,

> it is written there in black and white. Ethics is not, okay? It comes from within. And it changes over time, we see it in the world. What is ethical now was not ethical then, and we should keep up with that. We should be open to understanding the basis of what changes. And if we don't keep up, we'll get crowded out by other jurisdictions that permit something. We shouldn't just say that shouldn't be permitted and leave it at that and have Victorian attitudes.

"What do you mean Victorian?" I asked.

> Well, you can't be Victorian about it. At the last meeting, someone said, "We will create a Frankenstein." Those are antiquated views—as long as it is not unlawful, it can be done. If it meets criteria, and is properly monitored, and the parameters are set then okay.

But the "lawfulness" of something in Sri Lanka is largely unknown. He tells about "weak" regulation and "gray" areas. He laments the small likelihood of legislation emerging: The beleaguered civil war government has other priorities and insufficient awareness. Research cannot wait, he says, until the Ministry of Health makes regulations; it will never happen. So, he tells me, "it is important for ethics committees to try and work out modalities which might serve the needs of research, as a stop-gap . . . That seems to be the primary problem the committee has . . . Do you permit people to engage in research and be competitive, or am I worried that the Buddhist clergy will come and protest against me?" While he concedes that there is little or no public debate at present, "all it takes is a tiny thing, a little cinder, and it becomes huge." I play the devil's advocate: Would not something "huge" help his case, bring attention, awareness, focus, and prompt legislation? He smiles and shakes his head, pauses for a moment, then, "A public debate would not be a rational debate," he says softly, "these issues are very complex and there are very few politicians with the brains to sit down and understand it." Reflecting on the preoccupations of Sri Lankan legislators, he shook his head again and said he didn't think legislation would come for a long time.

> That is why ethics committees play an important role, because they set down certain guidelines which will be used and drafted if the government comes to make laws. They'll look at what is existing and use that. That is the heaviest

> burden the ethics committee caries with them. I can't see any bureaucrat sitting down to draft guidelines. The committee is the best possibility at the moment. The composition has doctors who are highly regarded, modern in their thinking, it is a diverse group and composed of people of all religions, communities, and ages.

The neuroscientist's comments echo Cristina's wish to see FERCAP lead not through agitation of the masses[11] but through the education and support of professionals. They also reveal a further "burden" on committees operating in the absence of governmental support.

Both the lawyer and the neuroscientist held that rather than law producing change, it was too fixed to adapt to changes in "society" over time. Ethics has a temporality, not just a location. When one of my Sri Lankan interviewees told me that the ethics review committee was "quite an old concept," I thought she was referring to the relatively early establishment of committees in Sri Lanka during the 1980s (Dissanayake et al. 2009). However, what she meant was quite different, referencing an International Court of Justice (ICJ) case on the contestation between Hungary and the Czechoslovak people's republic over the resources and control of the Danube. The judge in the case, a Sri Lankan, had used the following story as a way of explaining the long heritage of the concept of "sustainable development" in Asia:

> Long ago, I don't remember the period, monks were sent from India to Sri Lanka, to do preaching here. When the monks came, the king had gone hunting. They told him, "Don't kill animals. You must be the guardian of the people, the animals, the land water and air. You must not destroy or spoil them." The ruler agreed, and undertook to protect [them]. Now, the judge cited that incident. He said, "We don't have to look to the Stockholm declaration, we have the conventions already in our system. It is you who must search for them." We have that, already, in Asian culture.[12]

The sense that ethics was already somehow located in "culture" (Sariola and Simpson 2011, 518) led some interviewees to opine that it could not be codified. During an interview, a Sri Lankan doctor told me that, in his view,

> a code to implement ethical principles is absurd. It would be sad if it goes to that level. While you can have regulations and guidelines, sanction based [law] should not be there. Professional bodies and ourselves should enforce it.

While the focus in these examples has been Sri Lanka, the idea of legislating for ethics carries force elsewhere. During an interview with the chair of a committee in Taiwan, he explained that he believed research there had "progressed fast" because they had "used law regulations to do regulation." The advantage, as the chair saw it, was that this had ensured that ethics was "not only for moral problem[s]." Again, using the language of levels invoked by the Sri Lankan doctor above, he said that using legislation as a "level of regulation" above that of "moral issues" and turning ethics into "law issues" meant ethics could "live on the level of these issues," and the government could "use this power to push ethics." By elevating ethics to the "level" of law, the chairman said, investigators were made to take it seriously: "We believe research and ethics here will develop fast and live on a very high level."

While Coleman and the Taiwanese interviewee above have sought and framed ethics as a matter of law, Noah and the Sri Lankan doctor above both associate the law with an objectionable depersonalization, inadequate to the "aspirational" qualities they attribute to ethics. According to this line of critique, by setting "the minimum standards of conduct" (Aubert 1979, 34), the law instills "a morality of obligation, not one of aspiration" (Fuller 2000, cited in Aubert 1979, 34). Similarly, the USFDA summons an idea of ethics that goes beyond mere compliance with the law: "Responsible research is ethical, not just compliant . . . [b]ecause the regulations are the ethical floor, not the ceiling" (White 2011). Ethics, it seems, is expected to be something more than just compliance, or just law.

Ethics and the Law

"It's hard to imagine how Americans could fulfill their role as democracy advocates any better than helping the Japanese become jurors," wrote Robert E. Precht in his 2006 *New York Times* opinion piece where he recommended an exchange program in which "Americans can visit Japan and share their jury experiences and Japanese can also visit American courthouses and talk with American jurors." Just as the jury was seen as a turn toward democracy in Japan (a politics encapsulated in a form),[13] I have in this chapter unpicked the ethics committee's invocation of principles of representation, equality of view, and voice.

This proximity between law and ethics as modes of governing gave rise to Coleman and Noah's debate. Coleman reports that "a 1996 General Accounting

Office study found that IRBs are overburdened, underfunded, insufficiently prepared, and often too willing to rely on investigators' *good intentions* as the primary method for protecting subjects" (2003, 1147; emphasis added), a situation he finds untenable. Despite Coleman and Noah's disagreement on how it is that human subjects participating in research should be protected, I suggest that the critical insight here can be to the way in which the debate is cast. The poles of Coleman and Noah's debate reemerge throughout my ethnography: governance through external legal mechanisms or through inculcating and encouraging ethical behavior?

As much as these are the poles of Cristina's capacity-building activism, they are also substantive issues of legal anthropology, replayed out of debates on social control, in debates on the nature and use of research ethics committees. The ethics committee—in design and implementation—replicates the idea that law and regulation is about external structures of governance: one realm (ethics) that comments on another (biomedical research). Ethics, as we saw in earlier chapters, is presented as a set of behaviors brought in by FERCAP, codified in Standard Operating Procedures, rooms, and discussions. But the material in this chapter has explored the limits of seeing ethics as a codified behavior. In the mocking tone of the Sri Lankan interlocutors, this is not what ethics is at all. It does not belong, they argue, to a domain of compliance with the law, but sits as a personal orientation. While committee members may go along with the committee as a necessary and even useful device, ethics here does not extend from bureaucratic origins; it begins elsewhere. For these researchers and committee members, law is a domain outside of ethics into which ethics should not extend, not because the law is primary but because ethics is. To return to the legal imaginaries I discussed through Flear and Ashcroft at the start of this chapter, I suggest it matters how genealogies of ethics as a technique of democratic deliberative decision-making surface in dilemmas over the place of ethical conduct. When an ethics committee is likened to a jury, the imaginary of evidence of decision and of discussion brings with it the legitimating power of the law. In extension of Flear and Ashcroft's argument, then, here it is not the "role of imaginaries in mediating relations between law and biomedical technoscience" (2021, 1), but the imaginary of the law in the worlds of ethics as *it* mediates relations between researchers and prospective patients. When ethics committees became part of biomedical worlds, they were seen as taking oversight out of the sole hands of medical professionals, and bringing "society" into decision-making about medical research. But they remain highly institutional. In recognition of the reality that many committees *are* in institutions, the 2023 WHO Benchmarking tool includes a provision to "preserve the independence of REC members and chairs": Indicator 02.04 requires that "REC members and chairs may not be removed before the expiration of their terms unless they have been found to have substantially breached their duties" (World Health Organization 2023, 9). Yet as formalization and standardization sediment into practice, demarcating the ethical, my interlocutors still wonder about the capacity of a system to shape the everyday life of research projects. In the unresolved space between ethics and the law, there is at the same time a turn toward conscience not compliance, the pursuit of integrity and interiority I turn to now.

SEVEN
Locating Ethics

> People are the hard thing. If they don't have a quality culture, it's very difficult. People tend to do the same old thing. And they cannot change. It has to be there for a long time, starting when you're young perhaps.

Juntra was giving a lecture in Bangkok in late March 2010, a time at when the Thai "Red Shirts" (United Front of Democracy Against Dictatorship) had filled the city and would, in the weeks to come, occupy large parts of the capital's commercial center (Sopranzetti and Fabbri 2021). But quality trainings took place regardless, and Good Clinical Practice discussions filling King Chulalongkorn Memorial Hospital lecture halls as FERCAP took their workshops and sessions on tour. From the stage, Juntra had just facilitated a long discussion and good quality in research, presenting from her slides, walking up and down, keeping the energy in the darkened room high. She summed up the last half hour with a rather exasperated comment about how "people" tended to "do the same old thing," then paused and stood looking out at the scattered rows of workshop participants. She let a silence fall: People looked down. Did she mean them? Having seen this training before, I knew she wanted the workshop participants to reach a new understanding of what a quality culture looked like. Although the large lecture hall had no windows, she threw her left arm out in the imagined direction of the city center. "If we wanted to go to the market right now," she asked the room, "how would we get there?" Struggling with the change of topic, the room silently looked at her. "There are demonstrations, right?" she asked, and began to list what we would need to get to the market: We'd need information on where the roadblocks were, what routes we can take, a up-to-date map. Then, she'd look at the different risks of the possible routes and choose the best, the most efficient. "It might not be perfect," she warned, but "quality culture is the culture of your thinking: the shortest time, the cheapest way." Gesturing again at the university buildings around us, she continued:

> There is a quality culture of people working here: When they go home, they switch off the fan. If there is no quality culture, they wouldn't do this: "I don't care." Quality culture is about the whole organization, not about you. People say, "I use a piece of paper and then I throw it away." Quality culture is to reduce waste, it is an organization on top of your thinking. I use two sides [of paper]. Whatever you do, you have it in mind. It's very hard, hard to define quality. But you have to define what it is. I have to get quality culture into each person.

What is Juntra talking about when she says she wants to get quality "into" people? What is this thing "quality," which is not "about you" yet must be "inside" the person? For the past thirty years, scholars have attended to the language that has accompanied the growth of audit, not least the pressure that grows on the audited subject to monitor themselves. From critical engagement with "Best Value" (Miller 1998) and audit (Power 1994, 2022; Strathern 2000; Shore and Wright 2024), work is continuing to critically analyze how other terms such as "best practice" (Chong 2018) and "good quality" itself (Wahlberg 2018) shape social expectations, hopes, and acceptability. Quality and "best practice" have languished perhaps because of their apparent *obviousness*, being taken "at once as evidence of [themselves] and perceived as a layer added to others" (Strathern 2004, 10). The quality culture Juntra is speaking of also seems self-evident, and she certainly seems to think I should immediately grasp what she is attempting to instill. But what if we do not take quality to be a self-evident term, and seek to unpick why and how Juntra would try to get quality "into" people? What might this effort require, and what might be the result?

In this chapter, I explore different attempts to bring ethics review closer to being a wider way of living for committee members and researchers. Juntra's technique above is to make quality and ethics synonymous, and to locate ethics practice within an encultured individual. Moments like this one, where ethics comes to be thought through other regimes—duty, professions, systems of belief—present a pattern in the ethnography between external and internal measurements. So far, my analyses have brought forward the location of ethics within managerial and material objects: standards, minutes, rooms, protocols, decisions. Yet amongst these forms of technocratic dreaming exist visions of ethical subjectivity, narratives of conversion, and a belief in ethics. The "ethics" people locate in themselves and others is more difficult to describe than that which they locate in good minute-taking or in bullet-point standards. As Science and Technology Studies (STS) scholar Sheila Jasanoff puts it, "making codes is one thing; transforming them into forms of life, quite another" (2005, 175). This is the extension FERCAP members work, sometimes inchoately, toward.

Transforming ethics codes into forms of life draws the ethical into new conceptual relations and pushes it beyond peoples' work lives. Ethnographic accounts of personal and social virtues, moral knowledge, conformity, responsibility, and accountability remain apposite in this encounter with ethics formalized into the bureaucratic. Following when and where ethics becomes located in systems and when in an ineffable quality of self reframes central questions upon which extensive anthropologies of the twentieth century were written.[1] Quality, the term that leads the present chapter, exemplifies the phenomenon. Juntra's discussion above incorporates both an internal disposition ("the culture of your thinking") and something external that can be measured. It is a binary pervasive in much of the contemporary commentary on governance, as Simpson summarizes: "Within the rationality of neoliberalism, the objective is to re-position government such that it no longer governs the people but governs the governance by which people govern themselves" (2012, 157). Thus, we see ever greater use of techniques of surveillance, monitoring and expertise, at the same time as we see a push for people to empower themselves, take responsibility, and assert their autonomy (Rose 1991; Trnka and Trundle 2017). Useful though it may be politically, and evident though it is ethnographically, I suggest that this split between the interior and exterior is less useful analytically. A new term resurgent within the research ethics arena, "integrity," puts pressure on precisely this split, as it oscillates between seeking researchers who have integrity (carry it within themselves) and environments or institutions that support research conducted with integrity (Davies 2019). Again, we find ethics extending its reach: Despite fine-grained monitoring and promises of continuing review, it is still seeking ever greater territory over an ethics located within researchers themselves.

Quality

The idea of quality permeates training. We can trace its institutional life through the World Health Organization's TDR's Strategic Quality Management

(SQM) Unit. When she held the role,[2] Juntra not only favored the term "quality" but was in a position to push its use. "There is a clear need to implement the principles of strategic quality management in health research to prevent failure, maximize the utilization of available resources and ensure consistency and credibility of results," she and her colleagues wrote in *TDRnews*, the newsletter of TDR (Karbwang et al. 2010, 24). In an interview in 2010, I asked Juntra how she thinks about ethics and quality, trying to understand in what way they come to occupy the same frame. She used herself as the example through which to explain the relationship:

> If I give a lecture on the principle of good practice in ethical review, what is my measurement of you? How do I know you have learned? I can ask you, give you an exam or an exercise. But I have to define what I expect, what is my learning objective [. . .] A lot of [the] time [I] don't know what we're looking for, so it's difficult to measure. Same as going to the market—you're buying dinner, if you have a list, you go to this section, buy this, that, fast, and get what you want in a short time. If not, you buy things and you don't know what to do, [it] doesn't make a meal, [it] becomes junk. If you don't have anything in mind, [you] buy many things, [but you] don't get what you really need.

Juntra's recursive descriptions pass from the measurement of the activity (ethical review) to the measurement of the learner ("How do I know you have learned?") to the measurement of the training (Is the training good enough?) to the identification of learning objectives. Quality is potentially present through measurement at any of these moments: an orienting principle for designing and implementing the Survey, in addition to being the thing that Surveys seek in committees surveyed. Using language that recalls the images of fragmentation commonly used in descriptions of ethics capacity building, Juntra and her colleagues observed that

> until now, quality management was often fragmented. For instance, there was a quality check at the start of a new research project in the grant selection process, and another at the end through peer review publications. But during the balance of the research process, quality management was frequently left to researchers and their institutions. (Karbwang et al. 2010, 24)

During revisions to the Standard Operating Procedures for Survey teams—as we were working around a large table, many laptop screens open, people typing, talking, and getting up to stretch—Juntra used a metaphor to describe the way in which the group doing the revisions should *aspire to quality in their definitions of quality*. She drew their attention. "Do not just say 'I will make a pen,'" she said. "I will say:

> "I want a yellow one with a red bottom, five inches long." It's not [an attitude of] "any pen will do," we want *that* pen. And if we're talking about Surveyors, we need to define the quality of the Survey and the Surveyors. Otherwise it's just another routine thing.

Juntra would perhaps have got on well with anthropologist Clifford Geertz, for whom culture was "best seen not as complexes of concrete behavior patterns—customs, usages, traditions, habit clusters—[. . .] but as a set of control mechanisms—plans, recipes, rules, instructions [. . .]—for the governing of behavior" (Geertz 1973, 44; Strathern 1985, 111). An example of such control mechanisms for the governing of behavior are Standard Operating Procedures, described as "recipes" in Chinese ethics training documents (Figure 7.1). Surveyors take up the language of quality improvement with enthusiasm. At a FERCAP training prior to a Survey in Manila, April 2010, I heard this statement from a Surveyor: "We believe in continuous quality improvement. Therefore, there is no perfect EC, we will always find something, some weakness that we will make recommendations about." FERCAP Surveyors have passed this language on to committees seeking renewal of their recognition status.[3] On a visit to an IRB in Taiwan, I received an office tour, and the secretary handed me a thick folder filled with the documents from their recent Survey. The hospital's PowerPoint slides listed the IRB's Strengths, Weaknesses, Opportunities, and Threats (SWOT) analysis. Their W (weakness) was improving the continuing dialogue between the PI and IRB "to ensure the PI's positive attitude toward IRB functions and responsibility." Their T (threat): "Owing to tightened standards reinforced, the number of research protocols submitted to this IRB for reviewing may be reduced temporarily; for the long run, however, we believe that the sponsor and PI would recognize, appreciate and benefit from our continuous insistence on quality."

What interests me here is the "continuous insistence on quality": It is something that committees must always strive for, but chained as it is to the terms "continuous" and "improvement," it can never be arrived at. This is how

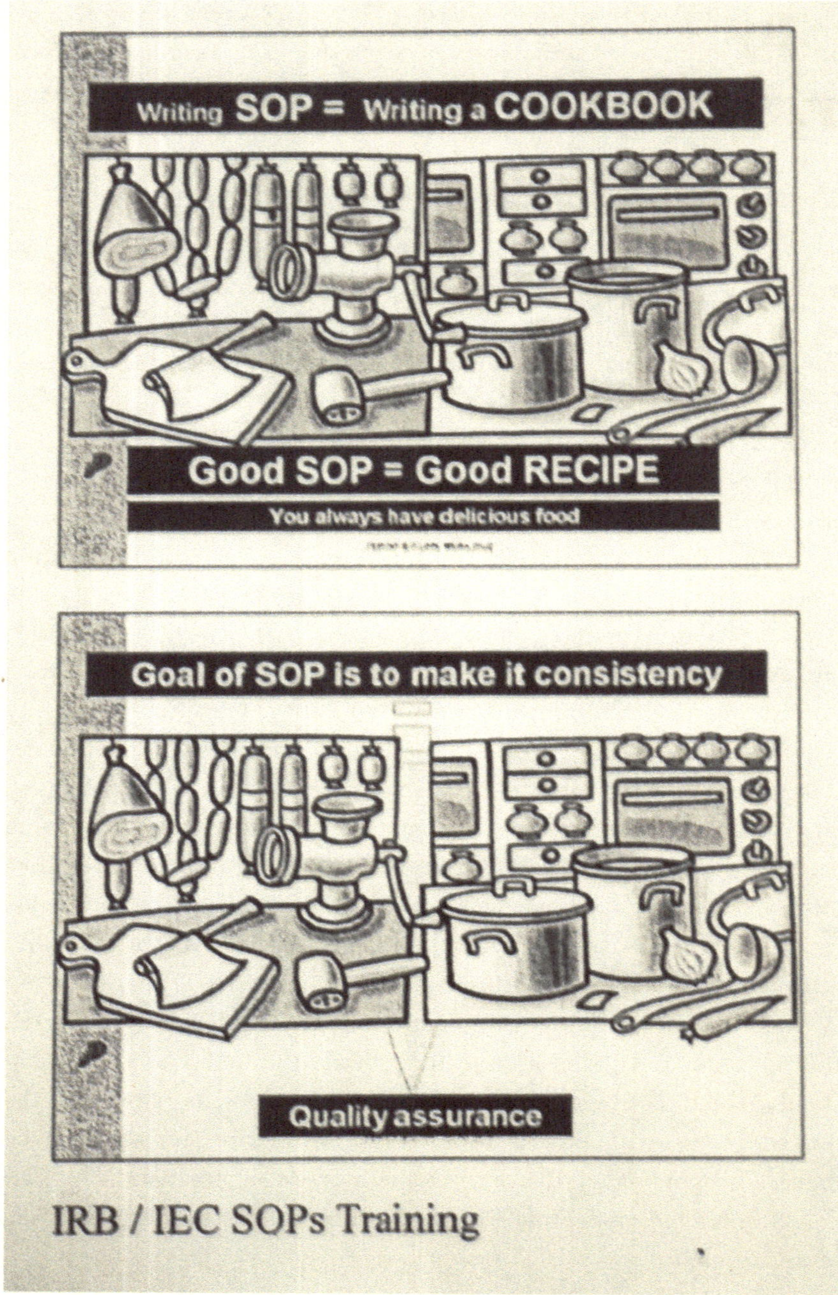

Writing SOP = Writing a COOKBOOK
Good SOP = Good RECIPE
You always have delicious food
Goal of SOP is to make it consistency
Quality assurance
IRB / IEC SOPs Training

Figure 7.1. A training manual for Chinese Research Ethics Committees, showing Standard Operating Procedures as recipes for quality assurance. Source: Author.

Surveys first appear: as efforts to see committees reach a certain standard, be recognized through the FERCAP/SIDCER program, and then continue to work toward re-recognition. But the introduction of higher standards and changes in regulations and guidelines suggests that this process may not easily be considered complete; indeed, if no committee is ever perfect, then their condition is one of infinite improvability. With the announcement that there is no perfect ethics committee, the sociality of this potentially infinite project is visible in the operation of the Survey. But it is also visible in trainings on running compliant clinical trials, as illustrated in this comment from a researcher in a Philippines GCP training:

> Should results of non-GCP compliant studies be published? It boils down to GCP. From the research protocol up to publication [. . .] Remember, there is no study that is perfect. Who can do a perfect study? Nobody except God probably. No investigator can claim that his study is perfect and fully, fully 100 percent. *Sapagkat kami ay tao lamang*, because we're just people.[4] We're just human beings. We're bound to make mistakes.

Refracting both quality and ethics, "perfection" returns the framing of standards to the ethnographic setting. Here, perfection is a property of the divine, a Catholic framing that aligns humanity with flaws, the potential for judgment and blame. The researcher explained how he had felt when a monitor came to visit his site during the conduct of a multi-sited clinical trial in the Philippines:

> The first time we were monitored we hated it. We were debating. "Why are you doing this?" we asked the monitor, "Your role here is to help!" But they did want to help—so in the end it becomes good, a good study. We were like that for the first visit, but then there was a second visit. [. . .] You start blaming each other in front of the monitor. There was a third visit, and by the fourth visit, we came to like the monitor.

Just as Surveyors declare there is no perfect committee, GCP trainers declare there can be no perfect study. This is, in part, because it is the same people who are doing both. The researcher above who initially hated his clinical monitor is a member of an ethics review committee. Their clinical experience informs committee decisions about clinical trials but, I suggest, it also shapes the way in which "ethics" is developed and implemented.

While my discussion so far has focused largely on ethics review committees themselves, the economics of research and narratives of personal and national productivity are never far away. One trainer told me that she aimed to motivate her students: "By the end of the session, [I want them to] think '[There are] many things I have to do! Many things in need of change.'" For Juntra, trainee attentiveness mattered. Amongst the attendees that week, she perceived a lack of willingness to see their "role in the system," leading her to grumble that there were few with the potential to become Surveyors. "Many have a fixed mindset . . . [T]hese are from some provincial hospital[s]. They are not going for FERCAP recognition, they will go for the national one. The research [their committee] sees is just local investigator, lots of case reports. If they continue to have this 'copy' attitude, they get further away from the principles." The conversation turned to her schooling in Chiang Mai, and a geometry class. The students had been asked to do a proof of something, that this added up to that, or this side of the equation meant this. She produced a proof, but it was not the one the teacher had taught. And she was told it was wrong, even though it worked as a proof. She said she still remembered that day, when they told her she was not good at following rules. This story, recounted in the context of of a training session, was offered as a perspective on her pedagogy and the personal ethics that suffused the sessions. She realized that day that she didn't like an educational system where you are taught to compete against others, and not taught to independently contribute something to wider society. Contribution, for her, is why there is an imperative for trainees to pay attention:

> You are contributing to your country, using resources properly. People who come and don't want to learn should feel ashamed, they are wasting their nation's resource. If I go and I don't pay attention, I feel guilty because the organization has paid for me. You should feel it *yourself.* I'd like that to happen to everyone. Shouldn't wait for people to evaluate you, but evaluate yourself. If I've been sleeping, I should feel bad.

Quality, like ethics, becomes a value to believe in, and something to be advocated for. Made deliberate, conscious, it can be practiced. In unknowing parallel to Lars Noah's argument that perfect documents mean nothing unless the researcher has "bought in" to the process (2004, 292), a Thai committee member commented, "Yes, I've done six months at Western IRB but unless you keep it in mind, the training is nothing. It is up to you."

Through these reflections, we can see how FERCAP's capacity-building work extends beyond documentation, Surveys, and training into an understanding of the research process and of one's role within it. "Before you accept responsibility," argued trainers, "you have to know what [your responsibility will be] about. If it's beyond your capacity, you have to gain that capacity first. You should ask, 'How can I best contribute?'" Good Clinical Practice merges ethics and responsibility together, as the trainer continued: "That's why in GCP you have to state very clearly what each [party's] responsibility is about. So the person can see, 'For me to take responsibility I need this training.'" This trainer's configuration of a prospective committee member looks for responsibility toward others (trial participants) in the framework of GCP, which in turn foregrounds responsibility for oneself. The trainer's closing comments carry the weight she intends: "That's what ethics is about. Even in daily life. It's about responsibility."

Professional Integrity

Ethics committees, Sarah Dyer and David Demeritt remind us, "are part of a wide sea-change in the governance of professional conduct. Until recently," they claim, "research ethics were treated as matters of personal and professional integrity" (2009, 47). Writing about "self-regulation" in medicine, Sylvia and Richard Creuss (2005) draw on the work of William Sullivan, a medical sociologist, using his words to conclude that "neither economic incentives nor technology nor administrative control has proved an effective surrogate for the commitment to integrity evoked in the ideal of professionalism" (Sullivan 1995, xvi). Looking at the United Kingdom, Duncan Wilson, a historian of biomedicine, has charted the factors that "fostered outside scrutiny of medicine," with an aim to show "how particular individuals fashioned themselves into 'ethics experts'" (2012, 195). "The new regimes of external oversight, like bioethics, were not simply the product of the conservative demands for audit and accountability," he writes, "but also depended on the presence of individuals and professional groups willing to define themselves as the new arbiters of best practice" (2012, 196). Laura Stark's analysis for the United States is similar, following "how the moral authority to decide how to treat research participants was relocated from professions to the state and reinvested in procedures rather than ethics principles" (2012, 7), although she suggests that "group review was invented, justified, and expanded less by 'outsiders' like bioethicists and activists than by researchers themselves" (2012, 7). As it professionalized (itself), bioethics kept intact the idea of the profession, to which research ethics is now returning. The limits of this external gaze are being felt most strongly in countries that have invested heavily in mechanisms that are designed as checks on professionalism. Speaking from the United States, Dr. Greg Koski began a webinar with the frustration that "there is little direct, measurable evidence that the heightened burden [of review] actually increases the effectiveness of protecting human subjects, or improves the quality of the research itself" (Koski 2011), a comment that prefigures a movement that turns scientific scrutiny upon research ethics committees to evaluate them not for their *efficiency* but their *effectiveness* (Fernandez Lynch et al. 2023). In his webinar, rather than expanding on the measures suggested by critics at the time such as Jeremy Sugarman (2004), Ezekiel Emanuel et al. (2004), Brenda Beagan and Michael McDonald (2005), among others, Koski concludes that the absence of "evidence" brings something else to the fore:

> We simply have to say, all right, if we're really talking about integrity, if integrity is what we're falling back on in hope that that's what is actually going to protect human subjects, [then] of course that's what Henry Beecher[5] says. [I] t's really the integrity, the well trained, well intentioned investigator, doing the right thing, that provides protection for human subjects, not a committee, not regulations. It's the individual integrity of scientists.

Pointing to the "Human Subjects Protection" regime as it has been built up in North America, Koski goes on to argue that responsibility for ethics in research has shifted to committees, with those he considers most central to ethical research—professional investigators—no longer taking responsibility for the ethics of their work. He turns to certification and examination as a solution, suggesting that becoming an "ethics professional" would enhance the felt responsibility of researchers. In contrast with Wilson's "ethics professionals," who stand outside the practice of medicine, these are the researchers who are being certified for their competence in ethics. Koski calls this a shift from a "culture of compliance to a culture of conscience," a move formulated during his tenure in the U.S. Office for Human Research Protections:

> Where we are today is in the compliance domain, where so much of what we do is driven by our desire to ensure that research is going to be reviewed and

> performed in compliance with regulations. Regulatory compliance is the floor for all Human Subject Protection. Because if you go below that you're breaking the law. That means you're a crook. And certainly this is not where we want to be, and yet this is where we stay 'cos it's the only thing we've known how to do. It's not where we want to stay. (Koski 2011)

The result of a move from a "compliance domain" to a "true performance domain," he says, would be trust: research that is trusted "not only by the participants but by society, sponsors, everyone" (Koski 2011):

> Under a professional system, investigators who fail to meet their responsibilities lose their privileges. If you don't do it right you don't get to do it at all. That seems to be a very powerful way to motivate people to do things right, it works in medicine, it works in law, and other fields, there's no reason it wouldn't work in research. [. . .] There would also have to be personal accountability. Rather than shutting down an IRB or suspending a[n] FWA. (Koski 2011)

An increase in personal accountability comes through mechanisms such as certification. I first heard about the widespread Certified IRB Professional (CIP) qualification (a North American professional certification) from Edith, a secretary of a committee in Taiwan. She told me that she had taken the exam but failed. "There are 250 questions on the exam!" she complained. When we first met, she was trying to decide whether to sit the test again. I asked her why she wanted it, and she paused. "To become a professional? When I'm in the IRB, I want to have the test, but it's been two years [since I was a WIRB fellow]. I can't remember the U.S. regulations," she told me.

> Just like IRB, this qualification is just for the name. In Taiwan, five people here have the CIP, and they tell others it is *very* difficult. Many tried and failed, even famous profs who have conducted clinical trials. [They] just thought "It's just about clinical trials and ethics." I think they failed 'cos CIP is about CFR, which is U.S. regulations. So, not very important for Asia[n] people. But if you say you have it, people will think you're good.

In the international currencies of certification, then, CIP is promoted by the American professional association Public Responsibility in Medicine and Research (PRIM&R). Originating in dinner groups of people trying to stay on top of burgeoning regulations in the 1970s when, as longtime PRIM&R board member Ada Sue Selwitz said "there was no such thing as a professional research administrator" (PRIM&R 2009), the organization has seen "management of [. . .] human subjects committees become not only an accepted but also a respected profession" (PRIM&R 2009). "PRIM&R are different from FERCAP," Edith told me:

> They really provide education, and they earn lots of money [through doing it]. One day can cost $600 USD! They know how to make money, they go to each state, they provide Ethics 101, 201. And they encourage the CIP. It costs $438. You need to prepare, study. No Americans fail, only foreigners, because of the language barrier.

Since the CIP was based on U.S. regulations, neither Cristina nor Juntra had taken the exam, and had told Edith it wasn't so relevant to research based in her country. But the logic of individual certification followed from committee recognition so clearly that FERCAP did, in 2008, try out what Edith called an "imitation" of the CIP. FERCAP's version was called CERP, Certification for Ethics in Research Proficiency. Based on "credentialing" and focusing "specifically on the individual" and their "current knowledge in an international and specialised area of practice" (Lee 2008), passing CERP would allow successful candidates to use the designation after their names. "But it didn't work," Edith told me, "nobody wanted to take it. There was a meeting in Taipei, but only a few people came. There were more speakers than audience!" Edith thought while it was a good idea, the low uptake was largely because it was not (yet) a formal requirement. This reminds us of something not made obvious in the direct comparison between the CIP and the CERP: that research ethics is not a profession in Asia in the same way as it is in the U.S. For all but the secretarial staff of committees, the role is a voluntary one, on top of existing duties or work.

Belief in Ethics

Deep within the technocratic operationalization of ethics, Forum participants and committee members talk about growth in capacity. But what does "ethical enough" look like? And who, or what, is making whom ethical? At a FERCAP Strategic Planning session in Shanghai, June 2010, meeting attendees were preparing PowerPoints for use in trainings. During the first session after lunch, Juntra was sitting at a computer, comparing versions of the FERCAP logo in order to select one for a standardized PowerPoint to be used across the network: "This one is nice, but the letters are not nice. When the proportions are wrong, it's not the logo anymore! It should be a flame, like this, it should go up." I took the opportunity to ask about the logo in more detail. "It is the flame of enlightenment," she told me, "to revive and fan a passion for ethics and research." Her description encapsulates how "ethics" can be simultaneously thought of as an international system of committees and a *state of mind*. "It's the same as when you change your paradigm," she told me. "This thing may be obvious for some person, but others can't see it until they cross that line." We were sitting opposite one another around a table at the workshop, and she put her hands on her laptop screen that formed a barrier between us. "It's hard to explain when you don't cross [gesturing to her side of the screen] when you're on this side [gesturing to my side of the screen]. However much I tell you, it doesn't mean anything until you cross the line." My face must have betrayed confusion, because she continued with another example. "Do you ride a bicycle?" I nodded.

> You can ride a bicycle now, but before you could, why [was it] so hard? Do you remember that first time? That moment, the first time you ride the bike, you remember. That's why I try to find examples, what does it mean, when you can't do it, you can't do it, you can't do it, then you suddenly can do [it]. Take that moment.

Some trainings were thought to produce this effect more than others. Cristina, who had been following our conversation, warned the others present not to expect the participants to reach this understanding immediately. "At the beginning the participants wouldn't care," she told me, "then they start to listen." Calling the workshop "transformative," she grinned at me: "You see them change." FERCAP trainings are not merely targeted at making students realize their own ignorance and seek to overcome it; rather, the aim is a transformation of attitude or, in Juntra's terms, "paradigm."

While I thought this sounded idealistic, many interviewees gave accounts that argued for an ethics beyond the slides and SOPs. During a lunch break on a GCP course in Chulalongkorn University, Bangkok, in April 2010, I was talking to Cathy, a committee member, about the presentations we had seen that morning. My head was full of the complexity of compliance, and Cathy nodded along, but after a pause, she pointed out something she thought I hadn't quite grasped. "There is one thing you haven't mentioned," she said: "the integrity of the researcher." Cathy argued that no rule could cover everything, "every aspect and every speech of the doctor to the patient." Pointing to the limits of ethics as a formalized, rule-bound conceptualization, she told me that "only the integrity of the doctor will control good or bad science and research." She hoped this understanding would be passed between members in her institution:

> When you are young staff, and you haven't come to an ethical issues course and you don't know much. Still, if someone told you, "This is the rule," even if you don't know yet you will not avoid a rule or do something against it or behind the backs of others. So first you recognize that it is a rule. Then someone says there are ethical issues, and if someone has a good integrity, to be a good doctor, they will go to the course. And start to understand it. That's when they start to understand what it means to be ethical; you *become* ethical not just in your rules but in your life and your mind.

What Cathy makes very clear is that there can be no rule that governs social interaction, for wherever we look—the conference, the room of the ethics committee, the Survey, and of course (most obviously) doctors and patients—the relationships cannot be reduced to rules. More is hoped for in this enculturation than rule-following; in my focus on standardization, I had—for Cathy—missed the point. "Regulators cannot do what integrity, and the culture of a faculty can do," she said, "people need to want to be good." Her reaction to the standardization we were learning about in our GCP sessions was to root action in the staff, not in the rules.

In FERCAP trainings, learning to see ethics, to really understand, is felt to lie beyond their implementation of activities and training committees. We have seen hints of this already, with a moral value placed on acting through *belief*, not through policing. Sri Lankan bioethics advocate Athula Sumathipala, for example, argues that researchers can be guided to do quality research "because they *believe* in the ethical framework," going on to tell researchers that they "should become an ethical researcher because you believe in it and not because somebody has started to police you" (2006, 78). This and other invocations of the idea of *belief* in an ethical framework interested me, as I had heard it elsewhere. At the opening of a Surveyor's training, one Surveyor described his transformation and how FERCAP had helped him "see" ethics in these terms:

> Well, before 2005, I'm just like you, some of you. I sit in the audience for the first time when Cristina came to [City X] to give a symposium on SOP. I was not an IRB member in that moment, so I had no idea, though I knew what it [ethics] was. Then I had a chance to learn a lot from Dr. Torres and Dr. Juntra. So thanks to them, we had the opportunity to visit WIRB for six months. And after that Cristina gave us a lot of chances to visit other IRB, a kind of field trip. So, we learned from the book then we learned from reality.

These moments, in conjunction with the language of "belief," prompted the single occasion on which I addressed ethics and religion directly with Cristina and Juntra. We were having lunch together in Bangkok between training sessions, and I asked about their experiences across the region with religion and ethics. Cristina responded:

> Each religion is thinking about the common good. No matter what your religion, it's about the good for the other person. In the Philippines, I say it's *not* about Catholic dogma. The idea in EC is to respect how a person thinks. *That's* autonomy. Respect his conscience, how he thinks. How you relate it to your belief system, well that is one area Asians are different—things are not in boxes.

In emphasizing the *distinction* between ethics and "Catholic dogma" Cristina was focusing implicitly on general principles abstracted from religions and applied in an ethics committee setting. Commentators point out the difficulty of separating religious and ethical thought, even down to the language used for concepts (Hongladarom 2004). At the same time as FERCAP members claim a space for ethics separate from the language of religion, they find it difficult. Ethics has merographic qualities, seemingly equally part both of the secular (medical) world and spaces of faith, fully encompassed by neither (Strathern 2018). Catholic Surveyors who attend churches while abroad on Surveys joke that "you can follow the same all over, you know where you are, it has SOPs!" bringing the formalistic Standard Operating Procedure language into the ritual of Latin mass. Buddhist teacher-pupil relationships bind with research ethics to produce personal quandaries framed in the language of research ethics. In Manila, I laughed with Taiwanese Surveyors who were former student and teacher over our snack options. As the local hosts introduced the snacks brought in to keep our energies up, the student offered to eat his teacher's *balut,* a boiled egg snack containing a partially developed, crunchy duck embryo. The offer, he joked, would spare his teacher the consequences of an "unethical act." Spilling over, discussions of what is right and wrong led to reflections on fairness, balance, empathy, compassion, and even semblances of conversion as committee members are brought to "see" ethics more clearly. To locate ethics ethnographically is to attend to how it is made sense of, even or perhaps especially where it takes on the language of belief.

Evaluating Ethics

The medical interventions that ethics committees assess are interventions on the body, oriented at relieving pain and bringing about healing. Ethics has been central to the practice of medicine since its inception, and the relationship of the two is subject to shifts in comprehensions over both what the body is and what it means to practice medicine toward a cure. Thus, an ethnographic approach that focuses on its extensibility must also read the time of ethics. Discussing Rosalind Rey's work on pain during the enlightenment, Talal Asad argues that "the secularization of pain signals not merely the abandonment of a transcendental language ('religious obsessions') but the shift to a new preoccupation—from the personal attempt at consoling and curing (that is, inhabiting a social relationship) to a distanced attempt at investigating the functions and sensations of the living body" (2003, 48, cited in Hirschkind 2010). I suggest that this "new preoccupation" is advanced in the kind of biomedicine to which research ethics committees attend, and particularly in countries newly adopting multi-sited clinical trials, with their requirements from sponsors and auditors. As Bob Simpson and Salla Sariola put it for an Australian sponsored trial in Sri Lanka, "doctors, who might otherwise follow their disposition as healers [. . .] are no longer operating in craft-mode but are recast as mechanical and meticulous monitors of the body and its functions" (2012, 565).

However, perhaps a "transcendental language" is not entirely abandoned. Ethics is capacious, after all. As it extends from bureaucratic requirements to quality management, professional standards and beliefs, an obsessional quality falls not for questions of faith but those arising in practices of quality assurance, audit, and monitoring. Much of what is described in this chapter is recognizable as self-management, where "the manager . . . gets internalized:

externally imposed control becomes internally generated motivation" (Martin 1997, 241, cited in Strathern 2004, 10). The internalization—a relocation—of control, and change into motivation—a conversion—has been widely discussed by scholars of audit and organizational theory, even framed as being "dependent on a compliant soul who will [. . .] seek to achieve the kinds of norms and standards expected of them in the ritual context" (Scott 2022, 33). However, there is a prior question that governance demands: In order to govern and in order to make people into what you want them to be, you must have an idea of what the people you wish to influence *already are*. You are working from an idea of what was long termed "human nature." For the Taiwanese Surveyor Dr. Sam, these ideas were regionally bound. We had just eaten breakfast at a noodle bar, and he was driving me to the hospital to meet up with the Surveyors. His job that day was to introduce ethics principles, and he explained that in his view these documents governed ideas of who someone really was: "America has Belmont, Europe has Helsinki. We have Confucius. It just depends if you want to do it or not." In his equation of the declarations of Belmont and Helsinki with Confucius, Sam is elevating them to the status of philosophies that provide resources through which to understand "ethics." However, in Sam's view, these documents revealed profoundly different reasons for having ethics committees in different places, focusing on the fusion of personal character and regulation. What he argued, as he approached this statement, is that Americans have a different idea of what rules are *for*:

> In U.S. [they] use IRB to limit and regulate research because [they] believe humans are bad, personality is bad. In Chinese, we believe the personality is good but sometimes we need to have regulations. So, we give a lot of regulations for people because everyone knows regulation is good for research subject[s]. But in our education system we already put ethical education in our primary schools, through to university.

In chapter 6 I showed that not everyone with whom I spoke agreed that law, as a separate realm of social control, is where ethics should lie. Interviewees in the preceding chapters have opined eloquently on ethics coming from "within," ridiculing the notion that ethics should take documented, fixed form. One scoffed at the idea that it ever could: "It's like saying someone is beautiful . . . How can you prove you are right?" While both Koski and this speaker are applying the standards of evidence to ethics, the former seeking proof that "ethics"—the committees and their procedures—are working, the "ethics" spoken of by the latter does not lend itself to such methods of proof. If, however, ethics is viewed as a set of measurable processes, then it *can* be proven. It is on this distinction that FERCAP's work hinges. It does not seek to prove it is "right" about the content of decisions. Instead, it audits, measures, codifies, and checks the processes. Providing evidence for an ethics review is the focus of the Survey; providing evidence for the efficacy of ethics review is a growing concern.

But the other focus made evident by Koski is the changed practitioners. FERCAP's objective is not merely to measure, reorder, and record; they seek to transform people by "putting ethics into them," "making them see," and eliciting a personal response. What the ethnographic moments presented reveal is the way in which these terms simultaneously rely on and collapse into one another. "Ethics" is slippery. What, for example, holds quality and ethics apart? In her ethnography of "best practice" in Chinese management consulting, the anthropologist Kimberly Chong argues for the achievement of best practice as an ethical orientation (2018). In the ethnography of this chapter, we see how both quality and ethics are hinged together through "belief," how ethics itself can be thought of as a form of belief or state of mind resulting in a transformation. The profession model encourages accountability to one's fellow professionals, something of which one is *already* a part. The mutual implication committees in the Survey take is another example of the way in which professionals can be constituted through others, becoming what one might call dividually professional. Such a model requires of them not only the enactment of a form of public accountability turned inward, but also a form of personal transformation, rendered most memorably in a description of a chairperson I heard during the 2009 conference: "A chair cannot tell people to be ethical if he or she is not ethical. You cannot be having an affair."

Anthropologists have been thinking about how people manage the moral implications of their social affairs since the inception of the discipline. Bryan Turner reflects that for French sociologist Émile Durkheim, "morality and moral force is always to be discovered in 'something that goes beyond the individual, and to the interests of the group he belongs to' (Durkheim 1992, 24)" (1992, xxxii). In her recourse to "moral force," this is what Cristina is pushing for. The good professional is a good compromise: It can accommodate both the scientific goal-oriented measurement as well as appeals to duty-based ethics.

Duty can be invoked in a way that employs the "moral force" of a (professional) community, be that the nascent community of FERCAP's ethical professionals or the biomedical professions from which most members of committees come. One way of reading the placement of ethics as a duty in her statement "if you don't do your duty then you're not a good professional" is to see that Cristina's ethics *is* professionalism, the separation collapsed. For all the work of externalizing ethics "outside" of medicine and the concomitant rise of audit, the idea of ethics is shifting back toward ethics as something located *within* the practicing professional.[6]

Taking a progression of professional *anthropological* codes as his material, Peter Pels has argued that the ethical code that attends to the ethos of self-auditing is aligned with the production of marketable selves (2000). The example of the CIP serves different "technologies of self" from those addressed to professional duties oriented toward a public domain. It is also the division that has implicitly structured the thesis, moving from ethics committees as an "external," recognizable form of governance to "ethics" as people's "internal" reactions and convictions. Drawing upon the philosopher Alastair MacIntyre ([1984] 2007), Pels reminds us of the concept of an ideal toward which every person would strive, which he suggests is missing from contemporary ethics. Where striving for ethics blurs with striving for quality, I suggest a dimension that MacIntyre's "lost element" pushes forward. Quality—especially in its "total quality management" mode—demands that when committees are surveyed, they commit to being "the best we can be," in a regime that recognizes no possibility of completion. The language enrolled is that of belief, as in the PowerPoint closing statement from a Taiwanese committee: "Our belief: To pass the accreditation of SIDCER is to affirm our IRB's unceasing improvement." Unceasing improvement harnesses ethics and hope in anticipation of and engagement with an infinite project, a project that is not just an abstraction. Inspired by the materiality of ethics it becomes anchored in specific futures, materialized in dreams toward which people work.

EIGHT

Dreams for an Ethics to Come

Research ethics, fashioned into a domain of expert knowledge with concomitant professionals, is a site of dreams for a better future. Explicit or not, this is part of capacity building's future orientation, summoned "because the future it works towards is seen as more desirable than the present" (Douglas-Jones and Shaffner 2021, 2). But during fieldwork I realized just how many different dreams fell under that umbrella, how many different paths people imagined would take them there. I found myself orienting my ethnographic attention "towards orientations" (Bryant and Knight 2019, 201), not least the "fragile and tentative ways in which the present is projected into the future" (Bryant and Knight 2019, 193). To consider the future orientations present in this chapter is to take seriously "the place of desire, fantasy and anxiety in the production of expert knowledge" (Boyer 2008, 43). While dreams might seem not to belong to bureaucracy, for the psychoanalyst Ben Kafka, it has ever been thus: Bureaucratic practice transforms the "insignificant, however briefly, however incompletely" into an "opportunity to fulfill fantasies of power and powerlessness, revenge and love" (2012, 144).

Desire, fantasy, and anxiety are not always confessed in interview settings. They can, however, play out in public, as initiatives to bring others along, or because those speaking of their personal envisaged futures consider them so obvious as to be unremarkable. In 2017, I traveled to Brussels for the closing conference of a large European research project called SATORI, Stakeholders Acting Together on the Ethical Impact Assessment of Research and Innovation. The event, held in a series of rooms named after European capital cities in a nondescript conference center, marked the end of the four-year study aiming to "develop a common framework of ethical principles and practical approaches" for research ethics (SATORI 2014).[1] I attended both out of curiosity about the project itself, and because it was a chance to meet up with

Cristina, who had been invited to travel from Manila to speak about FERCAP's work on the Globalization and Ethics Assessment panel. Conferences are familiar to the point of banality for academics. From time to time, anthropologists have turned their attention to their own ritual gatherings—and those of others—to analyze what it is that compels people to travel large distances, meet, and discuss. In their studies of professionalized communities and experts, scholars have found themselves, as I did, conducting fieldwork at conferences, listening to papers being given and break-time conversation shared (Mead and Byers 1968; Høyer Leivestad and Nyqvist 2017). As Cristina stood in the hall called "Europe A" laying out her network's activities, she framed them neatly within the panel's theme of globalization. Here, I saw FERCAP's work discussed in Europe and, for the first time, saw an explicit comparison with European initiatives to build capacity in ethical review. Various SATORI deliverables had been laboriously mapped onto national "European values," unsurprisingly demonstrating that while committees and review exist across most countries Europe, there are vast differences in how review is institutionalized and gulfs of disagreement about supposedly fundamental European principles (Shelley-Egan et al. 2016, 85). Coordinated by philosophers, funded by the European Union's Horizon 2020 program, one of the project's stated ambitions had been to develop an International Organization for Standardization (ISO) standard for European ethics review.

Founded in London in 1947 and today based in Geneva, the ISO regime is the product of seventy years of attempts to end "technical nationalism" (Yates and Murphy 2019). The standards it produces range from the correct running of phlebotomy laboratories to the right way to brew tea (ISO 2019), the latter now in its second edition. However, as the sociologist Lawrence Busch has pointed out, there has been a growing realization amongst standards bodies of "the difficulty of keeping standards for things and those for people apart" (2011, 26).

Given my experiences with FERCAP over the prior decade, SATORI's ISO ambition seemed both an absurdly fascinating proposal and a reflection of the scale of European ambitions for efficiency and identity tied up in funding grants. Reporting on the progress of their project, members of SATORI revealed wrestles with their uneasy assumptions: Surely a Europe-wide agreement on ethics review processes was possible? Surely the creation of Europe-wide standards for ethics was desirable? FERCAP seemed, from afar, to represent success in what the SATORI project was aiming at, albeit with nearly two decades of work to the European project's four. Cristina's presentation initially seemed to confirm the similarities: "Like Europe," Cristina asserted, opening her talk, "the Asia-Pacific is very similar in terms of its diversity, its social, cultural, and political systems, the developed and developing economies. We [FERCAP] had to situate ourselves within this particular context and address the diversities at the same time as we try to harmonize the practices of the research ethics committees." The European ISO initiative had partially failed; about this the philosophers were none too surprised. Questions posed to Cristina afterward revealed the curiosity of the audience (and their starting assumptions) about the success of her initiative: Did FERCAP start with European regulations and go from there? Were there Association of Southeast Asian Nations (ASEAN) regulations that they had used? Cristina's presence in Brussels was an indicator of FERCAP's international profile as well as a reflection of how few truly *sustained* initiatives there have been in ethics review capacity building. But the question I was left with, on the train to the airport that evening, was one of the place of standardization initiatives in ethical review. What, I wrote in my notebook, is the problem to which the standardization of ethics procedures is the solution?

Standardization is a dream pursued by European projects, with an ISO standard as an envisaged outcome. But as Cristina spoke of harmonization, something that is also present, as legal scholar Mark Flear precisely identifies, is the ICH "mission of 'harmonization for better health,'" which "set[s] and shape[s] an imaginary of the future" (2021, 5). That additional dimension is an implicit "judgment on the present state of health; there is something lacking and it is possible to make it *better* through harmonization" (Flear 2021, 7). This is a powerful imaginary. But other dreams circulate for the future of research ethics review. In this final chapter I juxtapose dreams review held by ethics committee members in Sri Lanka, the U.S., and Taiwan, reflecting on their relationship to policy priorities. At a remove from everyday capacity-building priorities like offices and paperwork, these dreams reveal more than the imagined systems or structures of an international research regime. Amidst risk assessments, balance sheets of benefits, and conflicts of interest, a vision of the world "as it could be" comes forth as a strong motivator in this ethnographic material. We are now familiar with Juntra's vision in which, through the work of her international Strategic Initiative, FERCAP incorporates good ethics as part of a system approach to clinical trials, themselves contributing to improved medical research and ultimately better quality of life for patients. As she put it herself, "when I close my eyes . . . I have energy because I want to see Ethics Committees in different countries recognized by criteria we set out. Every year I count and I am happy when it increases fast."

In Annelise Riles's view, this kind of collision of dreaming and technocracy is not as unexpected as one might think. Her key interlocutor in Tokyo, Sato, works on something called a Real Time Gross Settlement (RTGS) project within the Japanese finance sector that he hopes will have "effects on the character of *people* in the market" (Riles 2011, 175). Technocratic work goes hand in hand with dreams, says Riles, an act of small-scale personal utopianism predicated on a "distance between the world as others see it and the world as it could be" (Riles 2011, 178). Building on her work, Flear and Richard Ashcroft argue that imaginaries "govern, in part, by enabling and shaping certain political and policy conversations, while disabling others, which in turn helps to determine the selection and effectiveness of legal and regulatory tools, processes and discourses" (2021, 4). Of course, it matters where and how "individual dreams and aspirations take hold and acquire collective force only when key actors mobilize the resources for making their visions durable" (Jasanoff 2015, 25). But as I found, technocratic dreams reveal a desire for certain kinds of people, and the extensibility of ethics means it becomes easily available for thinking the ethical beyond the bureaucratic. Dreams are personal and presented as the outcomes of individual experiences, yet here they stand for more than themselves, for threads of future-making that recur or exceed the given instance. One move is to make ethics like other things: more like laboratory practice, more like standard measures that can be handled consistently around the world. Another is to seek a systems approach, with innumerable, interlocking, moving parts. Still others dream of a future in which ethics is no longer necessary, fully incorporated into the practices of doctors through changes to their biomedical training. I share these radically distinct dreams for ethics, the future and capacities for a world to come, because in them, we find futures where ethics is in some way resolved, completed, or perhaps even obsolete.

Dreams for Laboratories of Ethics

I met Dr. Bartholomew Shar, who served on an ethics committee in at the University of Ruhuna in southern Sri Lanka, several years before the 2017 SATORI conference in Brussels. A genetics researcher working extensively with laboratory data, his interests lay in the advancement of Sri Lankan science, and standards as a means of participation in global economies of research. I took the train that follows the country's coast with the Indian Ocean south from Colombo to Galle, and the next day made my way to the Medical Faculty to find him in his offices. During our interview, Dr. Shar told a story that intertwined ethics with his professional expertise in genetics, particularly lab-based research. If laboratory figures were wrong, he explained, there would be consequences for patients and public health policy in the country, and research itself would suffer. His position was that with the right procedures and standards, inaccurate figures could be fixed. Our conversation weaved back and forth, as his dream for laboratory standards in Sri Lanka seemed to make possible—and desirable—his second dream: standardization in ethics.

Once settled in his office, desk full of papers and filing cabinets, I started by asking Dr. Shar to describe what he did on his ethics committee. "Well, we take a file like this," he said, holding his hands four inches apart to indicate the large volume of paperwork. "I review in my area, how much blood needs to be collected, what is routine, volume and timing issues, transportation, genetics and social issues." The remit he has just reeled off is an expanding chute, beginning with a vial of blood and ending with "social issues." To illustrate, he links those "social issues" to a particular case, re-grounding the concerns of his committee:

> For example, a thalassemia[2] carrier. Someone comes with a proposal to detect, but are they going to inform those from whom they took the samples? The garment factory girls, they have a [thalassemia] prevalence of three percent or something, but when you really do have that prevalence data, what will you do? If you convey that they are a carrier, there is no counseling adequate. It affects marriages. Sri Lanka is . . . a very Asian country. Marriage and these things are very serious. Once you are having an affair, it seems you will marry, the social pressure is there. If you are married, even though probably there will be dispute[s], or you are not matching well, the majority choose to continue marriage even though it's hell. It's not like in your country, where it is not necessary to suffer for life. The question comes because of sociocultural differences between countries. When we consider ethics, it's similar to something hand in hand with human rights. Whether it's Australia, Africa, U.S., UK, I think research ethics should be the same internationally. It's a sort of standardization

> of research for an acceptable level. So, for example, if there's a lab diagnostic test, we have accreditation—it comes from the Sri Lanka accreditation board. I'm an assessor. If we accredit, the certificate will be accepted. It's ISO15189, the standard for medical quality of diagnostic tests for that lab. It means it's the same as any lab, anywhere in the world.

I have shared the entirety of Dr. Shar's answer above to show the transition within his story from thalassemia to diagnostic laboratories, via a standardized model of ethics. Dr. Shar was not simply making a *comparison* between the systematization afforded by ISO standards, he was making the processes of standardization *equivalent*, thus changing the capacity of those objects for variation. Put differently, in his view, a scientifically designed manner of measuring and controlling laboratory machinery had produced a desirable state of global interchangeability, accountability, and trust. Consider the things that an Ethics ISO would solve for him:

> [For the laboratories] we get international recognition and when you come to hospital, [you] don't have to worry about the quality of the service. If you have your own level of guidelines, or you differ from other countries, how much the gaps can be a problem, not be acceptable. Expect standard up to when [to] diagnose diabetes should be same, between U.S., UK, Sri Lanka. So, it's the same with ethics. If we try to stick to [our] own principles and guidelines, we'll try to avoid some aspects of guidelines practiced in other countries. This might be advantageous for our researchers in a way but considering internationalization and globalization, will it be acceptable internationally?

Again, in the crossing over of biomedical models (the diagnosis of diabetes) with the question of research ethics, Dr. Shar is applying principles from ISO training to what he regards as an equal problem of international standards. He went on to tell me how his training in laboratory standards had come about. A cabinet paper, presented under the Ministry of Science and Technology, had established a Sri Lankan accreditation board (SLAB), which received funding from a Swedish Government grant, Swedish International Development Cooperation Agency (SIDA), via the Swedish Board for Accreditation and Conformity Assessment (SWEDAC). Trainers from Sweden arrived and stayed in Sri Lanka for three weeks, assessing, guiding, and supervising. They offered qualifications, through an examination which Dr. Shar described as "continuous surveillance." "They were behind us when we were conducting assessments, walking without saying a single word. At the end of the day, they would say, 'These are the inadequacies.' They raised all the nonconformities, and we corrected all of these things." Dr. Shar qualified as a technical assessor and consultant. He began accrediting laboratories in September 2009, in accordance with ISO 15189, an international standard for the quality of laboratory testing.[3] But the mutual recognition that the training and assessment had ensured would expire. "You can do this, but next year, even in the next six months, you have to improve," he said. The acceptability of variation in laboratory accuracy and ethics fits his vision of how research in his country is changing:

> We are a fast-developing country. The next step is research. We need to characterize our patients, diseases, compare the therapeutic efficacy of drugs invented elsewhere. Lots of factors can influence each disease. Even for reference ranges we depend on a textbook. We chose the Western figures from these books—is it correct? We can see from experience [a blood measurement is] usually twelve to fourteen, but we don't know if it's nutritional, or due to ethnic difference.

The interview moved rapidly in the direction of his research, but for Dr. Shar, this was also ethics. I listened as he patiently explained how the availability of diagnostics limits his ability to publish. If he uses high-performance liquid chromatography (HPLC), an accepted method all over the world, he can send his work to journals. If he uses what is available—cellulose acetate Hb (hemoglobin) electrophoresis—he cannot. He worries about the accuracy errors of his uncalibrated machines, and insists on the need for external quality: "You don't know the value [of the machines] the external body does." Extrapolating from his experience with ISO quality review, Dr. Shar insisted that the ethics review committees should themselves be reviewed:

> I am sure if we're to say we're an ERC, to give approval on projects, we should also be reviewed. They'd have to see if we're doing it in a proper way. Sometimes researchers might find fault with members of committee. To be transparent, we need proper documents there. If it's in a document, we can say, if the checklist fits it'll be correct. If these things are uniformly maintained, one researcher won't be annoyed. If we come under the umbrella [they will say] if you're going to be our member, you need this. They give us the documents. That should be uniform to the country, region, globally eventually, one fine day, if you had

> applied to any ERB, if one granted, then all others should have granted. Should be uniform, nationally, then regionally, then globally.

Dr. Shar is describing much of what makes FERCAP successful: They do the work he desires—review committees, assess them, ensure the presence of documentation, and bring committees under an umbrella. Yet he takes the scaling a step further, locating uniformity within FERCAP and the links the capital's ethics committee had with "outside agencies." To these agencies he looked to "make sure we keep up with standards that [a] regulatory body would want. It's a big job providing technical know-how." His concern was that, without this, different committees would become known for their decision-making: "You might say Galle ERC [is] very strict but if [you] send [it] to Peradeniya, much more lenient, maybe a similar project [would be] given approval." This practice, known in the U.S. as "IRB shopping," is a topic with decades of discussion—without resolution (Malakoff 2002; Spellecy and May 2012; Spellecy et al. 2024). Dr. Shar had a plan for counteracting this effect: first, national standards, then international ones, a path of resolution through standard processes that would give rise to standard decisions. In the next dream, the standards and standardization take an equally expansive form.

Dreams for Trials as Planes

During the summer months of 2018, the British Standards Association (BSA) put out for consultation a new document called ACRES-QC S001. The acronym refers to a new Quality Continuum Standard for the Quality Management of Clinical Research Sites, created by the Alliance for Clinical Research Excellence and Safety (ACRES). Founded in 2012, ACRES is a nonprofit "multi-stakeholder collaborative" of actors aiming toward a global network that will, in their words, "enable sponsors, regulators, service providers, ethics committees, research sites, and patient subjects to be connected as never before, to share and more effectively use information across the entire clinical research enterprise, benefiting all stakeholders" (ACRES 2014). I first heard Dr. Greg Koski speak about ACRES as part of an online webinar held in December 2011.[4]

> I'm going to ask you to just suspend your disbelief for a minute and imagine the possibility of a global network that includes perhaps 120,000 clinical research sites, each one of which is fully accredited by independent accrediting agencies, according to international standards, standards that are established by the

> public working in conjunction with regulatory authorities, ethicists and others, so we have a truly global standard for quality and safety that's accepted around the world. Each of these accredited sites would be staffed by a fully trained and certified professional research team. These sites would be connected, interconnected through a very robust webpage information system that would allow real-time capture of important performance information but also important safety information so that we're continually watching to see how things are done, continually monitoring adverse events, pharmaco-vigilance, in order to truly do something that if there's an early signal for potential harm to research subjects with a class of drugs that we identify those before harm is done and take steps as appropriate to fix that. All of these independent sites would operate under a fully integrated and accredited human research protection program, the exact model for that we don't know but perhaps something that would involve various levels: a central review in combination with local review, not that there'd be dual ethical review, but perhaps a centralized ethics and scientific review that would work in tandem with local review to determine whether or not it's appropriate to do a study in a particular location. We'd start with the assumption that any research study that might be done globally in fact would be ethical everywhere that it's done and the only question would be not whether it's ethical or scientifically sound but that it be appropriate for the standards prevailing in local community and the resources available to do it. The model that I've just described to you in terms of a global network is in fact very much in the limelight these days through an initiative we started about two years ago, called ACRES, the Alliance for Clinical Research Excellence and Safety.

Koski continued, like Dr. Shar, developing an analogy by which his dream could be understood:

> ACRES is working to build this kind of global clinical research network based on a model that's derived from the global air transportation system. You know, back in 1945, the airlines realized that in order to be able to fly planes safely around the world, and get people to be comfortable flying on them, they were going to have to be able to have a global network of airports that allowed for planes to take off in Boston and fly to Brussels before they go on to Mumbai and Singapore and know that every place a plane was going to take off and land it was going to be handled through the same kind of SOPs and procedures that are accepted by all of the stakeholders to ensure that it's going to be done safely and it doesn't matter there's a system so there's no confusion about how its done.

> Over the years the organization known as IATA, the International Air Transport Association, has worked to build this kind of network and we know today that although the global airlines are every bit as competitive as the global Pharmas, you know. We know drug research today is very much an international endeavor. If we had a new system that was based on the model of professionalism that I've described before, with the adoption of standardized policy and procedures for safety, we'd have the opportunity to completely revolutionize the way clinical research is done around the world today.

The analogy is not unique. During the FERCAP Conference in 2008, Dr. Beat Widler, then working for Roche, gave a presentation on "Promoting Human Subjects through the Risk Management Approach." He opened with the familiar *Time* magazine slide ("From this image of perception"), moved to an image of Florence Nightingale ("to this assurance"), and followed with a slide titled "we need" and a photo of an American Airlines jet taking off, the logo of BAE Systems "JetEye" in the corner and sensors, lasers, control electronics, and control panels demonstrating the breadth of risk management in the aviation industry.

Where ethics shifted to measurement through Dr. Shar's analogy in the dream above, here it is elided with safety. The absence of ethics from the ACRES acronym is only part of the shift. In Dr. Koski's comparison with global air transport, as with Dr. Shar's comparison with ISO measurements, concerns are regarded as *so* analogous that differences between them are erased. Here, the unspoken concern alongside safety is trust: the trust of a public participating in clinical trials, thought lost. The real-time reporting of data and the safety of planes offers a working model. In his linkage of air transport and ethics, Koski is putting forward three principles: "technology, complete and accurate information, and trust."[5]

Through the accounts I have given of FERCAP's Survey work, objectivity has been sought, made, and manipulated as a technique both of scientific and of political power. However, the machines of objectivity in this dream create a network not of active people but of passive watching as the technology reports. While we cannot call Koski's dream "*small*-scale personal utopianism," it certainly supports Riles's claim that dreams sit alongside technocratic thought. An industry newsletter interview with Koski heralds the ideal of global systems interoperability:"Systems engineers are creating a global technology network using off-the-shelf equipment" (Olds 2014). Koski knows that "integrity" of researchers has previously been the focus of a stack of reports on the conduct of research by the U.S. Institute of Medicine (IOM 1989, 1992, 1993, 2009). Much of what he recommends has been said before:

> Individual scientists in cooperation with officials of research institutions should accept formal responsibility for ensuring the integrity of the research process. They should foster an environment, a reward system and a training process that encourage responsible research practices. (IOM 1992, 13)

Yet *integrity* is hard to measure: What standardized test can chart something that only offers hope because of its exteriority to the logic of audit?

Dreaming the Dead

A radically different imagined future comes from interviews with ethics committee members at the Tzu Chi General Hospital in Hualien, Taiwan. As we spoke, they offered an alternative to ethics committees, which tied closely to the education of doctors. In this future, it was not enough to just educate medics in research ethics, it was necessary to intervene in their formation as physicians, from the very beginning. One interviewee began by lamenting the quality of research that was being done, suggesting that the doctors were "well intentioned" but quite "thoughtless" when it came to patient comfort and safety: "Someday we will produce better doctors, our Silent Mentor Program will help with that." I asked some follow-up questions about this program, mostly pursuing my interest in the relationship between ethics review and how researchers were regarded. I learned that in the early 1990s, Taiwan faced a massive shortage in cadavers for medical training purposes. Students were struggling to learn gross basic anatomy. Then, in 1995, a person who "felt she had received a lot from society" donated her body. This act did not go unnoticed by the hospital's Buddhist founder, Master Chen Yen, who, according to my interviewee, said:

> If we could utilize a program as [an] interface to bring out the best of medical students and inspire face to teach students best and use the program to educate people in society that every phenomenon has meaning: getting born, getting sick, and getting death has meaning.

When Edith, the ethics committee secretary observing the interview, saw my interest in the Silent Mentor Program, she arranged for me to visit the unit and have meetings with several of the program coordinators. The visit took place the following day. I was greeted by representatives sharply dressed in navy blue and white. The tone was professional—I was a welcome international guest who had come to find out about the innovative cadaver donation program. The corridors on the perimeter of the second floor were bright and airy. A kind of mummification process meant that cadavers could be kept in a central temperature-controlled room, which my guide, Sam, revealed by drawing a curtain. I was given a view of the darkened space in which embalmed bodies, wrapped in white, rested on narrow metal shelves. There was an extended moment of reverent silence as we gazed in, and Sam closed the curtains again. In a low voice, Sam told me that students come here, and in a tone indicating surprise said, "They even talk to them." We walked the perimeter, looking at the posters and poems, statements by donors and letters from students. Su Chen was one of the Silent Mentors whose extraordinary life caught my eye.

> Teacher was sold by her stepfather to a Taiwanese opera group. Since then, she had been making living by performing at the temples and theaters. Her graceful movement and beautiful voice won her the leading role. At the age of seventeen, she was forced to give up her career and become the mistress of a Taiwanese Mafia Boss. Unfortunately she needed to bear the financial responsibility to support her husband's luxury lifestyle. Working diligently, she gradually expanded her green onion stall into a market with six hundred stalls. After her friends and husband took over her business forcefully, she indulged herself in excessive drinking. Since becoming a Tzu Chi volunteer, she had found the new meaning of life and wished to encourage the frustrated people by her story. She determined to be a silent mentor and to keep on helping others.

Why had the students found out about Su Chen's life in this detail? Why were the walls lined with photographs of donors and the stories of their lives? Why did the organization insist on non-anonymous donors?

Students are required, in the summer before the course, to learn about donors' lives through home visits to the families. Then a memorial blessing ceremony is held, where the four medical students stand opposite the family members, around the anatomy table where the body is placed. Buddhist nuns lead the ceremony with chants. "The body is open so that the family can take [a] last look," Sam told me. "You hear the crying and mourning. At the time, students face great pressure." During the dissection classes, the stories and pictures that the students have gathered are projected on screens and classes begin with "students respectfully and humbly greeting the cadaver." They are encouraged to think of the cadaver as a teacher, and some students address the body directly. Writing in the *British Medical Journal*, Steven Lin and colleagues describe the program:

> The actual dissection course lets students connect their "teachers" to their biographical profile, which rests at the dissection table to serve as a constant reminder of the underlying human story. This custom also promotes mindfulness of the teacher's life experience that may manifest physically. Meeting donors and learning about their lives fosters humanistic values in students, such as gratitude and respect in light of the donors' selfless giving. (Lin et al. 2009, 1439)

At the end of the corridor in Hualien, I was shown into the Great Body Teacher Memorial Hall. The lights came on as the doors opened, illuminating rows of small crystal boxes, crafted in the shape of the Hall of Still Thoughts by a master Taiwanese craftsman. "The ashes of Silent Mentors are placed here. Students sometimes come and visit them," Sam told me. "They come to visit the silent mentors and thank them; some tell me that they confide their difficulties and feel that the silent mentor will continue to look over their shoulder as they work."

In an interview following my tour, the clinical director of the Silent Mentor Program who had taken the English name George explained some of the reasoning behind the program to me in this way:

> There are two parts to being a doctor, one part is a healer, the other is being a professional. It's based on a social contract, between medical society and the whole society, that is medical professionalism . . . [T]he base of medical professionalism has three points. To practice with skill, knowledge, and with morality to service others. However, morality and service are becoming weaker and weaker. How do you design a curriculum to help students learn morality and service to others?

He and other members involved in ethics review repeatedly told me about a change in doctor-patient relationships. Barbara, the lay member on the committee from chapter 5, considered it part of her role on the IRB to "change the atmosphere between medical people and patients." "Because right now," she said, "the relationship sounds like more commercialized—I pay you, you use me. It used to be friends, family doctor [. . .] So have to change relation—doctor, nurse, patient, family. They should be friends, like family." Barbara thought this change in attitude had been in part inspired by research practices. "They think it should be more cold blood, more science style, more powerful." Part of George's solution to designing a course to "help students learn morality" was the Silent Mentor Program, which he described as containing a "hidden curriculum": "We need more good doctors, not more famous or fame making doctors. So, we want to train the student to respect, not just by lecture or television, but by this kind of role model." The role model was the Silent Mentor themself.

Toward the end of an interview with one of the program coordinators, he brought me back to the reason I was in Hualien at all: ethics committees. He had been using a PowerPoint presentation designed for an international audience to help me understand how he saw the relation between the Silent Mentor Program, spirituality, and modern medicine. As he explained to me:

> To study medicine is a kind of spiritual practice. So physicians have to reflect how to contribute to society. If every physician can learn this, there is no need for the IRB. I'd like to use the surgical department, I'd really wish we can, by this foundation, train more and more good surgeons and serve the society and make IRBs unnecessary.

The link between training and the obsolescence of the committee illustrates a different place of hope for the future of ethical research, which falls not in audit but another kind of watching. By transferring the ethics to the researchers, the committee would write itself out of existence. George hopes to replace a committee with a person through a process that renders the external cadaver internal, intended to govern and censure reactions. It anticipates a future, invisible patient who will be the recipient of the trainee doctor's care. What comes to the fore is the question of what an ethical subject is, and what regulation becomes in such a regime. I am reminded of Riles's discussion of the introduction of the Real Time Gross Settlement (RTGS) system in Japan, during which, she tells us, debates raged over the correct involvement of the state in financial markets. Deregulation, in her story, was "framed as putting an end to state interference in the market," but, she says,

> in practice it entailed not so much an end to state intervention as a transformation of the role of the state, from a visible quotidian force to a less visible but arguably far more consequential role of shaping the very nature, preferences

> and objectives of the private actors who populated the market. This is deregulation as transformation rather than disappearance. (Riles 2011, 186)

What Sam's dream reveals is a version of ethics that, like Sato's hope for more rational actors, is directed at altering those who practice, so that through them changes come about. In the comment by the Silent Mentors trainer, he is innovating toward making ethics committees obsolete.

In the introduction to this book, ethics review was portrayed as a weakness in the wider system of biomedical research. From George's point of view, the starting point is the relationship between doctors and patients. I have argued that at the same time as FERCAP is pushing for legal regulation and the systematization of ethics, it is also inspired by the turn toward professionalism in the West, encouraging the creation of an ethos of responsibility. George has a very similar objective, only that he is not orienting the responsibility toward bureaucracy but toward the cultivation of that responsibility in the student. The final dream is the closest we have come in this study of ethics to the patient: The Silent Mentor becomes the archetypal patient, all patients. We might ask, does this "really work"? Does it actually change the attitudes, and more importantly, the behavior of students as they go on to become doctors? While these would be good questions for further research, they are also revealing in themselves. What is interesting to me about the Silent Mentors example was that it *suspended* the monitoring of people and moved the site of that monitoring into their professional personas, through their training. That the dream *existed* was the point.

Dreams of Different Stories

It matters what stories are used to convey the stakes of research ethics. As discussed in chapter 1, for years the majority of training materials contained stories from the United States, with limited examples of experiences that committees in the Asia-Pacific might recognize (Pratt et al. 2014). In her history of research ethics in Holland, Noortje Jacobs observes that history "is used to *justify* the existence of strict oversight mechanisms for human experimentation" (2022, 5), in her case, the invocation of publics as a means of reining in the medical profession. Histories also sustain: Writing about the continued "cultural resonance" of the study in Tuskegee over the "Guatemala story,"

Susan Reverby and Amy Moran-Thomas tell us that "collective relationships and persistence matter—and can be all too necessary—for how history becomes known" (2024, 566). They argue "it was not the facts of the case alone, but also the ways that people and institutions created relationships and practices around them over time that shaped its place in memory" (Reverby and Moran-Thomas 2024, 566). We can describe what they are reaching for in Tess Lea's terms, as a policy "hauntology": a series of "reverberations" (Lea 2024, 3) across settings, and through time, that become—or don't become—the stories told in lecture halls and conference venues.

Recognizing that the stories that don't get told matter, the Forum began to produce casebooks of challenges encountered by committees in the region. The first collection was published in 2012 as the FERCAP/SIDCER *Handbook of Case Studies Ethical Issues in Health Research.* The opening case takes us back to the beginning of this book, and the responsibilities of local committees relative to clinical trials and clinical monitors:

> 18 November 2012. Company ABC is the sponsor for a Phase III trial on an investigational new drug for treatment of tuberculosis. Site YZ has already recruited 60% of the patients for the study. Today, the clinical monitor who is currently on site for the routine monitoring visit calls the sponsor to seek advice. During the review of the study documents/investigator file, he noted that the renewal of the approval of the local REC was not on file. When he asked the principal investigator (PI) he was told that the new approval had not yet been received. The last approval covered the period 15/09/2011 to 30/09/2011. (FERCAP/SIDCER 2012, 9–10)

This first casebook was followed in 2016 with another collection of *Perspectives on Ethical Review* dedicated to Dr. Angela Bowen, founder of Western IRB, who had supported the WIRB fellowship program (2002–2009) and the subsequent Middleton Foundation for Ethical Studies Global Fellows Program (2013). As casebooks were developed by the fellows of different programs, they were distributed at the FERCAP Conference. As downloadable pdfs hosted on FERCAP's website, the collections act as pedagogical resources, but also as regional works of self-description. The second edition, for example, aimed to "demonstrate that perspectives matter: perspectives from varying research protocol types that ethics committees regularly address, perspectives from specific settings and cultural background, but mostly perspectives out of which ethical issues and challenges arise and are addressed" (Karbwang Laothavorn 2016). Atoy Navarro, FERCAP's long-term research fellow who had done much of the editorial work, including anonymizing and editing cases, told me that seeing different committees and watching the Survey in action over his years of coordination had given him cause to reflect on the differences he encountered. "The idea," he said, "is to get to know an idea of the context of the countries in terms of how do they go about ethical issues? Concepts like justice, autonomy, and beneficence, but what do these concepts mean for these countries?" He shares a background in history with Cristina, and explained to me that "histories give you a broader contexts on why these things are happening." He told me:

> In the Philippines, when we talk of ethical issues, it'll always be rooted in how the Spaniards or Americans did health research. The first ethical issues will always be rooted in a colonial experience. For Japan, their particular context is from World War II, they have ethical issues that may be traced, connected to World War II Japanese experiments. If you look at Korea, Dr. Hwang is a product of how they do academic atmosphere and culture in Korea. There, everyone needs to discover, and so there is a lot of research and not much . . . basically there are particular contexts why.

Atoy's final comment, "a context why," gives context as reason. It is not that contexts contain cultures, but that cultures form the ground for ideas of contexts. It is this that, I suggest, aids FERCAP in sidestepping "cultural difference" for "common goals." What is held constant—the similarity—is that there will always be a context, that there *are* contexts is what is alike. This is what Atoy reveals when he brings "context" forward as the rationale for a casebook. "You cannot have a black and white view of things when you don't understand the context, the country," he said of Surveyors.

> Some trials which would in one country be considered risky might be seen to be beneficial to the population, depending on the context. There's not a universality of particular instances and issues. [There] should be contextualization according to country. For example, FERCAP cannot just get people to sit and comment on how an EC do their job without knowing the country context.

He allows the fact that there are "contexts why" to stand as the figure against a ground of "cultural difference." When Cristina says that the "FERCAP experience is about a common goal" (Torres 2011, 52) she is choreographing commonality. In this shift from "cultural difference" to "context," we are subtly encouraged to focus on what is held in common over differences—in Nick Seaver's riff on Strathern, "the nice thing about context is that everyone has it" (Seaver 2015, 1101). Bringing about a dream of casebooks with examples drawn from and relevant to research happening in the committees FERCAP works with is acknowledgment of this.

Capacities for Worlds to Come

Not all the dreams presented in this chapter constitute what Rebecca Bryant and Daniel Knight call "fragile" projections of the present into the future (2019, 193). They are a complicated mix of dream and speculation, with varying degrees of action tied to bringing specific futures into being. Celebrating the tenth anniversary of FERCAP, the chairperson Kenji Hirayama declared that the first decade of FERCAP was "dreaming of our final products that will benefit our own societies and communities. To make this dream come true, EC/IRB quality is essential and at the same time we will need more human resources in the region" (2011, 5). Thinking with and in time is familiar to committee members, because committee work is, in itself, an act of anticipation (Douglas-Jones 2019). While the ethics committee represents a recognizable form of governance, standing "outside" and "above" the actions which it is supposed to regulate (Strathern 1985), it is also a temporally distinct mode of governance. When committee members sit assessing a protocol—its likely implications for participants, its likely contribution to knowledge—all of this occurs in a state of anticipation: ethics of the kind the committee practices happens before research becomes action.

Desire for certainty gives rise to desire for bureaucracy. In Lea's summary of Holly High's work on development programs in Laos, "peoples' desire solicits and completes structural formations . . . enabling criticism and hope to coproduce one another" (High 2014, 175–76, cited in Lea 2021, 67). Struggling to bracket uncertainty about future research, the dreamers borrow from one domain in another, pushing systems of knowledge together in the hope that what works for one type of knowing will work for another. We can see that Dr. Shar's dream of an ISO ethics—made vivid through his analogy with the standardization of laboratory procedures for blood sampling techniques—offers a kind of "natural world" planning for ethics. Stefan Timmermans and Steven

Epstein remind us that "the need for standards emerged when production processes and goods crossed geographical boundaries" (2010, 74). So, what do dreams of the calculability of ethics leave out, eliminate, mangle, as they aim to see like "governing agents" (Kipnis 2008, 282)? Cathy and Sam, experienced practitioners in their research domains and familiar with their colleagues, see regulation as secondary to the desire of a researcher to be good, to behave well. If we were to envisage a pendulum swinging between a monitoring given to the committee and ideas of scientific integrity, then in these dreams, it swings back toward an integrity that responsibilizes the individual scientist and prefigures the policy-led re-institutionalization of integrity within the global project of science. Thus, taking such dreams seriously can allow us to trace patterns in dreaming, offer us maps of where ethical action is thought to be inculcated in the worlds beyond the doors of the committee's review.

CONCLUSION
Committee Worlds

The network at the heart of this book emerged from a tumultuous time in the globalization of research around the turn of the century. Pressure had built amongst scholars of bioethics and medical anthropology to a examine the consequences of the fact that "most of the concepts and international regulatory principles in use continue to be derived from Western cultural values (Hess 1995, 2007; Nader 1996; Harding 2006)" (Strathern et al. 2007). Volumes like Catherine Myser's *Bioethics Around the Globe* collected examples, studying bioethics as a social force taken up by different actors in different settings in a "comparative anthropology" (Myser 2011, xix) of cases. Myser argued that studying the "evolution, cultural meanings, and social functions of bioethics" would allow researchers to consider whether the making of bioethics in their settings would "in the end undermine the ethics enterprise and avowed social justice goals" (Myser 2011, xxxiv). When I set out to understand the role FERCAP was playing in bioethics capacity building, I was prepared for bioethical incommensurability. I expected questions without answers and committee compromise, and I expected ethnography would be necessary for exploring these disjunctions, struggles between the ideals of collaborative partnerships and their funded realities. In short, I anticipated that different ideas of both ethics and personhood would have a significant role, in the necessary contrast between abstracted principles and local attempts to work with them. They did, but not in the ways I expected.

Had I remained with a single committee over the course of my fieldwork, I would no doubt have seen committees discussing—say—consent its local relationship to understandings of science (Jayasinghe et al. 2023). Had I followed a particular trial, I would have seen more strongly the influence of national histories of research, expectations of collaboration, and the personal character of approval (Widger et al. 2022). Had I worked within a single nation state, I would perhaps have seen the way bioethics as a discipline could be enrolled to express university rivalries (Simpson 2011, 47) or the long years of political and social work that have gone into creating national networks, standards, and even legislation. The lives of these national networks and their "regulatory orientations" matter (Sleeboom-Faulkner 2025, 89). They are increasingly being written up for publication by those directly involved, and further work remains to be done on the distinct positions that ethics committees have come to occupy within the national health regulatory systems of each of the countries where FERCAP works. Such analyses will complement our advancing understanding of how some places gain what Margaret Sleeboom-Faulkner terms "regulatory immunity," a combination of reputation and insider-ness that allows countries to "attract scientific collaboration" (2025, 92). Any of these would have been important projects.

Instead, by staying with an NGO, my work became an exploration of how committees both belong to and are used as an entry point into wider research governance capacity building. One of the afterlives of that era of distrust was the construction of my distributed field site. It was built by internationally mobile researchers, whose abstracted principles were the languages of standards, quality, and audit they used to make a case for "local" capacity. This field is made up of those who support committees who, Juntra contended, could review differently—and more appropriately—than those in "Geneva." I have described the skills and techniques used by the NGO to create, interpret, and present research ethics in ways that had purchase precisely for their appearance of "no culture" (Traweek 1992, 162). Their experiences and priorities offer a history of the present, in which total quality assurance, principles of audit, and practices of benchmarking have been summoned as devices through which capacity in research ethics—as part of wider systems—is built. For ethnographers, there is a temptation to see technologies like Standard Operating Procedures and meeting minutes as too familiar or too boring for study. But unless we offer such bureaucratic devices the sustained depth of ethnographic attention, we fail to see the achievements and complexities involved in the development of research infrastructures. Only if we "refine our craft" (Mathur 2017, 8) to the demands of bureaucratic policy can we can follow the emergence and adoption of ideas of continuous improvement, and see how the infrastructures of ethics in its bureaucratic form—particularly quality and audit—work on people, through comparison, inspiration, competition, and cooperation. By asking what worlds the committee carries with it, I have been led to reformulate earlier academic attention to different localized versions of bioethics into one that centers the priorities of a field. Instead of venturing into what they regarded as the unresolvable terrain of bioethics, the network focused on processes. While never articulated as such, they did not go into battle with the philosophical elements of bioethics that consider Standard Operating Procedures the work of "clerks." But nor did they stand for the dismissal of a leadership team of Thai and Philippine women. They lit upon standards and audit as carrying the power of the universal—established as successful through ICH-GCP—and with space within it for national variance. As biomedical researchers, those with whom the worked found standards, quality assurance, and compliance more familiar than philosophy. Unlike bioethics, procedures are measurable, auditable, and accreditable. These are, without doubt, bureaucratic worlds.

In this conclusion, I step back from the labor and politics of committee decisions to return to the questions of what worlds committees bring with them, and what worlds they bring into being. I draw together five worlds I see as particularly consequential—Capacities, Form, Standards, Capital, and Integrity—for what they might teach both policy makers and ethnographers of policy. Because the members of research ethics committees we have met in this book care deeply about research ethics and its role in research, their questions are foundational: How to run a committee that *protects* those who participate in biomedical research? How do you convince researchers of the importance of ethical considerations in research? How to make decisions about global research, weaving together Standard Operating Procedures, strategic quality management, and committee meetings as sites of knowledge politics? And in a now more than twenty-year story of coordinated nongovernmental action, FERCAP's Bangkok-anchored activity has successfully motivated volunteer time and created extensive networked relations, initiating activities across thirteen different countries, dedicating energy, resources, and time to the bureaucratic—and personal—transformations that populate these pages.

Worlds of Capacities With(in) Reach

"And how is *our* ethics?" was one of the first questions asked of me in my research. I was speaking to Renuka, a Sri Lankan researcher from the southern city of Galle during the project-run workshop in Colombo. "And how is *our* ethics?" was a confronting question of comparison. With her arms folded over her sari, Renuka was asking for an evaluation, but she was also questioning the position of a novice ethnographer who wanted to "study ethics review" in her country. While on the surface her question was asking me to draw contrast between the "ethics" of the UK, the country from which I had just told her our research funding and event was originating, and that of postcolonial Sri Lanka, in whose capital city we stood, she was also asking who I was to set up a comparison in the first place. That day, I had no answer for Renuka. I was barely a week into my field research but, as I wrote in my stressed out fieldnotes that day, I didn't think of myself as playing *that particular* comparative game. I was neither an expert in research ethics nor a capacity builder trying to make Sri Lankan ethics committees "better." Renuka's pointed question might have prompted me to embark on a series of my own comparisons using the implicit units of the question: nation states and the "cultural and socio-political differences" FERCAP recognizes. I could have asked how ethical review in Sri Lanka differed from that in the UK, or how the colonial structures of biomedicine, from the blazing white clocktower of Colombo's medical faculty to the secondary status of Ayurvedic medicine, shaped deliberations in ethics review. I could also have fallen into step with the presumed, implicit categories, comparing the operation of ethics review committees within their national legal and regulatory frameworks. Not answering her question meant I reached instead for an "epistemic unsettlement" (Sunder Rajan 2021, 57) and analytically refused a comparison that holds steady the category of the nation state. Like Cal Biruk, who struggled between the roles of ethnographer and demographer, I was aware of my discipline's awkward relationship to evaluative improvement. In proximity to medicine (and collaboration) anthropology is often looked to for explanatory power over issues of "cultural difference" (Biruk 2018, 209). By refusing both position of assessor of the ethics review practices I encountered and that of the external comparator, I found myself able to ask different questions of the construction of regionality and the place of difference in FERCAP's work.

While posed to me in the field, "And how is our ethics?" is not a question for me to answer as an ethnographer. For readers seeking knowledge of the status of ethics compliance across different countries, my refusal to perform an analysis resulting in national comparisons with respective rankings will frustrate. But in the foregoing chapters, I have offered something else instead: an analysis of the kinds of comparisons that are active and ongoing, the comparisons that make regionality, networks, and the kind of capacity-building work that FERCAP does possible. I argue that this, too, is skilled work. Ethnographers are never the only ones making analytical moves, comparisons, and analogies (Walford and Krøjer 2017). "And how is our ethics?" is a question members of FERCAP *have for one another*, a comparative question that becomes enactment and takes on a constitutive power in the sociality of the FERCAP network. It relies on an easy background cartography of national comparisons to make some places, as I discussed in chapter 1, more central to ethics stories, other places more peripheral (Jensen 2007). Members of FERCAP use comparison to shape the social world of the network. In turn, comparison-as-organization operates by removing the focus from comparison itself.

In its most earnest form, "And how is our ethics?" undergirds the ever-incomplete work of capacity building. As my colleague Justin Shaffner and I have previously argued, it is *part* of capacity building's promissory character that it draws participants into a present continuous, the "ing" of continuous action (Douglas-Jones and Shaffner 2021). Fitting imperceptibly smoothly with the continuousness of quality assurance, capacity building's promise means that the task that can—should—never be complete. While scholarship has discussed how ethics review itself *anticipates* future action (Hedgecoe 2020, 15), I argue that the distinct temporality of anticipation also shapes the NGO's approach to building ethics review systems. My fieldwork overlapped with FERCAP's decade of greatest growth. First recognitions were soaring, and there was an electric buzz to Conference life. In bar charts counting FERCAP's "recognized" committees, the "new recognitions" shoot up almost every year from 2005 to 2015, dropping off after 2015.[1] The "renewal" count rises in the same pattern at a delay of three years, peaking with forty-five re-recognitions in 2017 (Chokevivat 2019, 1149). In its combination of capacity building and quality assurance, FERCAP creates a "vernacular timespace" (Bryant and Knight 2019, 194) in which "the future 'activates' the present" (2019, 34). The anticipatory character and forward momentum in the marriage of capacity building and total quality assurance exists in relation and response to another kind of timespace: the flow of ever-changing policy. In the time since my main fieldwork ended, core documents within the NGO's repertoire have been revised and updated. The Declaration of Helsinki, a "living document responsive to changing ethical norms" (Bierer 2025, 19), now asks researchers and ethics committees to "actively consider how their decisions contribute to or mitigate systemic inequalities," a new acknowledgment that research ethics "must extend beyond the protection of participants within discrete contexts" (Lindholm et al. 2025). At the same time, the framework of WHO Benchmarking invites institutions to compare themselves with standards beyond the region. Capacity and its scope are not fixed, but change with the "living documents" that inform its work.

As Renuka's question stayed with me, I came to ask myself how it was possible (and seemingly necessary) for an NGO founded with the explicit intent of growing Asia-specific ethics committees, with their knowledges of place, people, and the research that would be of benefit to them, to be so committed to standardized processes. These chapters have shown how "ethnography destabilizes portraits of the Global South as merely a network of host communities for Northern scientists or volunteers or a laboratory for Northern experiments" (Biruk 2021, 13). Having capacity in this book was, from the outset, introduced by Juntra as a response to a paternalism that sought "evidence" that committees in the countries where she worked could do ethics review. She argued that they could do it in ways more meaningful to those who would be participants in research—with knowledge of people and place. This orientation toward capacity building—and its agency—contrasts with the figures that feature in critical collections of capacity building. This capacity building has not been rhetorically enrolled to justify extractive "partnerships" in research (Wendland 2016), nor to offer training in a narrow medical technique. In contrast with critiques of the way the language of capacity building neutralizes and becomes self-evident, members of FERCAP do not see capacity building as an apolitical exercise. The foregoing chapters make evident that members see and strive to make explicit the labor involved for committee members and committee staff. FERCAP is willingly enrolled in institutional arguments so that standards can be deployed to acquire physical space for offices, training programs for staff, fellowships abroad, and the costs of attending networking conferences. The volunteers who are both doing capacity building and participating in it are not visiting for a summer, returning to medical training programs in the U.S. They meet up for short periods, but repeatedly over years. In contrast with the "silences, pointed questions, muttered anxieties, whispered complaints" that Betsey Brada (2023, 168) describes as U.S. Americans descend on Botswana to "build capacity," this capacity building rests on narratives, rhetorics, and strategies of regionality that actively manage hierarchies and differences that would destabilize the "common goals."

Worlds of Form

At the same time, this capacity building also recognizes the politics of having an audience beyond itself. As I discuss below, using the "rhetorical strategy" (Brada 2023, 168) of capacity building has worked not just to ensure funding over many years, but to make training appealing to committee members and their universities or hospitals. It has "argue[d] for and promise[d] a particular vision of the world" (Brada 2023, 168). That vision is a world in which the committee operates in a knowable way, and in a way that can be audited. In the chapters of this book, I have suggested that paying attention to the form the committee takes is to recognize its embedded ideas of representation, equality of voice, and expertise. It is also to recognize it as a social technology, devised to draw on biomedical knowledge whilst at the same time compensating for a perceived absence of biomedical ethics. I have shown that the form of the committee is a contested construction, organizing and creating the conditions for decisions. Rather than staying with principles and their application, I have followed the work of the network into the making and assessment of standards for committee process and quality of review. Analytically, this has brought up a new set of considerations for what a committee *as a form* carries: about people, discussion, evaluation, even the character of politics. In "not doing bioethics," in refusing the endless deliberation attributed to encounters with philosophy, in insisting that ethics committees must make a decision, FERCAP chooses process. Unable to observe every discussion, knowing the infinite permutations of research projects, it has chosen standards as proxies. Through recasting committee work in another form—Standard Operating Procedures—it is able to make interventions through its sufficient flexibility: SOP 1.2.1.2.2 can, and did, become 1.2.1.2.2.1. Without an ethnographic body of literature on how Standard Operating Procedures are efficacious, and their social life as they slip powerfully yet quietly from managerial space to managerial space, what more can be said of this apparently technocratic reduction?

Form matters for anthropologists. Jacob Copeman and Alice Street argue that Marilyn Strathern's insistence "on the persuasiveness of form allows us to discern more fully the underside of disciplinary power: its capacity to empower the subjects it produces at the same time as it delimits the forms of action that are possible" (Copeman and Street 2014, 213). If, as they suggest, we complement Foucauldian understandings of power and borrow the aesthetic gaze more strongly into the anthropology of policy, we can see not only how the form of documents persuade, but also how the social formations they bring about do, too. *Being seen* has had consequences beyond single committees or the formation and consolidation of the network. Pushing from its nonstate position, FERCAP has achieved what Timothy Mitchell called NGO's "state effect" (1999), that is, making the state "visible by emphasizing that they are not the state" (Bernal and Grewal 2014, 7). As FERCAP's recognition was used to establish committees, it prompted conversations within nation states about why *its* standards were being used, and what the role of national health systems and regulatory authorities ought to be. In Taiwan, as Wen-Hua Kuo writes, when the Department of Health outsourced IRB accreditation to the Taiwan Joint Commission on Hospital Accreditation, "some IRBs complained about the redundancy of this accreditation, since they had already met international standards" (2018, 13). In 2013 revisions to India's research regulatory environment went through under considerable pressure, including the new requirement that "all ethics committees [were] to be registered with the Drugs Controller General India (DCGI) before reviewing and approving a clinical trial" (Sariola et al. 2019, 215). In the aftermath, the Forum of Ethics Review Committees of India (FERCI), a forum encouraged by FERCAP and run by its members in India, "put up standard SOPs on its website and these could be used by IECs to develop their own SOPs" (Bhide et al. 2016, 3). However, Shruti Bhide and colleagues—pharmacologists and members of ethics committees—looked to the Indian government to "declare what would be considered acceptable SOPs so that the IECs can all function according to one standard" (Bhide et al. 2016, 3).

These developments are what Kenji Hirayama, on the occasion of FERCAP's tenth anniversary, explicitly hoped for, perhaps necessarily as part of consolidating the NGO's legitimacy outside, not instead of, state authority. Outlining the coming decade from 2011, what he termed the "second phase of quality management of ECs/IRBs in the region," he wrote that "we are strongly proposing that each country establish a national accreditation system to improve its quality that their society can rely on. We will support such efforts to establish national accreditation systems" (Hirayama 2011, 55). If earlier eras of anthropology attempted to address the elusive problem of "the machinery by which group decisions are reached" (Richards 1971, 1), then I have sought to show how one of those machineries—committee work—has been coupled to biomedicine and established as a now global passage point for research. It shows how, by asking what worlds the committee carries with it, we gain understanding of the policies, politics, and international mobility that comes with learning the craft of this machinery. Hirayama's future-oriented claim points in a direction visible throughout this book: The capacities FERCAP has built are not only those of the conduct of ethics review, but also its assessment. In explicitly not positioning itself as a replacement or substitute for national powers, the NGO is nonetheless setting an expectation that committees should be assessed, introducing the form of "recognition" or accreditation to these bureaucratic processes. That process begins with the world of standards.

Worlds of Standards

Establishing and improving standards by which ethics committees operate is framed by key interlocutors as an ethical objective in itself. At the outset of this book, the backdrop of globalizing research was urgent and fraught. Cristina took over as FERCAP coordinator in 2004, a few short years after the Forum's founding, and later reflected that her first visits to "our partner countries made [her] realize the urgency of the work to build an ethical review infrastructure that we could promote" (Torres 2011, 44). With the creation and publication of the 2000 "Silver Book," which established standards for committees, and the accompanying "Blue Book" (WHO/TDR 2002), which established standards for assessing them, Juntra and her colleagues enacted what Andreas Folkers calls a constitutive dimension of "infrastructural" power, not only making a committee knowable, but shaping and "even making up the actors and objects it assembles" (2024, 507). This claim on standards first had to be created, then disseminated, forming communities of practice around them as they went. The people involved are printed directly into the Standard Operating Procedures that orient the Survey through which their committees are reviewed: Version 4.0 downloads slowly, as the final page is a composite of ten different end-of-Survey photographs, over two hundred people lined up in formation, Juntra, Cristina, or both of them amidst the sea of faces (Navarro et al. 2020). The faces are researchers, secretaries, chairs, and committee members, learning ethics review as part of the enterprise of good clinical practice. And some of them asked themselves, "Why should the techniques applied to other parts of the research process, laboratories, data formats, not apply also here, for ethics?"

Many ethnographers share the unease Stefan Timmermans and Steven Epstein identify when faced with standards, unsure whether where to position themselves on a narrative spectrum that posits standards "somewhere between glorified globalization and dark dehumanization" (2010, 83). Ethnographic sensitivity to difference produces wariness, and ambiguous relationships to how "local erasure allows new manipulations to take place such as calculation and commodification" (Timmermans and Epstein 2010, 83). FERCAP's work recognizes explicitly that "no single model for ethical review is appropriate for all countries or all research situations globally" (Karbwang Laothavorn 2016). In Cristina's reflections on "The FERCAP Experience," written for the tenth anniversary of the network's founding, she writes that "respect for cultural and socio-political differences is important" (Torres 2011, 52). Her point is that members of the network focus on the common task of improving ethical review, "rather than on their political and cultural differences" (Torres 2011, 52). As a result, she tells us, "they begin to see each other as friends and co-workers despite their divergent political and cultural background. Asia is a land of contrast and diversity but the FERCAP experience is about a common goal" (Torres 2011, 52). This is a description that writes against ("despite") divergent backgrounds, foregrounding similarity. It is well established "guidelines, rules, regulations and laws to enforce standards reinforce their creators' values" (Graham 2021, 262). By *not* being focused on cultural specificities, FERCAP cultivates a proximity to the comprehension of difference through their distance from it: To use Annelise Riles's phrase, difference is left in the gaps (2001). It becomes possible for a network to operate regionally: As James Scott, scholar of large projects of modernity, would argue, "the lack of context and particularity is not an oversight": It is a necessity that allows for planning (Scott 2020, 346).

Standard Operating Procedures are a device of networking, replication, and regionalization. In the first decades, SOPs were the basis for establishing committees in the absence of national legislation, or other "spheres" of regulation (Wahlberg et al. 2013). If SOPs can be wrestled into view as a social device, a shared format and language through which committees convene, then they can be generatively seen in Joan Fujimura's terms as a standardized package (1992). But SOPs have also allowed for something else. Working with those that would improve research ethics capacity bureaucracies, I observed an inarticulate sense of disarray giving rise to a longing for *systems* that would unify and deal with an ever-fragile assemblage of discrete parts, all of which must work together to generate publishable scientific knowledge.[2] Anna Tsing pointed out long ago that universals are perceived as belonging to some and not to others, with universal reason belonging to colonial power and the particular to the colonized. In her phrasing, "the particular is that which cannot grow" (2005, 9). In this book, being able to evidence compliance is a form of (social) capital: It is a way to grow. When committees approach FERCAP to undergo the SIDCER Recognition Program, it is in part to make themselves legible—nationally and internationally—through an increasingly global industry of verification and accreditation, certification and authentication. In their summary of what standards can do, Timmermans and Epstein remind us that if "standardization is a soft form of regulation (Brunsson and Jacobsson 2000) it can also be viewed as a soft form of stratification, employed by myriad stakeholders to elevate some at the expense of others" (2010, 84).

In the pages of *Committee Worlds* I have described the merged character of capacity building's development orientations with audit principles, reflecting FERCAP's desire to establish itself in that "niche" of standard setting. Rather than *shaping* capacity building through audit and metrics informed monitoring-and-evaluation mechanisms (Gimbel et al. 2018), the capacity itself is to be auditable, and to see and think as an auditor. In following how research ethics has been made into an accompanying infrastructure to biomedicine, I have come to understand that it is not only a *standardized* package (Fujimura 1992), allowing for collaboration across sites of the making of knowledge. It is, in this book, also a version of what Steven Sampson calls a "compliance package" (2015, 2021). On the surface, what Cristina, Juntra, Atoy, and hundreds of volunteers have been creating from their headquarters in Bangkok are wholly distinct from the trajectory of research ethics in the United States. There, as Sarah Babb has argued, a corporate model has emerged as ethics committees have transformed "from collegial bodies into compliance bureaucracies" (2020, 108). Compensating for "limited federal oversight" (2020, 116), compliance bureaucracy offers an appealing "rationalizing structure" (2020, 109) with AAHRPP enrolled in the mix. In contrast, FERCAP operates across many nation states, with committees predominantly made up along the "collegial" model. Yet support of committees meeting standards makes them auditable in the absence of, or anticipation of, an auditor. When they began their work, there was no legal pressure to force the presence of "compliance," although many countries have, during the years of FERCAP's work, adopted what the WHO Benchmarking guidelines would call "legal provisions" (World Health Organization 2023b, 1). Instead, as Cristina put it, since her audience are doctors, academics, and regulators, the network has pushed morally for a compliance with the highest possible standards. And FERCAP itself has positioned itself both as the trainer in "the need to comply" and as the entity to whom committees demonstrate compliance, that demonstration to others "lead[ing] to new relations" (Sampson 2021, 127). In place of compliance officers, FERCAP has creatively positioned the "us" of FERCAP as both the external observer and, through its membership, that which is observed. In 1994, Michael Power argued that "what is audited is whether there is a system which embodies standards and the standards of performance themselves are shaped by the need to be auditable . . . Audit becomes a formal 'loop' by which the system observes itself" (1994, 36–37, cited in Strathern 1996, 8). Through the FERCAP initiatives in SOPs and quality assurance, committee members experience a new version of ethics review, one that makes them legible through the "loop" of compliance.

As we have seen, recognition is clearly desired by committees—as Cristina said in the opening pages of this book, "our audiences are doctors, academics, regulators." Appealing to "moral force," Cristina is also working on the latent desire in bureaucracy, both the appeal to the doctor's professional ethics above and also to the appeal of standards and recognition themselves (Lea 2021). In her analysis of global science regulation as a sphere with "'agency' or 'life' in the practices of those that use it, including scientists, entrepreneurs, medical experts, patients, officials and politicians," Margaret Sleeboom-Faulkner reminds us that seeing regulation through a performative lens allows us to recognize that it is an "activity entailing strategy, politics, and competition for resources" (2025, 24). Introducing standards for committee operation allows them to self-evaluate, introducing the opportunity for recognition allows them to *perform* and potentially to attract international research. In their book, where it is the Sri Lankan laboratory that must meet global standards, Salla Sariola and Bob Simpson write that "like some landing strip for a latter-day cargo cult, the conditions for the successful reception of this new form of wealth creation had to be built in anticipation" (2019, 113). Noting the metaphor, Noémi Tousignant lays emphasis on the way that "it was not the weakness of regulatory mechanisms in Sri Lanka that proved attractive to the company [the private trial sponsor] but their apparent robustness" (Widger et al. 2022, 3). Recognition trophies, certificates, and accreditation gold seals demonstrate this robustness.

Following Babb's foregrounding of compliance, then, this book adds another version of a compliance regime: a version that *anticipates* through compliance as much as it *keeps up* though compliance. I have shown an enactment of compliance with a nonnational, ambiguous auditor, whose authority comes not from efficiency, the wealth of time to review ever more complex federal regulations, but from longstanding relationships, familiarity, and a belief in "moral force." What compels this version of compliance, I argue, is the desire not to attract research but also to *defend*: competence in review as itself proof of protecting research participants. In this book, this observation of the system by itself is peopled, ambitious, and highly networked, and through decades of work with standards, they have anticipated and made themselves ready for the Benchmarks that arrived twenty years later.

Worlds of Capital

When the new WHO Global Clinical Trials Forum first convened in 2023, its inaugural emphasis was on "the importance of promoting equity in clinical trial capability" by "strengthening the clinical trial global ecosystem" and "strengthen[ing] country capacities to conduct clinical trials" (WHO 2022). Ethics review was explicitly raised as an area requiring "coordination and streamlining" (WHO 2023), and, in the publication from the gathering, set as one of the "four broad pillars supporting the clinical trial ecosystem" (Moorthy et al., 2024, 124). Since the COVID-19 pandemic, significant attention has been paid to "sustainable clinical research infrastructure," with the need for "trialists, funders, communities, and organizations in the Global South [to] share an equal leadership role for prioritization, trial design, and analyses," while dedicating funds "for national clinical research infrastructure" (Moorthy et al., 2024, 124). Participants emphasized the "the importance of promoting equity in clinical trial capability" by "strengthening the clinical trial global ecosystem" and "strengthen[ing] country capacities to conduct clinical trials" (WHO 2022, 2). In the diagram accompanying the publication, research ethics is one of the four pillars on which such capability rests, supported by the Benchmarking tool (World Health Organization 2023b) that had been a decade in the making. Cristina was part of its construction, one of a thirteen-member international expert group alongside academic and practitioner colleagues, drawing on her knowledge of what committees struggle with.[3] The "tool" is described by scholars at USAID's Medicines, Technologies, and Pharmaceutical Services (MTAPS) program as a "game changer for strengthening national regulatory capacity" (Guzman et al. 2020), and one of its developers, Simão, emphasized the consultation process as "extensive": "I mean we had like 100 virtual meetings and we went through consultation with 1,100 comments" (Branigan 2019). The tool brings an explicitly "systems"-oriented approach to the management of global research, and regulatory systems in particular. The user guide explains that:

> The primary purpose of the tool is to enable countries to evaluate their existing capacities in ethics review and monitoring, identify strengths and limitations and develop plans for improvement. The tool is not intended to be used as a means of "grading" or "ranking" countries or the entities being assessed. Rather, the goal is to assist countries in ensuring that their systems comply with international norms. (World Health Organization 2023a, 1)

Benchmarking belongs to the same universe of "total quality management" and "continuous quality improvement" that we have seen throughout this book. It is not alien to the field, having been used to ask and delimit "what makes clinical research in developing countries ethical" (Emanuel et al. 2004) in the aftermath of the debates that opened this book. Benchmarking's power, critical scholars tell us, is "bound up in the mechanics and effects of ranking and quantification, which in turn generate a form of 'constructed objectivity' that acts back upon the reality it aims to describe" (Broome and Quirk 2015, 821). When the assistant director-general for Drug Access, Vaccines, and Pharmaceuticals at WHO, Mariângela Batista Galvão Simão, was interviewed about it, that sense of objectivity is present in her argument that it is "more transparent; it's very structural. Just by having the parameters by which you will be assessed already helps the structures to get organized" (Branigan 2019).

It is explicitly "intended to be adaptable to systems in which there a few RECs nationally or regionally . . . as well as systems in which many RECs operate throughout the country" (World Health Organization 2023b, vi). When I spoke to Atoy about it in early 2025, he was enthusiastic about its potential. Not only does the Benchmarking checklist now open the Survey, it allows committees, he said, to "self-assess not just against other committees in Asia, but in the rest of the world." Early publications agree: Reflecting on the potential use of the Benchmarking tool, researchers recommend "a systems thinking approach guided by implementation science . . . [to] help translate the benchmarking findings into formulation of actions for facilitating changes" (Shi et al. 2023, 13).

Warning ethnographers not to gloss audit as a singular global phenomenon, the anthropologist Andrew Kipnis, who studied performance auditing in Zouping, China, reminds us that anthropologists are well positioned to "critique the scientism that is widespread in audit cultures" (2008, 286). Ordinarily it is numbers—the metrics of global health—that anthropologists develop critical relationships with in the course of their fieldwork. However, I suggest metrics logics are present in the background of how capacity in research ethics has been conceptualized. Just as scholars have interrogated how numbers are made, used, and limited (Biruk 2018), the seemingly more *qualitative* version of measurement, benchmarking, needs equal attention. While the tool may not be intended to be used in its competitive genre, with neither "grading" nor "ranking" as the goal, it is difficult not to see its deployment as "classification of relative performance or value" and, with André Broome and Joel Quirk, as a "distinct mode of governance in world politics" (2015, 820). To borrow Greg Koski's image of the single broken thread, the Benchmarking tool systematizes the threads and decides which will form the pattern.

Adam Hedgecoe has rightly argued that if researchers assume isomorphism between different committees—with distinct governance roles, practices, habits, contexts, and kinds of research under review—we fail to recognize both the differences between systems of research governance and the dissimilarities between committees within one country or jurisdiction (2012, 81). I have argued that what we see in FERCAP's work, and the scale of its intervention, is strategic isomorphism that consciously manages difference into a place where it is part of, but does not interrupt the possibility of, compliance with the standards. The similarity is being sought and produced, as FERCAP's rollout of the SIDCER Survey advances a compliance regime in the absence of a single nation state. The differences or struggles I have discussed do not disappear; rather, in this leap to a global Benchmarking tool, its objectivity and neutrality only holds as long as all that is not contained in the tool becomes background.

Benchmarking has been explicitly labeled by governance scholars Broome and Quirk as "governing from a distance" (2015), in an echo of Nicholas Rose's description of neoliberal thought. However, as Andrew Kipnis reminds us, distance is a characteristic of numerous modes of governance, and it matters how distance is put to use. Perhaps the distance here is to ethics itself, following Mark Flear's critique of mistaking ICH-GCP, which was a *technical* standardization document, for an ethics standard. Following guidelines "focusing global harmonization on safety, quality and effectiveness—technical matters," he argued, "marginalizes other kinds of harm (social, political, environmental)" (2021, 10). What does not come into the guidelines becomes less visible. For scholars and practitioners alike, is important to ask after the goal of the benchmarking, and to be attentive to the "extra effects of the practice in addition to reaching the goal" (Harding 2006, 151). Because Flear's critique has a further relevant claim, and that is the "reduction of 'better health' to 'safe, quality and effective pharmaceuticals' may also shift attention and resources toward them, and away from non-pharmaceutical interventions" (Flear 2021, 10). As benchmarking of regulatory regimes advances, and FERCAP prefaces its Survey activities with its "indicators," living up to these benchmarks may have a cost.

Worlds of Integrity

At the start of the century, distrust permeated the internationalizing arena of biomedical research. Bioethics debates, trainings, experts, and committees flourished. And alongside these often loud discussions, researchers and clinicians worked to build systems around concepts they recognized—quality assurance—and could measure. In this book I have shown one of the afterlives of that distrust, constructed in the name of a higher ethical imperative that research must continue: the adoption of standards, an anticipatory compliance regime, and benchmarking practices into committee worlds. A longstanding concern in research ethics is the role that detailed rules have on "ethical thinking" (Molyneux and Geissler 2008, 692). It is ethical thinking from the funding of research to the choice of research design, selection of participants, and everyday conduct that is still tied to actions that protect participants. Internationalization of research continues to be contentious. Emma Kowal's analysis of a piece of groundbreaking global science—the use of next generation sequencing on ancient DNA—shows the international operation of ethics. In her story, "ethics" emerges initially at the point of publication, as a Danish researcher is attempting to publish in *Nature* and cannot answer the now standard question of whether he had "secured ethical approval for the study." Specifically, whether "anyone in Australia [had] given approval" (Kowal 2023, 80). The ethics appears initially to hinge on whether the work is "archaeological" or "biological." In an account that spans rock star scientists, prestigious institutions, headline-grabbing findings, journal inquiries, and archaeological versus biological classifications, there is also the significance of the physical—and epistemic—location of an ethics committee (Kowal 2023, 82). In this case, it is not they who take center stage, but the rock star researcher and their personal "epiphany of ethical enlightenment" (Kowal 2023, 73).

Kowal is asking how the ghosts of science can be lived with, a question tuned to her setting of Indigeneity and genomics. It is a provocative question highly pertinent for the field of research ethics, and one of the "hauntings" of this world of policy (Lea 2024). Through its trainings and the history of its composition, the ethics committee carries with it histories of abuse in research, anticipating the possibility for harm. At the same time, its assessments valued for their "local knowledge" are also enmeshed in "local" relations, institutional settings, and, to date, a trust that researchers will do as they say they will do. Ethics review is uncomfortably located temporally—for some, the review is too early, and ethical matters really arise in the moment of research, in the unexpected and sometimes critical situations of data collection. For others, it is too late, arriving after the formulation of the research project and its questions, the selected participants and the acquisition of funding. The international interventions that FERCAP's initiatives have made in building capacity for committees bring to the fore the competing, implicit beliefs about how and where the kernel of ethical behavior should lie.

Alongside the development of standards, auditing, and compliance in 2005, a collaboration began between the U.S. Office of Research Integrity and the European Science Foundation, as "a modest effort to expand a U.S. Office of Research Integrity outreach program to Europe" (Mayer and Steneck 2011, v), with the first World Conference on Research Integrity taking place in 2007. Rather than delegating to *committees* the work of making scientific research trustworthy through review and anticipation, the swing toward research integrity repositions ethical conduct as an orientation of the researcher within a system. In this sense, ethics extends; it spills over into peoples' lives, to show how trainings evoke a sense of the necessity for trainees to come, as they put it, to *believe* in ethics. Former students explain how the trainings helped them "see," experience a moment of revelation. By tracing the work that Cristina, Juntra, and hundreds of volunteers dedicate years to, I have given this oscillation a different kind of framing. By attending to ethics as it is codified, secularized into management and the seemingly neutral form of Standard Operating Procedures, we see ethics as set of policies given institutional life and form. Ethics committees are central, legitimated focus points for discussions about biomedical ethics, and sites to which these discussions have been delegated. Woven into the narratives of duty and virtue offered by trainers and trainees are the displaced values of infinite improvement, glossed as continuous quality and re-displaced through appeals to operationalization, offering a bracketed continuity through which discussions about the where, why, and how of ethics can be paused, and "simply" put into action.

Conclusion

I opened this book with a vignette that I see as encapsulating the meeting of two worlds. Cristina's world was one where medical researchers could be convinced, persuaded by "moral force" that biomedical research needs research ethics committees, its practitioners need an understanding of ethics, and that there is a role for them in building that system in their own working worlds. The world of Dave, the U.S. American academic, is one where the force of law and regulation has led to a pressured IRB landscape, with a growing need for committees to ensure compliance in ethics review. For both Cristina and Dave, the stakes are high.

The Forum of Ethics Review Committees of the Asia-Pacific, the storytellers of this book, describe their own "grassroots" transformation in the practice of research ethics in hundreds of universities and hospitals across the Asia-Pacific region, mapping and making landscapes of collaboration and collegiality that did not and could not previously exist. I have aimed to show the density of relations, the friendships, and the long histories of relationship that have carried this capacity-building work forward. As research continues to grow in the region, ethics review committees will come under ever greater pressure: It is institutions that must ensure that they have the resources to do their work. The policies are the results of relationships and have the power to sustain new webs of practice. The events in this book cover twenty-five years, during which conversations about research ethics have shifted. Taking a longitudinal view, it is work oriented toward a more just world, in which research of importance to their settings happens, and where the committees at their hospitals and institutions are well equipped to review. As policies play out over time, documents replace other documents, and there is an ongoing labor of both informing and keeping up with changes. Keeping up might mean joining a series of Zoom calls, responding to new proposed guidelines, creating and maintaining fora for conversation, or scouring the latest literature. But anticipating looks like getting ready, making use of "technologies of governing" such as standards and compliance regimes, attending conferences, and doing the local and national work of networking ethics into policy and even law.

As Elizabeth Dunn reminds us, ethnographic work is essential for scholars who are "interested not just in theories of management but in managerial practices as they were implemented in context—incompletely, in modified ways, and in the face of resistance, transformation and subversion by those who are its objects" (2004, 23, cited in Kipnis 2008, 285). In this book, I have followed the professional lives of two women, whose work in the largely male spaces of medicine and ethics has fostered an expansive community of participation, crossing national borders and strategically demonstrating how research ethics could—and in their view, should—be done. Staying alongside these changes with our interlocutors is the longitudinal gaze that anthropologists of policy can offer to the study of policies that shift practices in more than their settings of origin. Joy Y. Zhang and Saheli Datta Burton write that "science, as a systematic and methodological social production of knowledge, is ultimately about power. Governing science is about the means and ends of steering that power" (2022, 1). In the arc in this book from bioethics to benchmarking, ethnographic work has illustrated the centrality of proximity to practice, and the need for ethnographic attention to how context matters in its very acts of elision. I have sought to bring readers along, summoning

Andrea Ballestero's openness of wonder (2019, 199) into the worlds of Standard Operating Procedures, audit, and ethics. For as much as committees are the products of policy, they also make and enact it, and it is from their forms of expertise and knowledge that committees of the future may yet make their own committee worlds.

Notes

Introduction

1. The WHO ICTRP is not in itself a registry for clinical trials. Of the seventeen registries that, at the time of writing, meet the WHO Registry Network's criteria for "content, quality, validity, accessibility, unique identification, technical capacity and administration" seven are in the Asia-Pacific region.

2. Of these, PABIN is active.

3. Although see Kaur and Choy (2014) for a critical perspective, Dubinksy (Dubinsky 2021) for a practitioner's perspective, and Kuo (2008) for an STS analysis of the role played by discussions of race in the establishment of the original ICH-GCP.

4. With a nod to Cal Biruk's Fieldworker Among the Demographers (Biruk 2018).

5. The final loop occurred when my own funders, the Economic and Social Research Council, audited my compliance toward the end of my scholarship, asking for an accounting of my own institutional ethics approval in the UK.

Chapter 1

1. TDR Global uses the same metaphor to describe how its scientific community is formed: "Picture a single tapestry thread that can be woven into many rows. Naturally, this single thread has its limitations as it cannot create pictures or patterns on its own. If you add more threads, carefully weaving the thin fibres, the tapestry transforms into a colourful picture or beautiful design with intricate details. TDR Global is exceptional in the same way as the colourful patterns on a tapestry because we are a combination of many unique individuals. Each member has their own expertise, culture and background, creating a bigger, more powerful picture. Despite the complexity of the bigger picture, it connects us all in our shared field of interest" (TDR Global 2025).

2. April 22, 2002, "At Your Own Risk" was *Time* magazine's cover story.

3. Drane points out that universalizing (among Westerners) also occurs, and that within what is known as Western bioethics "different orientations and divergent views co-exist and compete with one another"; it is not as though "Ibero-American bioethics is [. . .] a self contained unified theoretical system providing a single, coherent perspective" (1996, 560).

4. Another instance of fractality, where social hierarchies within committees transfer without difficulty onto hierarchies between countries.

5. Alberto Corsín-Jiménez offers us a description of this process through his own writing: "You may be reading this and thinking 'this is not very interesting.' If that is so, you are in fact re-proportioning your ideas against mine by 'sizing down' my views" (2003, 16). He attributes the movement in the proportioning to capacity: "You are . . . *moving integrally* through such orders with a *sense of capacity* (and the term is not arbitrary, for capacities are magnitudinal categories)" (2003, 17).

6. FERCAP did stop working in mainland China after changes to the "NGO Law" in 2016 (see Wilhelm et al. 2021).

7. These requirements—in settings without committees—have on occasion led to the "the fabrication and retrospective issuance of ethics review certificates" (Li 2025, 3).

Chapter 2

1. The image is a fake, a composite of two images. It is unclear whether Dr. Sam realized this, but it does not change the meaning of this choice of picture. See Stentor Danielsen for a review of the email hoax to which the photo was originally attached (Danielsen 2002).

2. A Kantian derived "duty based ethics" is strategically taken up by the network within the Asia-Pacific region for its Confucian resonance (Torres 2011).

3. In their introduction to the volume on hospitality Matei Candea and Giovanni Da Col observe that Mandarin already has terms for precisely this position: *Keguan*, 客观 the concept of "objective" or to view things as outsiders would (2012, S6).

4. Chinese, Taiwanese, Thai, and South Korean committees use their own languages for documentation, and FERCAP regards it as a strength that they do not require committees to translate all of their records into English, a costly and time-consuming exercise that would potentially exclude committees with few resources.

5. 眼睛長在頭頂上 *yǎnjīng zhǎng zài tóudǐng shàng*, an idiom meaning that one regards others to be beneath one's notice (Sally's translation).

6. As Daniel Miller remarks (2003, 61) for the Best Value quality control final meetings he observed, the use of PowerPoint is one of a number of factors that mediate the construction and aesthetics of the final document (Riles 2001, 114–42).

7. The organization is applying to itself the same standards it expects for its ethics committees: Decisions must be based on evidence.

8. The image of perspectives not only comprising the object under study but also holding both it and themselves in balance is one that jumps between the committee's assessment and the assessment of the committee's assessment.

9. It is a further example of what Casper Bruun Jensen and Brit Ross Winthereik term audit's epistemological pluralism: "One gets to know more by examining more cases, and to know more by adopting new perspectives on existing cases" (Jensen and Winthereik 2013, 165).

10. The restaurant specializes in "imperial court cuisine" and was a popular place to take foreign guests.

11. Later documents, specifically *Preserving Public Trust* (Institute of Medicine 2001), discuss the development of standards for the accreditation of IRBs, "one spawned from the PRIM&R effort and the other developed through a contract between NCQA and the VA" (Institute of Medicine 2001, 32).

12. Indeed, the 2023 review of IRBs by the U.S. Government Accountability Office cited U.S. officials arguing that while AAHRPP accreditation is recognized as the hallmark of quality in the field, they did however note "limitations with the AAHRPP accreditation process, including that the process focuses on policies and paperwork and does not include auditing IRB meetings or decisions or interacting with research participants" (Dicken 2023, 38).

Chapter 3

1. In 2005, the Nuffield Council on Bioethics described "difficulties faced" by RECs in Kenya and noted that "the REC has limited office space in a hospital and a university, with no facilities for communication, photocopying or for keeping records. Although there are computers, there is no Internet connection and no access to a resource centre. This makes it difficult for members to perform literature searches or to familiarise themselves with specialised subjects under review" (Nuffield Council on Bioethics 2005, 52).

2. This did not always meet with the intended success. As one Surveyor remarked of a full board meeting we observed, "[The layperson] asked, does using these [contraceptive] pills lead to cancer? And instead of cancer, the secretary wrote abortion!" Nobody on the committee noticed, but the Surveyors did.

3. The first took place in Manila, the Philippines, from October 21 to 25, 2001, as an International Training Course on Ethical Research (Chokevivat 2019, 1147).

4. Steven Shapin and Simon Schaffer note that the word "laboratory" arrived in English usage in the seventeenth century, carrying with it apparently hermetical overtones: The space so designated was private, inhabited by secretists (Shapin and Schaffer 2011, 335).

5. I am not suggesting that the "achievement" of space is unique to Asian contexts; rather that as we saw above, hospitals and universities may need convincing. A parallel of the significance of "taking" space for ethics is found in the language of Sarah Auerbach's report on an Amherst alumnus, Ezekiel Emmanuel, a bioethicist who took up a role at the U.S. National Institutes of Health: "Emanuel [. . .] took one look at the government-issue green-hued rooms where NIH scientists did their work and [said] 'That's not the right environment for bioethicists.' Emanuel created a central common space. Under a giant conference table, he placed an Oriental rug, and on the walls, he hung 'real art,' he says, including African masks from his many travels to that continent. Emanuel tore down walls to expand the bioethics department's territory, and he has colonized other NIH institutes to add faculty to his department" (2009).

Chapter 4

1. The further repercussions of which I discuss in chapter 7.

2. Whom we met first at the Regional Collaborative Workshop, in the introduction.

3. Finding ways to ensure "appropriate expertise" from all areas is indeed a challenge in developing world settings and is acknowledged by documents such as the Nuffield discussion paper (Nuffield Council on Bioethics 2005, 48).

4. Sometimes they find themselves caught up in loops, where in order to research problems of informed consent, their own research regulations require them to obtain informed consent from participants, in order to talk with them about why informed consent may not be suitable.

5. It was subsequently published with that phrasing (WHO 2011).

6. This point is developed in work by scholars whose work focuses on such forms of alterity (Crook 2007).

Chapter 5

1. Laura Stark uses her transcript material on IRB meetings in the U.S. to arrive at a similar finding, arguing that "IRB members use latitude each time they apply a regulation, which might make the range of possible decisions seem nearly limitless. Yet the ways in which IRB members go about making decisions is systematic because of the constraints of their social configuration" (2012, 66).

2. Used here with the U.S. American meaning rather than the British: to put the protocol aside and return to it in the next meeting.

3. Chandeep referenced the Challenger disaster as an iconic case of "groupthink." For an academic account, see Vaughan (1997).

4. A historical perspective connecting twentieth- and twenty-first-century arguments about censorship and groupthink, such as those raised by Katz (2007), Hamburger (2004), would be fascinating but is beyond my scope here.

5. Tagalog slang for a group of friends or peers. With thanks to Atoy Navarro for translation assistance.

6. Western IRB, based in Olympia, Washington, has had significant interaction with FERCAP and ethics committees in the Asian region through its WHO-funded developing countries training program. See Introduction.

7. See Dennis Thompson (1993) for the counterargument that conflicts are usually not illegitimate; indeed, they are frequently necessary and desirable.

8. I suggest this (re)complicates the individuality of the models from which notions of COI are drawn (see also Hess 2006).

Chapter 6

1. Citizen Participation in East Asian Legal Systems, September 22–23 2006. Cornell Law School, Ithaca NY.

2. Concern with judgment applies to both the ethics committee and to the Survey. At times during analysis, the two would become confused in my mind, the styles,

traits appearing to blur. This was a result of how each was spoken about in the field: "We are not police!"—a phrase uttered by Surveyors who have not come to investigate potential (past) crimes of the ethics committee but to help, in the hope that this spirit of cooperative support will encourage committees to be open about their difficulties. "We are not police!"—a phrase uttered by ethics committees who cannot, through lack of time and resources, pursue the investigators, check up on them as they proceed with their research. Occasionally, commentators would begin by addressing their comments to the Surveyors but end by speaking about the working of the ethics review committee. In the study of an audit of an audit, attention to how the two were conceptually kept apart and where they collapsed into each other was a constant challenge.

3. Indeed, efficiency was one of the key drivers in a recent study into the presence of PIs during IRB meetings in the U.S. (Taylor et al. 2016).

4. Although Stark writes that that a more "radical" move is to invite investigators to meetings, "an unwitting return to an internal NIH strategy [...] phased out 40 years ago" (2007, 784). While the persuasive influence of PIs may have been removed, her recent work clearly delineates strategies by which committee members persuade one another through reference to different types of authority: professional, personal, and publicly available information.

5. For example, Mahidol University, Thailand, has a Change History document, which reports changes prior to the Survey, including "9. Section 7.5 has been revised: (1) clinical investigator and ancillary staff may be called to EC meeting but are not allowed to stay during EC discussion" (Mahidol FTM ECS-004-05, December 2011).

6. A case of a famed scientist who fabricated and falsified data, fraudulently claiming to have created the world's first human embryonic stem cells.

7. Sri Lankan English in which "getting" includes reference to the thing that is acquired, in this case, the information missing from the application.

8. Another example of the way in which language shapes and shifts arenas: Is this management speak? Or is it ethics? More importantly, the speaker's concern with "risk and benefit" of the social dynamics of having a director as a chairperson illustrates how the balancing of research risks and benefits that ethics committees are required to do is suddenly made to apply to how committees are themselves arranged.

9. When we spoke in May 2010, Sri Lanka's thirty-five-year-long civil war had recently ended, and the priorities of the legal system were weighted toward its aftermath.

10. The committee (1954–57) made proposals that prompted the now famous mid-twentieth-century debate between Professor Hart and Lord Devlin (Cane 2006). The debate was also the origin of much of the "harm"-based discourse.

11. They also echo the debate between Walter Lippmann and John Dewey (Marres 2005, 217), in which we are reminded that "issues call a public into being." Sheila Jasanoff (2005) makes this point symmetrically, arguing that political cultures shape how

science is conducted at the same time as changes in science and technology create styles and modes of political culture.

12. In 1997 Justice Weeramantry, a Sri Lankan, was serving as vice president of the ICJ, and the contribution is recorded in the ICJ Gabčíkovo-Nagymaros Project (Hungary/Slovakia) ("Separate Opinion of Vice-President Weeramantry" 1997).

13. Although for critique of the form the jury has since taken in Japan, see Kage 2017.

Chapter 7

1. Ethnographers have spent a century focused on the allocation and attribution of blame, responsibility, and moral questions, amongst them Mary Douglas ([1992] 2005), E. E. Evans-Pritchard ([1937] 2009), and Max Gluckman (1972).

2. Responsible for the quality of TDR-supported studies.

3. Committees must be re-Surveyed every three years.

4. Lecturer's translation, taken from a popular Tagalog love song.

5. Henry Beecher (1966) wrote a key paper revealing ethical problems in American research.

6. Compare, for example, the Reith Lectures of Ian Kennedy (1993) and Onora O'Neill (2010), the former using them to argue for the place of outsiders in establishing standards doctors must meet, the latter using them to claim that systems designed to ensure public accountability simply deepen the mistrust they seek to remedy.

Chapter 8

1. As part of the scoping study for a project concerned with the implementation of the Danish Code of Research Integrity, I participated in SATORI's workshops along the way. In Ljubljana, Slovenia, I took notes on the ideas of standardizing ethics (January 31 and February 1, 2017).

2. A group of inherited blood disorders affecting the production of red blood cells. Occurring at a high frequency throughout South Asia, the disease poses significant challenges in terms of public health.

3. https://www.iso.org/standard/56115.html: "Can be used by medical laboratories in developing their quality management systems and assessing their own competence. It can also be used for confirming or recognizing the competence of medical laboratories by laboratory customers, regulating authorities and accreditation bodies."

4. The audio was made available through Xtalks, an online archive, and what quotes I use were transcribed from there.

5. This is a triangulation Alberto Corsín Jiménez (2011) observes in the work of Samuel DiPiazza and Robert Eccles (2002) on corporate ethics and reporting *and* Max Gluckman (1972) on African divination and the allocation of responsibility. He rightly remarks that anthropologists have long puzzled over these concerns.

Conclusion

1. A significant part of this plateau was no longer being able to operate in China, following the 2016 "Foreign NGO Law," which impacted the operation of international NGOs in the country (Wilhelm et al. 2021).

2. Despite the similarity such terms have with language anthropologists have used to describe "world systems" (Wallerstein 2011) and fragmented realities (Clifford and Marcus 2010; Tyler 2010), claims of "fragmentation" originate and circulate within the field; they are a description generated by the field itself, not my analysis. Part of the challenge of an ethnographic account of this kind is that the language used to describe the world by those with whom one works resembles (even takes on) certain of the problems of the history of anthropological and sociological thought.

3. Other figures who appear in this book also took part: For example, Carl Coleman, whom we met in chapter 4 in Shanghai, was responsible for drafting it alongside Juliati Dahlan at the Indonesian National Agency of Drugs and Food Control.

References

AAHRPP. 2022. "AAHRPP Accredits Three More Research Organizations, Including First Hospital in Japan." December 23. https://www.aahrpp.org/education-news-and-events/press-releases/2022/12/22/aahrpp-accredits-three-more-research-organizations-including-first-hospital-in-japan.

AAHRPP. 2023. "AAHRPP Accredits Two More Research Organizations, Including Another in China." AAHRPP Education News & Events. March 31. https://www.aahrpp.org/education-news-and-events/press-releases/2023/03/31/aahrpp-accredits-two-more-research-organizations-including-another-in-china.

AAHRPP. 2021. "AAHRPP History and Future: Yesterday, Today and Tomorrow." http://www.aahrpp.org/docs/default-source/default-document-library/aahrpp-history-and-future-(final).pdf.

AAHRPP. 2024. "Application and Annual Fees." AAHRPP Get Accredited. May 5. https://www.aahrpp.org/accreditation/get-accredited/application-and-annual-fees.

AAHRPP. 2010. "History of Innovation at the Catholic Medical Centre." *AAHRPP Advance.*

ACRES. 2014. "ACRES." ACRES Global. August 31. http://web.archive.org/web/20140831114752/http://www.acresglobal.net.

Aellah, G. J. 2021. "Everyday Life in a Site of Transnational Medical Research in Western Kenya: An Ethnographic Study." London School of Hygiene & Tropical Medicine. https://researchonline.lshtm.ac.uk/id/eprint/4663266.

AHRI (Armauer Hansen Research Initiative). 2023. "The Pan-African Bioethics Initiative Network (PABIN) Kick-off Meeting Held in Addis Ababa—Armauer Hansen Research Institute." November 12. https://ahri.gov.et/2023/11/12/the-pan-african-bioethics-initiative-network-pabin-kick-off-meeting-held-in-addis-ababa/.

Anderson, Warwick. 2017. "Postcolonial Specters of STS." *East Asian Science, Technology and Society: An International Journal* 11 (2): 229–33. https://doi.org/10.1215/18752160-3828937.

Angell, Marcia. 1988. "Ethical Imperialism?" *New England Journal of Medicine* 319 (16): 1081–83. https://doi.org/10.1056/NEJM198810203191608.

Angell, Marcia. 1997. "The Ethics of Clinical Research in the Third World." *New England Journal of Medicine* 337 (12): 847–49. https://doi.org/10.1056/NEJM199709183371209.

Ansari, Salik. 2023. "Supporting a Member Secretary of an Ethics Committee." *Asian Bioethics Review* 15 (4): 361–63. https://doi.org/10.1007/s41649-023-00255-4.

Applied Clinical Trials. 2016. "AAHRPP Accredits Four Research Orgs." December 22. https://www.appliedclinicaltrialsonline.com/view/aahrpp-accredits-four-research-orgs.

Asad, Talal. 2003. *Formations of the Secular: Christianity, Islam, Modernity*. Stanford University Press.

Assor, Yael. 2021. "'Objectivity' as a Bureaucratic Virtue." *American Ethnologist* 48 (1): 105–19. https://doi.org/10.1111/amet.12999.

Aubert, Vilhelm. 1979. "On Methods of Legal Influence." In *The Imposition of Law*, edited by Sandra Burman and Barbara E. Harrell-Bond. Academic Press.

Auerbach, Sarah. 2009. "Feature: Come for Dinner, Stay for Life." *Amherst Magazine*. https://www.amherst.edu/news/magazine/issue-archive/2009summer/emanuel.

Babb, Sarah. 2020. *Regulating Human Research: IRBs from Peer Review to Compliance Bureaucracy*. Stanford University Press.

Babb, Sarah. 2021. "The Privatization of Human Research Ethics: An American Story." *European Journal for the History of Medicine and Health* 78 (2): 392–411. https://doi.org/10.1163/26667711-bja10005.

Ballestero, Andrea. 2019. *A Future History of Water*. Duke University Press.

Ballestero, Andrea. 2012. "Transparency Short-Circuited: Laughter and Numbers in Costa Rican Water Politics." *PoLAR: Political and Legal Anthropology Review* 35 (2): 223–41. https://doi.org/10.1111/j.1555-2934.2012.01200.x.

Bastian, Michelle. 2014. "Finding Time for Philosophy." In *Women in Philosophy: What Needs to Change?*, edited by Katrina Hutchison and Fiona Jenkins, 215–30. Oxford University Press. https://doi.org/10.1093/acprof:oso/9780199325603.001.0001.

Bastian, Michelle. 2018. "Philosophy Disturbed: Reflections on Moving between Field and Philosophy." *Parallax* (4): 449–65. https://doi.org/doi.org/10.1080/13534645.2028.1546723.

Battaglia, Debbora. 2012. "Arresting Hospitality: The Case of the 'Handshake in Space.'" *Journal of the Royal Anthropological Institute* 18 (s1): S76–89. https://doi.org/10.1111/j.1467-9655.2012.01762.x.

BBC. 2002a. "Jury Trials 'Facing Fresh Threat.'" *BBC News Online*, April 16. http://news.bbc.co.uk/2/hi/uk_news/politics/1932917.stm.

BBC. 2002b. "Anger at Jury Reform Plans." *BBC News Online*, July 14. http://news.bbc.co.uk/2/hi/uk_news/politics/2126712.stm.

BBC. 2007. "Terror Trial Lawyer Defends Jury." *BBC News Online*, February 19. http://news.bbc.co.uk/2/hi/uk_news/6376833.stm.

Beagan, Brenda, and Michael McDonald. 2005. "Evidence-Based Practice of Research Ethics Review?" *Health Law Review* 13: 62–68.

Beecher, Henry K. 1966. "Ethics and Clinical Research." *New England Journal of Medicine* 274 (24): 1354–60. https://doi.org/10.1056/NEJM196606162742405.

Bell, Kirsten, and Ll Wynn. 2023. "Research Ethics Committees, Ethnographers and Imaginations of Risk." *Ethnography* 24 (4): 537–58. https://doi.org/10.1177/14661381209838 62.

Benatar, S. R. 2002. "Reflections and Recommendations on Research Ethics in Developing Countries." *Social Science & Medicine* 54 (7): 1131–41. https://doi.org/10.1016/S0277-9536(01)00327-6.

Bernabe, Rosemarie de La Cruz; Cox Née Dawkins, Shereen & Gispen-de Wied, Christine C. 2025. "Gaps in the Ethical Governance of Pharmaceutical Clinical Trials in Europe." *Frontiers in Medicine.* doi: 10.3389/fmed.2024.1507021.

Bernal, Victoria, and Inderpal Grewal, eds. 2014. *Theorizing NGOs: States, Feminisms, and Neoliberalism.* Duke University Press.

Bhanu Mehta, Pratap. 2006. "Self-Interest and Other Interests." In *The Cambridge Companion to Adam Smith*, 1st ed., edited by Knud Haakonssen, 246–69. Cambridge University Press. https://doi.org/10.1017/CCOL0521770599.010.

Bhide, Shruti S., Sharmila V. Jalgaonkar, Janhavi V. Katkar, et al. 2016. "Impact of Recent Regulatory Notifications on an Institutional Ethics Committee." *Indian Journal of Medical Ethics* (4) (October). https://doi.org/10.20529/IJME.2016.061.

Bhosale, Neelambari. 2014. "Protection of Human Research Participants: Accreditation of Programmes in the Indian Context." *Indian Journal of Medical Ethics*, January. https://doi.org/10.20529/IJME.2014.015.

Bhutta, Zulfiqar Ahmed. 2002. "Ethics in International Health Research: A Perspective from the Developing World." *Bulletin of the World Health Organization* 80 (2): 114–20.

Bierer, Barbara E. 2025. "Declaration of Helsinki—Revisions for the 21st Century." *JAMA* 333 (1): 18. https://doi.org/10.1001/jama.2024.22281.

BioSpectrum Asia. 2019. "Three Research Organizations Acquire AAHRPP Recognition." Industry. BioSpectrum Asia Edition. March 25. https://www.biospectrumasia.com/news/30/13093/three-research-organizations-acquire-aahrpp-recognition.html.

Biruk, Cal. 2018. *Cooking Data: Culture and Politics in an African Research World.* Duke University Press.

Biruk, Cal. 2021. "The Politics of Global Health." *PoLAR: Political and Legal Anthropology Review* 44 (2): e161–80. https://doi.org/10.1111/plar.12431.

Bowen, Angela J. 1997. "The Contribution of an Independent Ethics Committee to Quality Assurance in Clinical Trials." *The Quality Assurance Journal* 2 (4): 161–65. https://doi.org/10.1002/(SICI)1099-1786(199712 0)2:4<161::AID-QAJ41>3.0.CO;2-U.

Boyer, Dominic. 2008. "Thinking through the Anthropology of Experts." *Anthropology in Action* 15 (2). https://doi.org/10.3167/aia.2008.150204.

Brada, Betsey Behr. 2023. *Learning to Save the World.* Cornell University Press.

Branigan, David. 2019. "WHO Benchmarking Tool Made 'More Transparent' In Evaluating Regulatory Authorities—Health Policy Watch." *Health Policy Watch: Independent Global Health Reporting* (blog), February 5. https://healthpolicy-watch.news/who-benchmarking-tool-made-more-transparent-in-evaluating-regulatory-authorities/.

Brazelton, Mary Augusta. 2022. "Health for All?: Histories of International and Global Health." *History Compass* 20 (1): e12700. https://doi.org/10.1111/hic3.12700.

Brives, Charlotte, Frédéric Le Marcis, and Emilia Sanabria. 2016. "What's in a Context? Tenses and Tensions in Evidence-Based Medicine." *Medical Anthropology* 35 (5): 369–76. https://doi.org/10.1080/01459740.2016.1160089.

Brodin, Mark S. 1990. "Accuracy, Efficiency, and Accountability in the Litigation Process—The Case for the Fact Verdict." *University of Cincinnati Law Review* 19: 15–112.

Broome, André, and Joel Quirk. 2015. "Governing the World at a Distance: The Practice of Global Benchmarking." *Review of International Studies* 41 (5): 819–41. https://doi.org/10.1017/S0260210515000340.

Brown, Hannah. 2015. "Global Health Partnerships, Governance, and Sovereign Responsibility in Western Kenya." *American Ethnologist* 42 (2): 340–55. https://doi.org/10.1111/amet.12134.

Brown, Hannah, Adam Reed, and Thomas Yarrow. 2017. "Introduction: Towards an Ethnography of Meeting." *Journal of the Royal Anthropological Institute* 23 (S1): 10–26. https://doi.org/10.1111/1467-9655.12591.

Brown, Mark B. 2009. "Three Ways to Politicize Bioethics." *The American Journal of Bioethics* 9 (2): 43–54. https://doi.org/10.1080/15265160802617811.

Brunsson, N., and B. Jacobsson, eds. 2000. *A World of Standards.* Oxford University Press.

Bryant, Rebecca, and Daniel M. Knight. 2019. *The Anthropology of the Future.* 1st ed. Cambridge University Press. https://doi.org/10.1017/9781108378277.

Busch, Lawrence. 2011. *Standards: Recipes for Reality.* MIT Press.

Callon, Michel, and Bruno Latour. 1981. "Unscrewing the Big Leviathan: How Actors Macro-Structure Reality and How Sociologists Help Them to Do So." In *Advances in Social Theory and Methodology: Toward an Integration of Micro- and Macro-Sociologies*, edited by Aaron Victor Cicourel and Karin Knorr-Cetina, 277–303. Routledge. https://doi.org/10.4324/9781315763880.

Callon, Michel, and Vololona Rabeharisoa. 2008. "The Growing Engagement of Emergent Concerned Groups in Political and Economic Life: Lessons from the French Association of Neuromuscular Disease Patients." *Science, Technology, & Human Values* 33 (2): 230–61. https://doi.org/10.1177/0162243907311264.

Camic, Charles, Neil Gross, and Michèle Lamont. 2011. *Social Knowledge in the Making.* University of Chicago Press.

Candea, Matei, and Giovanni Da Col. 2012. "The Return to Hospitality." *Journal of the Royal Anthropological Institute* 18 (s1): S1–19. https://doi.org/10.1111/j.1467-9655.2012.01757.x.

Cane, Peter. 2006. "Taking Law Seriously: Starting Points of the Hart/Devlin Debate." *The Journal of Ethics* 10 (1–2): 21–51. https://doi.org/10.1007/s10892-005-4590-x.

Castro, Leonardo D. de. 1999. "Is There an Asian Bioethics?" *Bioethics* 13: 227–35.

Champney, Freeman. 1952. "Individual and Group: Reviewed Work 'Is Anybody Listening?' William H. Whyte, Jr." *The Antioch Review* 12 (3): 383–84.

Chau, Adam Yuet. 2019. "Hosting as a Cultural Form." *L'Homme* (231/232): 41–66.

Chokevivat, Vichai. 2019. "Improving Protections of Human Research Volunteers by SIDCER/FERCAP Recognition Program." *Journal of Health Science of Thailand* 28 (6): 1143–54.

Chokevivat, Vichai. 2011. "The FERCAP Story: A Decade of Fruitful Collaboration with Partners in Ethical Health Research." In *FERCAP @ 10: In Commemoration of a Decade of Capacity Building in Ethical Health Research in the Asia-Pacific Region*, edited by Atoy M. Navarro and Cristina E. Torres, 6–10. Thailand: Forum for Ethical Review Committees in the Asian and Western Pacific Region.

Chong, Kimberly. 2018. *Best Practice: Management Consulting and the Ethics of Financialization*. Duke University Press. https://doi.org/10.1215/9781478002376.

CIOMS Working Group on Good Governance Practice for Research Institutions. 2023. "International Guidelines on Good Governance Practice for Research Institutions." Council for International Organizations of Medical Sciences (CIOMS). https://doi.org/10.56759/hslk3269.

Citraningtyas, Theresia, Elspeth MacDonald, and Helen Herrman. 2010. "A Second Tsunami?: The Ethics of Coming into Communities Following Disaster." *Asian Bioethics Review* 2 (2): 108–23.

Clapp, Justin T., Katharine A. Gleason, and Steven Joffe. 2017. "Justification and Authority in Institutional Review Board Decision Letters." *Social Science & Medicine* 194 (December): 25–33. https://doi.org/10.1016/j.socscimed.2017.10.013.

Clarke, John, David Bainton, Noemi Lendvai-Bainton, and Paul Stubbs. 2015. *Making Policy Move: Towards a Politics of Translation and Assemblage*. Policy Press.

Clifford, James, and George E. Marcus. 2010. *Writing Culture: The Poetics and Politics of Ethnography*. University of California Press.

Coleman, Carl. 2003. "Rationalizing Risk Assessment in Human Subject Research." *Arizona Law Review* 45 (897): 1137–87.

Coleman, Carl. 2004. "Why Have IRBs at All?" *Journal of Legal Medicine* 25 (3): 295–301. https://doi.org/10.1080/01947640490496999.

Copeman, Jacob, and Alice Street. 2014. "The Image After Strathern: Art and Persuasive Relationality in India's Sanguinary Politics." *Theory, Culture & Society* 31 (2–3): 185–220. https://doi.org/10.1177/0263276413500321.

Corrigan, Oonagh. 2003. "Empty Ethics: The Problem with Informed Consent." *Sociology of Health & Illness* 25 (7): 768–92. https://doi.org/10.1046/j.1467-9566.2003.00369.x.

Corsín Jiménez, Alberto. 2013. *An Anthropological Trompe L'Oeil for a Common World*. 1st ed. Berghahn Books. https://doi.org/10.3167/9780857459114.

Corsín Jiménez, Alberto. 2010. "How Knowledge Grows: An Anthropological Anamorphosis." Open Anthropology Cooperative. https://openanthcoop.net/2010/06/01/how-knowledge-grows/.

Corsín Jiménez, Alberto. 2003. "The Form of the Relation, or Anthropology's Enchantment With the Algebraic Imagination." http://hdl.handle.net/10261/98307.

Corsín Jiménez, Alberto. 2011. "Trust in Anthropology." *Anthropological Theory* 11 (2): 177–96. https://doi.org/10.1177/1463499611407392.

Crane, Johanna T. 2010. "Unequal 'Partners': AIDS, Academia, and the Rise of Global Health." *Behemoth* 3 (3). https://doi.org/10.1524/behe.2010.0021.

Crawley, Francis P. 1997. "Considering Quality in Ethics: Designing QA Systems for Ethical Review and Informed Consent." *The Quality Assurance Journal* 2 (4): 159–60. https://doi.org/10.1002/(SICI)1099-1786(199712O)2:4<159::AID-QAJ51>3.0.CO;2-O.

Creuss, Syliva, and Richard Creuss. 2005. "The Medical Profession and Self-Regulation: A Current Challenge." *Virtual Mentor* 7 (4): 320–24. https://doi.org/10.1001/virtualmentor.2005.7.4.oped1-0504.

Crook, Tony. 2007. "'If You Don't Believe Our Story, at Least Give Us Half of the Money': Claiming Ownership of the Ok Tedi Mine, PNG." *Journal de La Société Des Océanistes* (125) (December): 221–28. https://doi.org/10.4000/jso.939.

Danielsen, Stentor. 2002. "Shark 'Photo of the Year' Is E-Mail Hoax." *National Geographic News*, August 15. http://news.nationalgeographic.com/news/2002/08/0815_020815_photooftheyear.html.

Daston, Lorraine. 1992. "Objectivity and the Escape from Perspective." *Social Studies of Science* 22 (4): 597–618.

Daston, Lorraine, and Peter Galison. 1992. "The Image of Objectivity." *Representations* 40 (October): 81–128. https://doi.org/10.2307/2928741.

Davies, Sarah R. 2019. "An Ethics of the System: Talking to Scientists About Research Integrity." *Science and Engineering Ethics* 25 (4): 1235–53. https://doi.org/10.1007/s11948-018-0064-y.

Dicken, John. 2023. "Institutional Review Boards: Actions Needed to Improve Federal Oversight and Examine Effectiveness." United States Government Accountability Office. https://www.gao.gov/assets/gao-23-104721.pdf.

Dickson, David. 2002. "WHO and Industry Combine to Form Ethics Body." *Nature Medicine* 8 (7): 645. https://doi.org/10.1038/nm0702-645a.

DiPiazza, Samuel A., and Robert G. Eccles. 2002. *Building Public Trust: The Future of Corporate Reporting*. John Wiley & Sons.

Dissanayake, V.H.W., R. D. Lanerolle, and N. Mendis. 2009. "Research Ethics and Ethical Review Committees in Sri Lanka: A 25 Year Journey." *Ceylon Medical Journal* 51 (3): 110. https://doi.org/10.4038/cmj.v51i3.1254.

Douglas, Mary. 2005. *Risk and Blame: Essays in Cultural Theory*. Digital pbk. ed. Reprint, Routledge.

Douglas, Cristina, and Barbara Pieta. 2024. "The Political Life of Research Ethics Committees and What It Means for Ethnographic Research." *Medicine Anthropology Theory* 11 (2): 1–11. https://doi.org/10.17157/mat.11.2.8135.

Douglas-Jones, Rachel. 2015. "A 'Good' Ethical Review: Audit and Professionalism in Research Ethics." *Social Anthropology* 23 (1): 53–67. https://doi.org/10.1111/1469-8676.12099.

Douglas-Jones, Rachel. 2019. "Getting Inside Ethical Review: Anxious Bureaucracies of Revelation, Anticipation and Virtue." *Critical Public Health* 29 (4): 448–59. https://doi.org/10.1080/09581596.2019.1591615.

Douglas-Jones, Rachel, and Justin Shaffner, eds. 2021. *Hope and Insufficiency: Capacity Building in Ethnographic Comparison*. Berghahn Books.

Drane, J. F. 1996. "Bioethical Perspectives from Ibero-America." *Journal of Medicine and Philosophy* 21 (6): 557–69. https://doi.org/10.1093/jmp/21.6.557.

Dubinsky, P. Michael. 2021. "History." In *The Fundamentals of Clinical Research*, 1–10. John Wiley & Sons, Ltd. https://doi.org/10.1002/9781119772682.ch1.

Dubois-Flynn, Geneviève. 2006. "CIHR Guidelines for Health Research Involving Aboriginal Peoples." In *The Regulation and Organization of Research Ethics Review*, edited by Trudo Lemmens and Tom Archivald, 61–62. Brown Book Company Ltd.

Dumit, Joseph, and Emilia Sanabria. 2022. "Set, Setting, and Clinical Trials: Colonial Technologies and Psychedelics." In *The Palgrave Handbook of the Anthropology of Technology*, edited by Maja Hojer Bruun, Ayo Wahlberg, Rachel Douglas-Jones, et al., 291–308. Springer Nature. https://doi.org/10.1007/978-981-16-7084-8_15.

Dunn, Elizabeth. 2004. *Privatizing Poland: Baby Food, Big Business and the Remaking of Labor*. Cornell University Press.

Durkheim, Émile. 1992. *Professional Ethics and Civic Morals*. 2nd ed. Taylor and Francis.

Dyer, Sarah, and David Demeritt. 2009. "Un-Ethical Review? Why It Is Wrong to Apply the Medical Model of Research Governance to Human Geography." *Progress in Human Geography* 33 (1): 46–64. https://doi.org/10.1177/0309132508090475.

Eckstein, Sue. 2004. "Policy Brief: Efforts to Build Capacity in Research Ethics: An Overview." *Sci Dev. Net*, June 1. https://web.archive.org/web/20110523031709/http://www.scidev.net/en/middle-east-and-north-africa/policy-briefs/efforts-to-build-capacity-in-research-ethics-an-ov.html.

Ellis, Gary. 1994. "Perspectives from OPRR." In *Changes and Choices for Institutional Review Boards: The Inclusion of Women and Minorities, and Other Emerging Issues in Research*, 31–32. Public Responsibility in Medicine and Research.

Emanuel, Ezekiel J., Anne Wood, Alan Fleishman, et al. 2004. "Oversight of Human Participants Research: Identifying Problems to Evaluate Reform Proposals." *Annals of Internal Medicine* 141 (4): 282–91.

Emanuel, Ezekiel J., David Wendler, Jack Killen, and Christine Grady. 2004. "What Makes Clinical Research in Developing Countries Ethical? The Benchmarks of Ethical Research." *The Journal of Infectious Diseases* 189 (5): 930–37. https://doi.org/10.1086/381709.

Engel, Nora, Ine Van Hoyweghen, and Anja Krumeich, eds. 2014. *Making Global Health Care Innovation Work*. Palgrave Macmillan U.S. https://doi.org/10.1057/9781137456038.

Engel, Nora, and Ragna Zeiss. 2014. "Situating Standards in Practices: Multi Drug-Resistant Tuberculosis Treatment in India." *Science as Culture* 23 (2): 201–25. https://doi.org/10.1080/09505431.2013.837875.

Epstein, Steven. 2023. "The Meaning and Significance of Lay Expertise." In *The Oxford Handbook of Expertise and Democratic Policies*, edited by Gil Eyal and Thomas Medvetz, 76–102. Oxford University Press.

European Medicines Agency (EMA). 2022. "Regulatory Harmonisation of Clinical Trials in the EU: Clinical Trials Regulation to Enter into Application and New Clinical Trials Information System to Be Launched." January 25. https://www.ema.europa.eu/en/news/regulatory-harmonisation-clinical-trials-eu-clinical-trials-regulation-enter-application-and-new-clinical-trials-information-system-be-launched.

Evans-Pritchard, Edward E. 2009. *Witchcraft, Oracles, and Magic Among the Azande.* Clarendon Press.

Ezrahi, Yaron. 1990. *The Descent of Icarus: Science and the Transformation of Contemporary Democracy.* Harvard University Press.

Fan, Ruiping. 1997. "Self-Determination vs. Family-Determination: Two Incommensurable Principles of Autonomy." *Bioethics* 11 (3–4): 309–22. https://doi.org/10.1111/1467-8519.00070.

Farmer, Paul. 2003. *Pathologies of Power: Health, Human Rights, and the New War on the Poor.* University of California Press.

FERCAP. 2024. "The SIDCER-FERCAP Recognition Program." SIDCER-FERCAP. https://www.sidcer-fercap.org/pages/about-the-program.php.

FERCAP/SIDCER. 2012. *The FERCAP/SIDCER Handbook of Case Studies on Ethical Issues in Health Research.* Pathumthani, Thailand. https://www.sidcer-fercap.org/file/23973.pdf.

Fernandez Lynch, Holly, Elisa A. Hurley, and Holly A. Taylor. 2023. "Responding to the Call to Meaningfully Assess Institutional Review Board Effectiveness." *JAMA* 330 (3): 221. https://doi.org/10.1001/jama.2023.8457.

Flear, Mark L. 2014. "Clinical Trials Abroad: The Marketable Ethics, Weak Protections and Vulnerable Subjects of EU Law." *Cambridge Yearbook of European Legal Studies* 16 (January): 75–107. https://doi.org/10.1017/S1528887000002561.

Flear, Mark L. 2021. "Expectations as Techniques of Legitimation? Imagined Futures through Global Bioethics Standards for Health Research." *Journal of Law and the Biosciences* 8 (2): 1–30. https://doi.org/10.1093/jlb/lsaa086.

Flear, Mark L. 2009. "The EU's Biopolitical Governance of Advanced Therapy Medicinal Products." *Maastricht Journal of European and Comparative Law* 16 (1): 113–37. https://doi.org/10.1177/1023263X0901600106.

Flear, Mark L., and Richard Ashcroft, eds. 2021. "Law, Biomedical Technoscience, and Imaginaries: Law, Biomedical Technoscience and Imaginaries." *Journal of Law and the Biosciences* 8 (2): 1–6. https://doi.org/10.1093/jlb/lsaa088.

Folkers, Andreas. 2024. "Risking Carbon Capital: Reporting Infrastructures and the Making of Financial Climate Risks." *Economy and Society* 53 (3): 504–26. https://doi.org/10.1080/03085147.2024.2348316.

Friesen, Phoebe, Aimi Nadia Mohd Yusof, and Mark Sheehan. 2019. "Should the Decisions of Institutional Review Boards Be Consistent?" *Ethics & Human Research* 41 (4): 2–14. https://doi.org/10.1002/eahr.500022.

Friesen, Phoebe, Luke Gelinas, Aaron Kirby, David H. Strauss, and Barbara E. Bierer. 2023. "IRBs and the Protection-Inclusion Dilemma: Finding a Balance." *The American Journal of Bioethics* 23 (6): 75–88. https://doi.org/10.1080/15265161.2022.2063434.

Friesen, Phoebe, Rachel Douglas-Jones, Mason Marks, et al. 2021. "Governing AI-Driven Health Research: Are IRBs Up to the Task?" *Ethics & Human Research* 43 (2): 35–42. https://doi.org/10.1002/eahr.500085.

Fujimura, Joan. 1992. "Crafting Science: Standardized Packages, Boundary Objects and 'Translation.'" In *Science as Practice and Culture*, edited by Andrew Pickering, 168–211. University of Chicago Press.

Fuller, Lon. 2000. *The Morality of Law.* Edited by Yaakov Elman and Israel Gershoni. Yale University Press. https://doi.org/10.12987/9780300191653.

Ganguly, Sumit. 2018. "Ending the Sri Lankan Civil War." *Daedalus* 147 (1): 78–89. https://doi.org/10.1162/DAED_a_00475.

Gearing, Fred. 1962. *Priests and Warriors: Social Structures for Cherokee Politics in the 18th Century.* Vol. 93. American Anthropologist Association Memoir.

Geertz, Clifford. 1973. *The Interpretation of Cultures: Selected Essays.* Basic Books, Inc.

Gimbel, Sarah, Baltazar Chilundo, Nora Kenworthy, et al. 2018. "Donor Data Vacuuming." *Medicine Anthropology Theory* 5 (2). https://doi.org/10.17157/mat.5.2.537.

Gluckman, Max. 1972. "Moral Crises: Magical and Secular Solutions." In *The Allocation of Responsibility*, edited by Max Gluckman, 1–50. Manchester University Press.

Gluckman, Max, ed. 1972. *The Allocation of Responsibility.* Manchester University Press.

Goodyear, M. D. E., T. Lemmens, D. Sprumont, and G. Tangwa. 2009. "Does the FDA Have the Authority to Trump the Declaration of Helsinki?" *BMJ* 338: b1559. https://doi.org/10.1136/bmj.b1559.

Gopalan, Nishakanthi, Robyna Irshad Khan, Henry J. Silverman, Jeremy Sugarman, and Vina Vaswani. 2025. "Enhancing Research Ethics Capacity in Asia: Fogarty International Center Supported Initiatives in India, Malaysia, Myanmar, and Pakistan." *Journal of Empirical Research on Human Research Ethics* (March). https://doi.org/10.1177/15562646251323133.

Graham, Janice. 2021. "Conclusion." In *The Social Life of Standards: Ethnographic Methods for Local Engagement*, edited by Janice Graham, Christina Holmes, Fiona McDonald, and Regna Darnell, 254–64. UBC Press.

Gregory, Chris. 2011. "On Money, Debt and Morality: Before Smith, Smith, After Smith." Keynote presented at the Debt Conference, CRASSH. https://sms.cam.ac.uk/media/1175000/.

Griswold, Jr., Charles L. 2006. "Imagination: Morals, Science, and Arts." In *The Cambridge Companion to Adam Smith*, 1st ed., edited by Knud Haakonssen, 22–56. Cambridge University Press. https://doi.org/10.1017/CCOL0521770599.002.

Grosfoguel, Ramón. 2007. "The Epistemic Decolonial Turn: Beyond Political-Economy Paradigms." *Cultural Studies* 21 (2–3): 211–23. https://doi.org/10.1080/095023806 01162514.

Günel, Gökçe. 2019. *Spaceship in the Desert: Energy, Climate Change, and Urban Design in Abu Dhabi*. Duke University Press. https://doi.org/10.1215/9781478002406.

Günel, Gökçe, and Chika Watanabe. 2024. "Patchwork Ethnography." *American Ethnologist* 51 (1): 131–39. https://doi.org/10.1111/amet.13243.

Guston, David H. 2006. "On Consensus and Voting in Science: From Asilomar to the National Toxicology Program." In *The New Political Sociology of Science: Institutions, Networks, and Power*, edited by Kelly Moore and Scott Alan Frickel, 378–404. University of Wisconsin Press.

Guzman, Javier, Erin O'Connell, Kate Kikule, and Tamara Hafner. 2020. "The WHO Global Benchmarking Tool: A Game Changer for Strengthening National Regulatory Capacity." *BMJ Global Health* 5 (8): e003181. https://doi.org/10.1136/bmjgh -2020-003181.

Hamadian, Lisa, and Allan K. Johansen. 2011. "Reviewing the Ethical Reviewers: The SIDCER/FERCAP Experience." In *FERCAP @ 10: In Commemoration of a Decade of Capacity Building in Ethical Health Research in the Asia-Pacific Region*, edited by Atoy M. Navarro and Cristina E. Torres. Thailand: Forum for Ethical Review Committees in the Asian and Western Pacific Region.

Hamburger, Philip. 2004. "The New Censorship: Institutional Review Boards." *The Supreme Court Review* 2004 (January): 271–354. https://doi.org/10.1086/scr.2004 .3536972.

Haraway, Donna Jeanne. 1997. *Modest_Witness@Second_Millennium.FemaleMan© Meets_OncoMouse: Feminism and Technoscience*. Routledge.

Harding, Sandra. 2006. *Science and Social Inequality: Feminist and Postcolonial Issues*. University of Illinois Press.

Have, Henk ten, and Bert Gordijn, eds. 2013. *Handbook of Global Bioethics*. Springer.

Hedgecoe, Adam. 2012. "The Problems of Presumed Isomorphism and the Ethics Review of Social Science: A Response to Schrag." *Research Ethics* 8 (2): 79–86. https://doi.org/10.1177/1747016112445437.

Hedgecoe, Adam. 2012. "Trust and Regulatory Organisations: The Role of Local Knowledge and Facework in Research Ethics Review." *Social Studies of Science* 42 (5): 662–83. https://doi.org/10.1177/0306312712446364.

Hedgecoe, Adam. 2020. *Trust in the System: Research Ethics Committees and the Regulation of Biomedical Research*. Manchester University Press.

Hedgecoe, Adam, F. Carvalho, P. Lobmayer, and F. Raka. 2006. "Research Ethics Committees in Europe: Implementing the Directive, Respecting Diversity." *Journal of Medical Ethics* 32 (8): 483–86. https://doi.org/10.1136/jme.2005.013888.

Herzfeld, Michael. 2012. "Afterword: Reciprocating the Hospitality of These Pages." *Journal of the Royal Anthropological Institute* 18 (s1): S210–17. https://doi.org/10.1111/j.1467-9655.2012.01773.x.

Hess, David J. 2007. "Crosscurrents: Social Movements and the Anthropology of Science and Technology." *American Anthropologist* 109 (3): 463–72. https://doi.org/10.1525/aa.2007.109.3.463.

Hess, David J. 1995. *Science and Technology in a Multicultural World: The Cultural Politics of Facts and Artifacts*. Columbia University Press.

Hess, Sabine. 2006. "Strathern's Melanesian 'Dividual' and the Christian 'Individual': A Perspective from Vanua Lava, Vanuatu." *Oceania* 76 (3): 285–96. https://doi.org/10.1002/j.1834-4461.2006.tb03058.x.

Heyman, Josiah. 2012. "Deepening the Anthropology of Bureaucracy." Edited by Akhil Gupta, Kregg Hetherington, and Matthew S. Hull. *Anthropological Quarterly* 85 (4): 1269–77.

High, Holly. 2014. *Fields of Desire: Poverty and Policy in Laos*. National University of Singapore Press.

Hirayama, Kenji. 2011. "FERCAP Beyond 10." In *FERCAP @ 10: In Commemoration of a Decade of Capacity Building in Ethical Health Research in the Asia-Pacific Region*, edited by Atoy M. Navarro and Cristina E. Torres. Thailand: Forum for Ethical Review Committees in the Asian and Western Pacific Region.

Hirschkind, Charles. 2010. "Is There a Secular Body?" SSRC The Immanent Frame. November 15. https://tif.ssrc.org/2010/11/15/secular-body/.

Ho, Karen. 2009. *Liquidated: An Ethnography of Wall Street*. Duke University Press.

Hoeyer, Klaus, and Linda F. Hogle. 2014. "Informed Consent: The Politics of Intent and Practice in Medical Research Ethics." *Annual Review of Anthropology* 43: 347–62. https://doi.org/10.1146/annurev-anthro-102313-030413.

Hogle, Linda F. 1995. "Standardization across Non-Standard Domains: The Case of Organ Procurement." *Science, Technology, & Human Values* 20 (4): 482–500. https://doi.org/10.1177/016224399502000405.

Holden, Kerry, and David Demeritt. 2008. "Democratising Science? The Politics of Promoting Biomedicine in Singapore's Developmental State." *Environment and Planning D: Society and Space* 26 (1): 68–86. https://doi.org/10.1068/d461t.

Home Office. 2002. *Justice for All (CM 5563)*. TSO (The Stationery Office).

Hongladarom, Soraj. 2004. "Asian Bioethics Revisited: What Is It?, And Is There Such a Thing?" *Eubios Journal of Asian and International Bioethics* 14: 194–97.

Howell, Jude, K. R. Fisher, and X. Shang. 2020. "Accountability and Legitimacy of NGOs under Authoritarianism: The Case of China." *Third World Quarterly* 41 (1): 113–32. https://doi.org/10.1080/01436597.2019.1658520.

Høyer Leivestad, Hege, and Anette Nyqvist, eds. 2017. *Ethnographies of Conferences and Trade Fairs*. Springer International Publishing. https://doi.org/10.1007/978-3-319-53097-0.

Humphrey, Caroline. 1974. "Inside a Mongolian Tent." *New Society* 30 (630): 273.

ICH. 2010. "The Value and Benefits of ICH to Drug Regulatory Authorities—Advancing Harmonization for Better Health." International Conference on Harmonisation of Technical Requirements for Registration of Pharmaceuticals for Human Use.

ICH GCP. 2025. "Guideline for Good Clinical Practice E6(R3)." International Council for Harmonisation of Technical Requirements for Pharmaceuticals for Human Use. https://database.ich.org/sites/default/files/ICH_E628R329_Step4_FinalGuideline_2025_0106.pdf.

ICH GCP. 1996. "ICH Topic E6 (R1) Guideline for Good Clinical Practice." European Medicines Agency.

IIA (Institute of Internal Auditors). 2018. "Ethics: The IIA." Industry: The Institute of Internal Auditors. https://www.theiia.org/en/standards/what-are-the-standards/mandatory-guidance/code-of-ethics/.

Institute of Medicine. 2001. *Preserving Public Trust: Accreditation and Human Research Participant Protection Programs*. National Academies Press. https://doi.org/10.17226/10085.

IOM, Institute of Medicine. 2009. *On Being a Scientist: A Guide to Responsible Conduct in Research: Third Edition*. National Academies Press. https://doi.org/10.17226/12192.

IOM, Institute of Medicine. 1992. *Responsible Science: Ensuring the Integrity of the Research Process: Volume I*. National Academies Press. https://doi.org/10.17226/1864.

IOM, Institute of Medicine. 1993. *Responsible Science, Volume II: Background Papers and Resource Documents*. National Academies Press. https://doi.org/10.17226/2091.

IOM, Institute of Medicine. 1989. *The Responsible Conduct of Research in the Health Sciences*. National Academies Press. https://doi.org/10.17226/1388.

ISO. 2019. "Tea—Preparation of Liquor for Use in Sensory Tests."

Jacob, Marie Andrée, and Annelise Riles. 2007. "The New Bureaucracies of Virtue: Introduction." *PoLAR: Political and Legal Anthropology Review* 30 (2): 181–91. https://doi.org/10.1525/pol.2007.30.2.181.

Jacobs, Noortje. 2022. *Ethics by Committee: A History of Reasoning Together About Medicine, Science, Society, and the State*. University of Chicago Press. https://doi.org/10.7208/chicago/9780226819310.001.0001.

James, Wendy. 1975. "Councils in Action." *African Affairs* 74 (294): 119–20. https://doi.org/10.1093/oxfordjournals.afraf.a096564.

Jasanoff, Sheila. 2005. *Designs on Nature: Science and Democracy in Europe and the United States*. Princeton University Press.

Jayasinghe, Krishani, W.A.S. Chamika, Kaushalya Jayaweera, et al. 2023. "All You Need Is Trust? Public Perspectives on Consenting to Participate in Genomic Research in the Sri Lankan District of Colombo." *Asian Bioethics Review* (November). https://doi.org/10.1007/s41649-023-00269-y.

Jensen, Casper. 2007. "Infrastructural Fractals: Revisiting the Micro-Macro Distinction in Social Theory." *Environment and Planning D: Society and Space* 25: 832–50.

Jensen, Casper Bruun. 2021. "Material Itineraries: Southeast Asian Urban Transformations." *East Asian Science, Technology and Society: An International Journal* 15 (2): 124–34. https://doi.org/10.1080/18752160.2021.1917840.

Jensen, Casper Bruun, and Brit Ross Winthereik. 2013. *Monitoring Movements in Development Aid: Recursive Partnerships and Infrastructures*. MIT Press.

Jesani, Amar. 2009. "Ethics in Ethics Committees: Time to Share Experiences, Discuss Challenges and Do a Better Job." *Indian Journal of Medical Ethics* (2) (April). https://doi.org/10.20529/IJME.2009.022.

Kafka, Ben. 2012. *The Demon of Writing: Powers and Failures of Paperwork*. Zone Books.

Kage, Rieko. 2017. *Who Judges? Designing Jury Systems in Japan, East Asia, and Europe*. Cambridge University Press.

Kant, Lalit, and Roli Mathur. 2023. "Vasantha Muthuswamy (1948–2023)." *Indian Journal of Medical Research* 157 (2 & 3): 223. https://doi.org/10.4103/ijmr.ijmr_444_23.

Karbwang, Juntra. 2008. "SIDCER Network and IRB Recognition Programme." PowerPoint presented at the International Round Table, Rome, December 15. http://www.unicri.us/special_topics/clinical_research/round_table/.

Karbwang, Juntra, and Francis P. Crawley. 2007. "Need to Strengthen Ethics Committees." *SciDev.Net* (blog), November 14. https://www.scidev.net/global/opinions/need-to-strengthen-ethics-committees/.

Karbwang, Juntra, Francis P. Crawley, Melody Lin, and Elaine Esber. 2001. "Ethical Review and the Globalization of Clinical Trials: Defining Policy Through Action." https://nus.edu.sg/research/docs/librariesprovider3/references/who-defining-policy-through-action.pdf.

Karbwang, Juntra, Mihai Mihut, and Christine Halleux. 2010. "Quality Management: Research Needs Quality Management System." *TDRnews* 85 (May): 24–25.

Karbwang Laothavorn, Juntra. 2016. "Introduction: The Origin of These Perspectives." In *Perspectives on Ethical Review: A Casebook for Reflecting on Challenges and Aspirations for Improving the Role and Function of Ethics Committees and Ethical Review Systems*, edited by SIDCER.

Karbwang Laothavorn, Juntra. 2011. "SIDCER @ 10." In *FERCAP @ 10: In Commemoration of a Decade of Capacity Building in Ethical Health Research in the Asia-Pacific Region*, edited by Atoy M. Navarro and Cristina E. Torres. Thailand: Forum for Ethical Review Committees in the Asian and Western Pacific Region.

Kass, Nancy E., Adnan Ali Hyder, Ademola Ajuwon, et al. 2007. "The Structure and Function of Research Ethics Committees in Africa: A Case Study." *PLoS Medicine* 4 (1): e3. https://doi.org/10.1371/journal.pmed.0040003.

Katz, Jack. 2007. "Toward a Natural History of Ethical Censorship." *Law & Society Review* 41 (4): 797–810.

Katz, Jay. 1972. "Who Is to Keep Guard Over the Guards Themselves?" *Fertility and Sterility* 23 (8): 604–609. https://doi.org/10.1016/S0015-0282(16)39141-5.

Katz, Jay, Alexander Morgan Capron, and Eleanor Swift Glass. 1972. *Experimentation with Human Beings: The Authority of the Investigator, Subject, Professions, and State int heh Human Experimentaiton Process*. Russell Sage.

Kaur, Sharon, and Choong Yeow Choy. 2014. "Ethical Considerations in Clinical Trials: A Critique of the ICH-GCP Guideline." *Developing World Bioethics* 14 (1): 20–28. https://doi.org/10.1111/dewb.12004.

Kelly, Ann H. 2012. "The Experimental Hut: Hosting Vectors." *Journal of the Royal Anthropological Institute* 18 (s1): S145–60. https://doi.org/10.1111/j.1467-9655.2012.01769.x.

Kennedy, Ian. 1993. *Unmasking of Medicine: A Searching Look at Healthcare Today*. Routledge.

Kenworthy, Nora, Lynn M. Thomas, and Johanna Crane. 2018. "Introduction: Critical Perspectives on US Global Health Partnerships in Africa and Beyond." *Medicine Anthropology Theory* 5 (2). https://doi.org/10.17157/mat.5.1.613.

Kim, Leo. 2008. "Explaining the Hwang Scandal: National Scientific Culture and Its Global Relevance." *Science as Culture* 17 (4): 397–415. https://doi.org/10.1080/09505430802515023.

Kipnis, Andrew B. 2008. "Audit Cultures: Neoliberal Governmentality, Socialist Legacy, or Technologies of Governing?" *American Ethnologist* 35 (2): 275–89. https://doi.org/10.1111/j.1548-1425.2008.00034.x.

Konrad, Monica. 2012. *Collaborators Collaborating: Counterparts in Anthropological Knowledge and International Research Relations*. Berghahn Books.

Koski, Greg. 2008. "Empowering Stakeholders in Health Research: Defining Stakeholder Responsibilities Toward Implementing a Duty-Based Ethics." 8th FERCAP Conference, November 24–25.

Koski, Greg. 2011. "Human Research Subject Protection: A Time of Reflection, Renewal and Reform? No—It's Time to Redesign!" Webinar. Xtalks. https://web.archive.org/web/20120413124911/http://xtalks.com/xt0451irbservices.ashx.

Kowal, Emma. 2023. *Haunting Biology: Science and Indigeneity in Australia*. Experimental Futures. Duke University Press.

Kuo, Wen-Hua. 2018. "Turning Ethics into Institutions: The Techno-Politics of Human Research Regulation in Taiwan." *Science, Technology and Society* 23 (2): 289–306. https://doi.org/10.1177/0971721818762877.

Kuo, Wen-Hua. 2008. "Understanding Race at the Frontier of Pharmaceutical Regulation: An Analysis of the Racial Difference Debate at the ICH." *Journal of Law, Medicine & Ethics* 36 (3): 498–505. https://doi.org/10.1111/j.1748-720X.2008.297.x.

Lamont, Michèle. 2010. *How Professors Think: Inside the Curious World of Academic Judgment*. 1st pbk. ed. Harvard University Press.

Lampland, Martha, and Susan Leigh Star, eds. 2009. *Standards and Their Stories: How Quantifying, Classifying, and Formalizing Practices Shape Everyday Life*. Cornell University Press.

Latour, Bruno. 2004. *Politics of Nature: How to Bring the Sciences into Democracy*. Harvard University Press.

Latour, Bruno. 2005. *Reassembling the Social: An Introduction to Actor-Network-Theory*. Oxford University Press. https://doi.org/10.1093/oso/9780199256044.001.0001.

Laurie, Graeme T. 2023. "Bioethics in Northeast Asia." *Asian Bioethics Review* 15 (4): 357–60. https://doi.org/10.1007/s41649-023-00260-7.

Law, John. 2008. "A Comment on 'A Turn to Ontology in STS?'" Presented at the International Day Workshop Said Business School, Oxford, June 25. http://www.sbs.ox.ac.uk/research/sts/ events/Documents/JohnLaw.pdf.

Lawrence, David R. 2025. "Bioethics Transformed: 40 Years of the Value of Life." *Cambridge Quarterly of Healthcare Ethics* 34 (2): 144–55. https:// doi.org/10.1017/S0963180124000549.

Le Guin, Ursula K. 1989. *Dancing at the Edge of the World: Thoughts on Words, Women, Places*. Grove Press.

Lea, Tess. 2021. "Desiring Bureaucracy." *Annual Review of Anthropology* 50: 59–74. https://doi.org/10.1146/annurev-anthro-101819-110147.

Lea, Tess. 2024. "Policy Ecology as Concept and Method." *Critical Policy Studies*: 1–18. https://doi.org/10.1080/19460171.2024.2370581.

Lee, Hwei-Ling. 2008. "Certification for Ethics in Research Proficiency." In *FERCAP Conference Panel Discussion 2: Empowering Investigators for Ethical Health Research*. Bangkok, Thailand.

Lemmens, Trudo. 2006. "The Commercialization of Research and REC Review in North America." In *The Regulation and Organization of Research Ethics Review*, by Angela Long, A. Sasha Kontic, Elizabeth Cuéllar Barroso, and Daniel Brinza, edited by Trudo Lemmens and Tom Archibald, 31–33. Brown Book Company Ltd.

Lemonick, Michael, and Andrew Goldstein. 2002. "How Medical Testing Has Turned Millions of Us into Human Guinea Pigs." *Time*, April 22.

Leng, Chee Heng. 1999. "A Brief Review of the GFBR Meeting." Report 1. Bethesda, Maryland: Global Forum on Bioethics in Research. https://www.gfbr.global/wp-content/uploads/2015/08/First_report1.pdf.

Levinson, Daniel R. 2010. "Challenges to FDA's Ability to Monitor and Inspect Foreign Clinical Trials." OEI-01-08-00510. Department of Health and Human Services Office of the Inspector General. https://oig.hhs.gov/documents/evaluation/2542/OEI-01-08-00510-Complete%20Report.pdf.

Lewis, David, and Mark Schuller. 2017. "Engagements with a Productively Unstable Category: Anthropologists and Nongovernmental Organizations." *Current Anthropology* 58 (5): 634–51. https://doi.org/10.1086/693897.

Lezaun, Javier, and Nerea Calvillo. 2014. "In the Political Laboratory: Kurt Lewin's *Atmospheres*." *Journal of Cultural Economy* 7 (4): 434–57. https://doi.org/10.1080/17530350.2013.860045.

Li, Dan. 2025. "Ethical Governance in Chinese Universities: An Overview of Research Ethics Committees." *Ethics & Behavior* 35 (1): 1–12. https://doi.org/10.1080/10508422.2024.2301764.

Li, Tania. 2007. *The Will to Improve: Governmentality, Development, and the Practice of Politics*. Duke University Press.

Lin, S. C., J. Hsu, and V. Y. Fan. 2009. "'Silent Virtuous Teachers': Anatomical Dissection in Taiwan." *BMJ* 339 (dec16 2): b5001. https://doi.org/10.1136/bmj.b5001.

Lin, Wen-yuan, and John Law. 2019. "Where Is East Asia in STS?" *East Asian Science, Technology and Society: An International Journal* 13 (1): 115–36. https://doi.org/10.1215/18752160-6995634.

Lindholm, Oskar, Sakari Karjalainen, and Veikko Launis. 2025. "Chasing 'Vulnerability' Across Six Decades of the Declaration of Helsinki." *Monash Bioethics Review*, February. https://doi.org/10.1007/s40592-025-00235-4.

Lister, Sarah. 2003. "NGO Legitimacy: Technical Issue or Social Construct?" *Critique of Anthropology* 23 (2): 175–92. https://doi.org/10.1177/0308275X03023002004.

Littler, Katherine, Joseph Millum, and Douglas Richard Wassenaar. 2014. "The Global Forum for Bioethics in Research: Past, Present and Future." *South African Journal of Bioethics and Law* 7 (1): 5. https://doi.org/10.7196/sajbl.312.

Loff, Bebe. 2000. "Forum Develops Ideas for a Global Strategy for Bioethics Research." *The Lancet* 356 (9240): 1502. https://doi.org/10.1016/S0140-6736(05)73259-1.

Loff, Bebe, Karen Hofman, and Vasantha Muthuswamy. 2000. "Conference Report: The Global Forum for Bioethics in Research." *Indian Journal of Medical Ethics*, Global Forum on Bioethics in Research. https://ijme.in/articles/the-global-forum-for-bioethics-in-research-report-of-a-meeting/.

Loff, Bebe, Karen Hofman, and Vasantha Muthuswamy. 2001. "The Global Forum for Bioethics in Research: Report of a Meeting." *Issues in Medical Ethics* IX (1): 63–64. http://hdl.handle.net/20.500.12424/231757.

Lynch, Holly Fernandez, and Stephen Rosenfeld. 2020. "Institutional Review Board Quality, Private Equity, and Promoting Ethical Human Subjects Research." *Annals of Internal Medicine* 173 (7): 558–62. https://doi.org/10.7326/M20-1674.

Lynch, Holly Fernandez, Whitney Eriksen, and Justin T. Clapp. 2022. "'We Measure What We Can Measure': Struggles in Defining and Evaluating Institutional Review Board Quality." *Social Science & Medicine* 292 (January): 114614. https://doi.org/10.1016/j.socscimed.2021.114614.

MacIntyre, Alasdair C. 2007. *After Virtue: A Study in Moral Theory*. 3rd ed. University of Notre Dame Press.

Macklin, Ruth. 2001. "After Helsinki: Unresolved Issues in International Research." *Kennedy Institute of Ethics Journal* 11 (1): 17–36. https://doi.org/10.1353/ken.2001.0005.

Macklin, Ruth. 2004. *Double Standards in Medical Research in Developing Countries*. Cambridge University Press. https://doi.org/10.1017/CBO9780511495359.

Malakoff, David. 2002. "Agency Wants to Stop Shopping for Best Deal." *Science* 296 (5575): 1953. https://doi.org/10.1126/science.296.5575.1953.

Malcolm, Noel. 2004. *Aspects of Hobbes*. 1st pbk ed. Oxford University Press.

Maranta, Alessandro, Michael Guggenheim, Priska Gisler, and Christian Pohl. 2003. "The Reality of Experts and the Imagined Lay Person." *Acta Sociologica* 46 (2): 150–65. https://doi.org/10.1177/0001699303046002005.

Marcus, George E. 2008. "Collaborative Options and Pedagogical Experiment in Anthropological Research on Experts and Policy Processes." *Anthropology in Action* 15 (2): 47–57. https://doi.org/10.3167/aia.2008.150205.

Marres, Noortje. 2005. "Issues Spark a Public Into Being: A Key but Often Forgotten Point of the Lippmann-Dewey Debate." In *Making Things Public: Atmospheres of Democracy; [Exhibition at ZKM, Center for Art and Media Karlsruhe 20.03.—03.10.2005]*, edited by Bruno Latour, Peter Weibel, and Zentrum für Kunst und Medientechnologie Karlsruhe, 208–17. MIT Press.

Martin, Emily. 1997. "Managing Americans: Policy and Changes in the Meanings of Work and the Self." In *Anthropology of Policy: Critical Perspectives on Governance and Power*, edited by Cris Shore and Susan Wright. Routledge.

Mathur, Nayanika. 2017. "Bureaucracy." *Cambridge Encyclopedia of Anthropology* (November). https://www.anthroencyclopedia.com/entry/bureaucracy.

Mathur, Dr. Roli, Dr. Ankita Kar, Dr. Mirunalini Sundar, Anamika Kumari, and Ms. Subashini. 2023. *The Mother of Bioethics in India: Remembering Dr. Vasantha Muthuswamy*. Compiled by ICMR Bioethics Unit.

Mayer, Tony, and Nicholas Steneck, eds. 2011. *Promoting Research Integrity in a Global Environment*. World Scientific. https://doi.org/10.1142/8102.

Mbidde, Edward. 1998. "Bioethics and Local Circumstances." *Science* 279 (5348): 155. https://doi.org/10.1126/science.279.5348.155a.

Mbidde, Edward K. 1997. "Letter to Harold Varmus from Edward K. Mbidde." May 8. Jon Cohen AIDS Research Collection. https://name.umdl.umich.edu/5571095.0418.012.

Mead, Margaret, and Paul Byers. 1968. *The Small Conference: An Innovation in Communication*. Mouton de Gruyter.

Meinert, Lotte, and Susan Reynolds Whyte. 2014. "Epidemic Projectification: AIDS Responses in Uganda as Event and Process." *The Cambridge Journal of Anthropology* 32 (1): 77–94. https://doi.org/10.3167/ca.2014.320107.

Merz, Sibille. 2021. "Global Trials, Local Bodies: Negotiating Difference and Sameness in Indian For-Profit Clinical Trials." *Science, Technology, & Human Values* 46 (4): 882–905. https://doi.org/10.1177/0162243920963813.

MFES (Middleton Foundation for Ethical Studies). 2013. "About the International Fellows Program." October 19. https://web.archive.org/web/20131019102811/http://middletonfoundation.org/aboutfellows.html#.

Michael, Mike. 1996. "Ignoring Science: Discourses of Ignorance in the Public Understanding of Science." In *Misunderstanding Science? The Public Reconstruction of Science and Technology*, edited by Alan Irwin and Brian Wynne, 107–25. Cambridge University Press.

Mika, Marissa. 2021. *Africanizing Oncology: Creativity, Crisis, and Cancer in Uganda.* Ohio University Press.

Miller, Daniel. 1998. "Conclusion: A Theory of Virtualism." In *Virtualism.* Routledge.

Miller, Daniel. 2003. "The Virtual Moment." *Journal of the Royal Anthropological Institute* 9 (1): 57–75. https://doi.org/10.1111/1467-9655.t01-2-00004.

Mitchell, Timothy. 1988. *Colonising Egypt.* University of California Press.

Mitchell, Timothy. 1999. "Society, Economy, and the State Effect." In *State/Culture: State-Formation After the Cultural Turn,* edited by George Steinmetz, 76–97. Cornell University Press. https://doi.org/10.7591/9781501717789.

Mitchell, Timothy, and Anupama Rao. 2013. "Comparative Studies of South Asia, Africa and the Middle East: Mission Statement." *Comparative Studies of South Asia, Africa and the Middle East* 33 (2): 135–36.

Molyneux, C. S., N. Peshu, and K. Marsh. 2005. "Trust and Informed Consent: Insights from Community Members on the Kenyan Coast." *Social Science & Medicine* 61 (7): 1463–73. https://doi.org/10.1016/j.socscimed.2004.11.073.

Molyneux, Sassy, and P. Wenzel Geissler. 2008. "Ethics and the Ethnography of Medical Research in Africa." *Social Science & Medicine* 67 (5): 685–95. https://doi.org/10.1016/j.socscimed.2008.02.023.

Molzon, Justina A. 2005. "The International Conference on Harmonization Common Technical Document—Global Submission Format?" *Food and Drug Law Journal* 60 (3): 447–51. https://www.jstor.org/stable/26660289.

Montgomery, Catherine M., Patricia Kingori, Salla Sariola, and Nora Engel. 2017. "STS and Global Health." *Science & Technology Studies* (September): 2–12. https://doi.org/10.23987/sts.65369.

Moorthy, Vasee, Ibrahim Abubakar, Firdausi Qadri, Bernhards Ogutu, Wei Zhang, John Reeder, and Jeremy Farrar. 2024. "The Future of the Global Clinical Trial Ecosystem: A Vision from the First WHO Global Clinical Trials Forum." *The Lancet* 403 (10422): 124–26. https://doi.org/10.1016/S0140-6736(23)02798-8.

Morita, Atsuro. 2017. "Encounters, Trajectories, and the Ethnographic Moment: Why 'Asia as Method' Still Matters." *East Asian Science, Technology and Society: An International Journal* 11 (2): 239–50. https://doi.org/10.1215/18752160-3825820.

Mormina, Maru, and Romina Istratii. 2021. "'Capacity for What? Capacity for Whom?' A Decolonial Deconstruction of Research Capacity Development Practices in the Global South and a Proposal for a Value-Centred Approach." *Wellcome Open Research* 6 (May): 129. https://doi.org/10.12688/wellcomeopenres.16850.1.

Mourouguessine, Vimal, Nishanthi Anandabaskar, and Kagne Rajendrakumar Nivaratirao. 2022. "Experiences on the Path to Achieving SIDCER Recognition of an Ethics Committee." *Bangladesh Journal of Bioethics* 13 (3): 53–60. https://doi.org/10.62865/bjbio.v13i3.45.

Moyi Okwaro, Ferdinand, and P. W. Geissler. 2015. "In/Dependent Collaborations: Perceptions and Experiences of African Scientists in Transnational HIV Research." *Medical Anthropology Quarterly* 29 (4): 492–511. https://doi.org/10.1111/maq.12206.

Munro, Rolland. 2005. "Partial Organization: Marilyn Strathern and the Elicitation of Relations." *The Sociological Review* 53 (1_suppl): 245–66. https://doi.org/10.1111/j.1467-954X.2005.00553.x.

Muthuswamy, Vasantha. 2013. "Ethical Issues in Clinical Research." *Perspectives in Clinical Research* 4 (1): 9. https://doi.org/10.4103/2229-3485.106369.

Myser, Catherine, ed. 2011. "First Steps Toward a Comparative Anthropology and Sociology of Globalizing Bioethics: Reflecting on the Cultural Meanings and Social Functions of Bioethics." In *Bioethics Around the Globe*, 1st ed., xix–xxxiv. Oxford University Press. https://doi.org/10.1093/acprof:osobl/9780195386097.002.0008.

Nader, Laura, ed. 1996. *Naked Science: Anthropological Inquiry into Boundaries, Power, and Knowledge*. Routledge.

Navaro-Yashin, Yael. 2007. "Make-Believe Papers, Legal Forms and the Counterfeit: Affective Interactions between Documents and People in Britain and Cyprus." *Anthropological Theory* 7 (1): 79–98. https://doi.org/10.1177/1463499607074294.

Navarro, Atoy. 2012. "Background of the Handbook." In *FERCAP/SIDCER Handbook of Case Studies on Ethical Issues in Health Research*, by Forum for Ethical Review Committees in the Qsian and Western Pacific Region (FERCAP) and Strategic Initiative for Developing Capacity in Ethical Review (SIDCER), 3–7. Pathumthani, Thailand: FERCAP/SIDCER.

Navarro, Atoy, Juntra Karbwang-Laothavorn, and Kenji Hirayama. 2020. "SIDCER-FERCAP Survey Terms of Reference & Standard Operating Procedures."

NBAC (National Bioethics Advisory Commission). 2001. "Ethical and Policy Issues in Researc Involving Human Participants." 600702009–001. Report and Recommendations of the National Bioethics Advisory Commission. https://doi.apa.org/doi/10.1037/e600702009-001.

Nicholl, Jon. 2000. "The Ethics of Research Ethics Committees." *BMJ: British Medical Journal* 320 (7243): 1217.

Noah, Lars. 2004. "Deputizing Institutional Review Boards to Police (Audit?) Biomedical Research." *Journal of Legal Medicine* 25 (3): 267–93. https://doi.org/10.1080/01947640490496962.

Noah, Lars. 2002. "Informed Consent and the Elusive Dichotomy Between Standard and Experimental Therapy." *American Journal of Law & Medicine* 28 (4): 361–408. https://doi.org/10.1017/S0098858800002690.

Nuffield Council on Bioethics. 2002. "The Ethics of Research Related to Healthcare in Developing Countries."

Nuffield Council on Bioethics, ed. 2005. *The Ethics of Research Related to Healtcare in Developing Countries: A Follow-up Discussion Paper.* Nuffield Council on Bioethics. https://cdn.nuffieldbioethics.org/wp-content/uploads/HRRDC-short-guide.pdf.

O'Neill, Onora. 2010. *A Question of Trust*. The BBC Reith Lectures 2002. Cambridge University Press.

O'Reilly, Michelle, Mary Dixon-Woods, Emma Angell, Richard Ashcroft, and Alan Bryman. 2009. "Doing Accountability: A Discourse Analysis of Research Ethics

Committee Letters." *Sociology of Health & Illness* 31 (2): 246–61. https://doi.org/10.1111/j.1467-9566.2008.01132.x.

OHRP (Office for Human Research Protections). 2009. "Federal Policy for the Protection of Human Subjects ('Common Rule')." June 23. https://www.hhs.gov/ohrp/regulations-and-policy/regulations/common-rule/index.html.

Ong, Aihwa. 2016. *Fungible Life: Experiment in the Asian City of Life*. Duke University Press.

Ong, Aihwa. 2010. "Introduction: An Analytics of Biotechnology and Ethics at Multiple Scales." In *Asian Biotech: Ethics and Communities of Fate*, edited by Aihwa Ong and Nancy N. Chen, 1–55. Duke University Press.

Ong, Aihwa, and Nancy N. Chen, eds. 2010. *Asian Biotech: Ethics and Communities of Fate*. Duke University Press. https://doi.org/10.1215/9780822393207.

Ong, Jerome A., Atoy M. Navarro, and Mary Dorothy Dela Jose. 2019. "Introduction: A Festschrift for Cristina E. Torres." In *Social Sciences, Health and Ethics: Papers Celebrating Cristina E. Torres*. Manila: Department of Social Sciences, University of the Philippines.

Parker, Michael, and Patricia Kingori. 2016. "Good and Bad Research Collaborations: Researchers' Views on Science and Ethics in Global Health Research." *PLOS ONE* 11 (10): e0163579. https://doi.org/10.1371/journal.pone.0163579.

Parry, Richard Lloyd. 2009. "Trial by Jury Returns to Japan and the Lawyers Aren't Happy." *The Times*, February 28. https://www.thetimes.com/best-law-firms/profile-legal/article/trial-by-jury-returns-to-japan-and-the-lawyers-arent-happy-9vgfn2hhjr8.

Parums, Dinah V. 2024. "Editorial: The 2024 Revision of the Declaration of Helsinki and Its Continued Role as a Code of Ethics to Guide Medical Research." *Medical Science Monitor: International Medical Journal of Experimental and Clinical Research* 30 (December): e947428. https://doi.org/10.12659/MSM.947428.

Pater, Jessica, Casey Fiesler, and Michael Zimmer. 2022. "No Humans Here: Ethical Speculation on Public Data, Unintended Consequences, and the Limits of Institutional Review." *Proceedings of the ACM on Human-Computer Interaction* 6 (38): 1–13. https://doi.org/10.1145/3492857.

Pels, Peter. 2000. "The Trickster's Dilemma." In *Audit Cultures: Anthropological Studies in Accountability, Ethics and the Academy*, edited by Marilyn Strathern, 1. Routledge.

Pereira, Pratibha, and K. L. Bairy. 2012. "Accreditation of Human Research Protection Program: An Indian Perspective." *Perspectives in Clinical Research* 3 (2): 80. https://doi.org/10.4103/2229-3485.96455.

Petryna, Adriana. 2007. "Clinical Trials Offshored: On Private Sector Science and Public Health." *BioSocieties* 2 (1): 21–40. https://doi.org/10.1017/S1745855207005030.

Petryna, Adriana. 2009. *When Experiments Travel: Clinical Trials and the Global Search for Human Subjects*. Princeton University Press.

Pickering-Saqqa, Susannah. 2023. "Introduction: Researching Development NGOs." In *Researching Development NGOs*. Routledge.

Pitt-Rivers, Julian. 2011. "The Place of Grace in Anthropology." *HAU: Journal of Ethnographic Theory* 1 (1): 423–50. https://doi.org/10.14318/hau1.1.017.

Power, Michael. 2022. "Afterword: Audit Society 2.0?" *Qualitative Research in Accounting & Management* 21 (1): 2–6. https://doi.org/10.1108/QRAM-03-2022-0040.

Power, Michael. 1994. *The Audit Explosion*. Paper 7. Demos.

Pratt, Bridget. 2023. "A Multidimensional Account of Social Justice for Global Health Research." *Bioethics* 37 (7): 624–36. https://doi.org/10.1111/bioe.13186.

Pratt, Bridget, and Jantina de Vries. 2023. "Where Is Knowledge from the Global South? An Acount of Epistemic Justice for a Global Bioethics." *Journal of Medical Ethics* 49 (5): 325–34. https://doi.org/10.1136/jme-2022-108291.

Pratt, Bridget, Cassandra Van, Yali Cong, et al. 2014. "Perspectives from South and East Asia on Clinical and Research Ethics: A Literature Review." *Journal of Empirical Research on Human Research Ethics* 9 (2): 52–67. https://doi.org/10.1525/jer.2014.9.2.52.

Precht, Robert E. 2006. "Opinion: Japan, the Jury." *The New York Times*, December 1. https://www.nytimes.com/2006/12/01/opinion/japan-the-jury.html.

PRIM&R. 2009. "PRIM&R's History and Future." YouTube. Public Responsibility in Medicine and Research. https://www.youtube.com/watch?v=v1jz8tWTuw8.

Rao, Ursula. 2022. "Policy as Experimentation: Failing 'Forward' Towards Universal Health Coverage in India." *Social Anthropology/Anthropologie Sociale* 30 (2): 81–100. https://doi.org/10.3167/saas.2022.300206.

Rehnquist, Janet. 2001. "The Globalization of Clinical Trials: A Growing Challenge in Protecting Human Subjects." OEI-01-00-00190. Boston. https://oig.hhs.gov/reports/all/2001/the-globalization-of-clinical-trials-a-growing-challenge-in-protecting-human-subjects/.

Resneck, Jack S. 2025. "Revisions to the Declaration of Helsinki on Its 60th Anniversary: A Modernized Set of Ethical Principles to Promote and Ensure Respect for Participants in a Rapidly Innovating Medical Research Ecosystem." *JAMA* 333 (1): 15. https://doi.org/10.1001/jama.2024.21902.

Resnik, David B. 2021. "Standards of Evidence for Institutional Review Board Decision-Making." *Accountability in Research* 28 (7): 428–55. https://doi.org/10.1080/08989621.2020.1855149.

Reubi, David. 2012. "The Human Capacity to Reflect and Decide: Bioethics and the Reconfiguration of the Research Subject in the Britich Biomedical Sciences." *Social Studies of Science* 42 (3): 348–68. https://doi.org/10.1177/0306312712439457.

Reverby, Susan. 2013. *Examining Tuskegee: The Infamous Syphilis Study and Its Legacy*. 1st ed. University of North Carolina Press.

Reverby, Susan M., and Amy Moran-Thomas. 2024. "On the Appearance and Disappearance of Difficult Medical Histories: What Does It Take to Sustain Public

Memory?" *American Journal of Public Health* 114 (6): 564–68. https://doi.org/10.2105/AJPH.2024.307643.

Richards, Audrey. 1971. "Introduction: The Nature of the Problem." In *Councils in Action*, edited by Audrey Richards and Adam Kuper. Cambridge Papers in Social Anthropology, no. 6. Cambridge University Press.

Richards, Audrey, and Adam Kuper, eds. 1971. *Councils in Action*. Cambridge Papers in Social Anthropology 6. Cambridge University Press.

Riles, Annelise. 2001. *The Network Inside Out*. University of Michigan Press.

Rivera, Roberto, and David Borasky. 2009. *Research Ethics Training Curriculum*. 2nd ed. Family Health International.

Rose, Nikolas S. 1991. *Governing the Soul: The Shaping of the Private Self.* Routledge.

Rosemann, Achim. 2019. "Alter-Standardizing Clinical Trials: The Gold Standard in the Crossfire." *Science as Culture* 28 (2): 125–48. https://doi.org/10.1080/09505431.2019.1606190.

Rothman, David J. 2003. *Strangers at the Bedside: A History of How Law and Bioethics Transformed Medical Decision Making*. 2nd pbk. ed. Aldine de Gruyter.

Sampson, Steven. 2021. "Good People Doing Bad Things: Compliance Regimes in Organisations." *Journal of Legal Anthropology* 5 (1): 110–34. https://doi.org/10.3167/jla.2021.050105.

Sampson, Steven. 2022. "NGOs, NGO-Ing, and NGO-Graphy in Serbia." *Focaal* 93: 112–18. https://doi.org/10.3167/fcl.2022.930109.

Sampson, Steven. 2015. "The Anti-Corruption Package." *Ephemera* 15 (2): 435–43.

Sandler, Ronald, and John Basl. 2019. "Building Data and AI Ethics Committees." Accenture and Ethics Institute at Northeaster Institute.

Sankar, Pamela. 2004. "Communication and Miscommunication in Informed Consent to Research." *Medical Anthropology Quarterly* 18 (4): 429–46. https://doi.org/10.1525/maq.2004.18.4.429.

Sansone, Rosa, and Letizia Bonanno. 2025. "Introduction: Documents, State Affects, and Imaginings at Times of Bureaucratic Impasse." *The Cambridge Journal of Anthropology* 43 (1): 1–20. https://doi.org/10.3167/cja.2025.430102.

Sariola, Salla, and Bob Simpson. 2019. *Research as Development: Biomedical Research, Ethics, and Collaboration in Sri Lanka*. Cornell University Press.

Sariola, Salla, and Bob Simpson. 2011. "Theorising the 'Human Subject' in Biomedical Research: International Clinical Trials and Bioethics Discourses in Contemporary Sri Lanka." *Social Science & Medicine* 73 (4): 515–21. https://doi.org/10.1016/j.socscimed.2010.11.024.

Sariola, Salla, Roger Jeffery, Amar Jesani, and Gerard Porter. 2019. "How Civil Society Organisations Changed the Regulation of Clinical Trials in India." *Science as Culture* 28 (2): 200–22. https://doi.org/10.1080/09505431.2018.1493449.

SATORI (Stakeholders Acting Together on the Ethical Impact Assessment of Research and Innovation). 2014. "SATORI." SATORI Project. https://satoriproject.eu.

Schaffer, Simon. 2005. "Seeing Double: How to Make a Phantom Body Politic." In *Making Things Public: Atmospheres of Democracy*, edited by Bruno Latour and Peter Weibel, 196–202. MIT Press.

Schwartzman, Helen B. 1989. *The Meeting*. Springer U.S. https://doi.org/10.1007/978-1-4899-0885-8.

Scott, Caitlin. 2022. "Audit as Confession: The Instrumentalisation of Ethics for Management Control." *Critique of Anthropology* 42 (1): 20–37. https://doi.org/10.1177/0308275X221074834.

Scott, James C. 2020. *Seeing like a State: How Certain Schemes to Improve the Human Condition Have Failed*. Veritas pbk. edition. Yale University Press.

Seaver, Nick. 2015. "The Nice Thing About Context Is That Everyone Has It." *Media, Culture & Society* 37 (7): 1101–109. https://doi.org/10.1177/0163443715594102.

Selwyn, Tom. 2000. "An Anthropology of Hospitality." In *In Search of Hospitality*, edited by Conrad Lashley and Alison Morrison, 18–37. Taylor and Francis.

Semeniuk, Ivan. 2010. "A Shocking Discovery." *Nature* 467 (7316): 645. https://doi.org/10.1038/467645a.

"Separate Opinion of Vice-President Weeramantry." 1997. The Hague. https://www.icj-cij.org/sites/default/files/case-related/92/092-19970925-JUD-01-03-EN.pdf.

Shapin, Steven. 2008. *The Scientific Life: A Moral History of a Late Modern Vocation*. University of Chicago Press.

Shapin, Steven. 1992. "Why the Public Ought to Understand Science-in-the-Making." *Public Understanding of Science* 1 (1): 27–30. https://doi.org/10.1088/0963-6625/1/1/006.

Shapin, Steven, and Simon Schaffer. 2011. *Leviathan and the Air-Pump: Hobbes, Boyle, and the Experimental Life: Including a Translation of Thomas Hobbes, Dialogus Physicus de Natura Aeris by Simon Schaffer*. Princeton University Press.

Shelley-Egan, Clare, Philip Brey, David Douglas, et al. 2016. "Ethical Assessment of Research and Innovation: A Comparative Analysis of Practices and Institutions in the EU and Selected Other Countries." FP7 Deliverable Deliverable D1.1. U Twente. https://satoriproject.eu/media/D1.1_Ethical-assessment-of-RI_a-comparative-analysis-1.pdf.

Shi, Junnan, Xianwen Chen, Hao Hu, and Carolina Oi Lam Ung. 2023. "Benchmarking Drug Regulatory Systems for Capacity Building: An Integrative Review of Tools, Practice, and Recommendations." *International Journal of Health Policy and Management* 12 (1): 1–15. https://doi.org/10.34172/ijhpm.2023.8100.

Shore, Cris. 2024. "The Bureaucratization of Ethical Integrity: Research Ethics Committees and Imaginaries of Risk." *Anthropology Today* 40 (2): 8–10. https://doi.org/10.1111/1467-8322.12872.

Shore, Cris, and Susan Wright. 2024. *Audit Culture: How Indicators and Rankings Are Reshaping the World*. 1st ed. Pluto Press. https://doi.org/10.2307/jj.10819589.

Shrum, Wesley. 2005. "Reagency of the Internet, or, How I Became a Guest for Science." *Social Studies of Science* 35 (5): 723–54. https://doi.org/10.1177/0306312705052106.

Shryock, Andrew. 2012. "Breaking Hospitality Apart: Bad Hosts, Bad Guests, and the Problem of Sovereignty." *Journal of the Royal Anthropological Institute* 18 (s1): S20–33. https://doi.org/10.1111/j.1467-9655.2012.01758.x.

Shryock, Andrew. 2008. "Thinking About Hospitality, with Derrida, Kant, and the Balga Bedouin." 405–21. https://doi.org/10.5771/0257-9774-2008-2-405.

SIDCER-FERCAP. 2020. "SIDCER-FERCAP Survey Terms of Reference & Standard Operative Procedures." SIDCER-FERCAP Foundation. https://www.sidcer-fercap.org/file/92941.pdf.

Sim, Ida, and Don E. Detmer. 2005. "Beyond Trial Registration: A Global Trial Bank for Clinical Trial Reporting." *PLOS Medicine* 2 (11): e365. https://doi.org/10.1371/journal.pmed.0020365.

Simpson, Bob. 2012. "Building Capacity: A Sri Lankan Perspective on Research, Ethics and Accountability." In *Collaborators Collaborating: Counterparts in Anthropological Knowledge and International Research Relations*, edited by Monica Konrad, 147–63. Berghahn Books.

Simpson, Bob. 2011. "Capacity Building in Developing World Bioethics: Perspectives on Biomedicine and Biomedical Ethics in Contemporary Sri Lanka." In *Bioethics Around the Globe*, 1st ed., edited by Catherine Myser, 39–54. Oxford University Press. https://doi.org/10.1093/acprof:osobl/9780195386097.003.0003.

Simpson, Bob. 2003. "What Might an Anthropology of Contemporary Bioethics Look Like?" In *Medical Humanities: Between Macroethics and Microrealities*, edited by Bob Simpson, 5–20. Wellcome Trust. https://preview.wellcomecollection.org/works/p7yqfa7c.

Simpson, Bob, and Salla Sariola. 2012. "Blinding Authority: Randomized Clinical Trials and the Production of Global Scientific Knowledge in Contemporary Sri Lanka." *Science, Technology, & Human Values* 37 (5): 555–75. https://doi.org/10.1177/0162243911432648.

Simpson, Bob, Vajira H. W. Dissanayake, Rachel Douglas-Jones, and Salla Sariola. 2010. "Ethical Review, Remit and Responsibility in Biomedical Research in South Asia." *Indian Journal of Medical Ethics* (2) (April): 113–14. https://doi.org/10.20529/IJME.2010.042.

Sitthi-amorn, Chitr, and Ratana Somrongthong. 2000. "Strengthening Health Research Capacity in Developing Countries: A Critical Element for Achieving Health Equity." *British Medical Journal* 321: 813–17.

Sleeboom-Faulkner, Margaret. 2016. "'(East) Asia' as a Platform for Debate: Grouping and Bioethics." *Kennedy Institute of Ethics Journal* 26 (3): 277–301. https://doi.org/10.1353/ken.2016.0025.

Sleeboom-Faulkner, Margaret. 2019. "Regulatory Brokerage: Competitive Advantage and Regulation in the Field of Regenerative Medicine." *Social Studies of Science* 49 (3): 355–80. https://doi.org/10.1177/0306312719850628.

Sleeboom-Faulkner, Margaret. 2025. *Regulatory Violence: The Global Dynamics of Regulatory Experimentaiton in Biomedicine and Health.* Cambridge University Press. https://doi.org/10.1017/9781009461757.

Sleeboom-Faulkner, Margaret, and Prasanna Kumar Patra. 2011. "Experimental Stem Cell Therapy: Biohierarchies and Bionetworking in Japan and India." *Social Studies of Science* 41 (5): 645–66. https://doi.org/10.1177/0306312711409792.

Smith, Elise, and Emily E. Anderson. 2022. "Reimagining IRB Review to Incorporate a Clear and Convincing Standard of Evidence." *Accountability in Research* 29 (1): 55–62. https://doi.org/10.1080/08989621.2021.1880902.

Smith, Lynn E. 2008. "Reaching Beyond Regulations: The Pursuit of Accreditation for Human Research Protection Programs." *Monitor* (June): 67–70.

Sneath, David. 2019. "Everyday Hospitality in Mongolia: Obligation, Enaction and Projects of Governance." *L'Homme*, no. 231–32 (November): 67–88. https://doi.org/10.4000/lhomme.35537.

Sopranzetti, Claudio, and Sara Fabbri. 2021. *The King of Bangkok.* Translated by Chiara Natalucci. University of Toronto Press.

Spellecy, Ryan, and Thomas May. 2012. "More Than Cheating: Deception, IRB Shopping, and the Normative Legitimacy of IRBs." *Journal of Law, Medicine & Ethics* 40 (4): 990–96. https://doi.org/10.1111/j.1748-720X.2012.00726.x.

Spellecy, Ryan, Nathan Thompson, and Ann B. Nattinger. 2024. "A Proposal by the U.S. Food and Drug Administration for Reliance on Single Institutional Review Boards: Proceed Only With Caution." *Annals of Internal Medicine* 177 (3): 383–84. https://doi.org/10.7326/M23-2152.

Star, Susan Leigh. 1990. "Power, Technology and the Phenomenology of Conventions: On Being Allergic to Onions." *The Sociological Review* 38 (1_suppl): 26–56. https://doi.org/10.1111/j.1467-954X.1990.tb03347.x.

Star, Susan Leigh, and James R. Griesemer. 1989. "Institutional Ecology, 'Translations' and Boundary Objects: Amateurs and Professionals in Berkeley's Museum of Vertebrate Zoology, 1907–39." *Social Studies of Science* 19 (3): 387–420.

Stark, Laura Jeanine Morris. 2012. *Behind Closed Doors: IRBs and the Making of Ethical Research.* University of Chicago Press.

Stark, Laura. 2011. "Meetings by the Minutes: How Documents Create Decisions for Institutional Review Boards." In *Social Knowledge in the Making*, edited by Charles Camic, Neil Gross, and Michèle Lamont, 233–55. University of Chicago Press.

Stark, Laura. 2007. "Victims in Our Own Minds? IRBs in Myth and Practice." *Law & Society Review* 41 (4): 777–86. https://doi.org/10.1111/j.1540-5893.2007.00323.x.

Stark, Laura, Rachel Gross, Emily O'Brian, and Jesse Pullen. 2021. "What Is Compliance? How Audits Change Ethics and Organizational Fields." *Contemporary Sociology* 50 (4): 273–77. https://doi/10.1177/00943061211021083a.

Strathern, Marilyn. 1992. *After Nature: English Kinship in the Late Twentieth Century.* Cambridge University Press.

Strathern, Marilyn, ed. 2000. *Audit Cultures: Anthropological Studies in Accountability, Ethics and the Academy.* Routledge.

Strathern, Marilyn. 2011. "Binary License." *Common Knowledge* 17 (1): 87–103. https://doi.org/10.1215/0961754X-2010-040.

Strathern, Marilyn. 2004. *Commons and Borderlands: Working Papers on Interdisciplinarity, Accountability and the Flow of Knowledge.* Sean Kingston.

Strathern, Marilyn. 1996. "Cutting the Network." *The Journal of the Royal Anthropological Institute* 2 (3): 517. https://doi.org/10.2307/3034901.

Strathern, Marilyn. 1985. "Discovering 'Social Control.'" *Journal of Law and Society* 12 (2): 111. https://doi.org/10.2307/1409963.

Strathern, Marilyn. 1996a. "For the Motion (1) The Concept of Society Is Theoetically Obsolete." In *Key Debates in Anthropology,* edited by Tim Ingold, 60–66. Routledge.

Strathern, Marilyn. 1996b. "From Improvement to Enhancement: An Anthropological Comment on the Audit Culture." *Cambridge Anthropology* 19 (3): 1–21.

Strathern, Marilyn. (1991) 2004. *Partial Connections.* Updated ed. AltaMira Press.

Strathern, Marilyn. 2022. *Property, Substance, and Effect: Anthropological Essays on Persons and Things.* HAU Books.

Strathern, Marilyn. 2018. "Relations." In *Cambridge Encyclopedia of Anthropology,* edited by Felix Stein. http://www.anthroencyclopedia.com/entry/relations.

Strathern, Marilyn. 2005. "Robust Knowledge and Fragile Futures." In *Global Assemblages: Technology, Politics, and Ethics as Anthropological Problems,* 1st ed., edited by Aihwa Ong and Stephen J. Collier, 464–81. Wiley. https://doi.org/10.1002/9780470696569.

Strathern, Marilyn. (1988) 2001. *The Gender of the Gift: Problems with Women and Problems with Society in Melanesia.* 3rd pbk ed. University of California Press.

Strathern, Marilyn, Monica Konrad, Bob Simpson, and Margaret Sleeboom-Faulkner. 2007. "International Science and Bioethics Collaborations: Critical Appraoches to New Knowledge." Project Proposal, Economic and Social Research Council UK.

Strathern, Marilyn, Monica Konrad, Bob Simpson, and Margaret Sleeboom-Faulkner. 2007. "International Science and Bioethics Collaborations: Critical Appraoches to New Knowledge." Project Proposal, Economic and Social Research Council UK.

Sugarman, Jeremy. 2004. "Determining the Appropriateness of Including Children in Clinical Research: How Thick Is the Ice?" *JAMA* 291 (4): 494. https://doi.org/10.1001/jama.291.4.494.

Sullivan, William M. 1995. *Work and Integrity: The Crisis and Promise of Professionalism in America.* Harper Business.

Sumathipala, Athula. 2006. "Bioethics in Sri Lanka." *EMHJ—Eastern Mediterranean Health Journal* 12 (1): S73–79.

Sumathipala, Athula, and Sisira Siribaddana. 2005. "Research and Clinical Ethics after the Tsunami: Sri Lanka." *The Lancet* 366 (9495): 1418–20. https://doi.org/10.1016/S0140-6736(05)67581-2.

Sunder Rajan, Kaushik. 2021. *Multisituated: Ethnography as Diasporic Praxis*. Duke University Press. https://doi.org/10.1215/9781478022206.

Sunder Rajan, Kaushik. 2017. *Pharmocracy: Value, Politics & Knowledge in Global Biomedicine*. Environmental Futures. Duke University Press.

Svare, Bruce B. 2020. "A Cautionary Tale for Psychology and Higher Education in Asia: Following Western Practices of Incentivising Scholarship May Have Negative Outcomes." *Psychology and Developing Societies* 32 (1): 94–121. https://doi.org/10.1177/0971333619900043.

Sweeney, Fergus. 2011. "European Medicines Agency's Fergus Sweeney: Increasing Inspection Coverage in the Wake of GlobalisationVideo." https://www.pharma-iq.com/regulatorylegal/videos/european-medicines-agencys-fergus-sweeney.

Taylor, Holly A., Peter Currie, and Nancy E. Kass. 2016. "A Study to Evaluate the Effect of Investigator Attendance on the Efficiency of IRB Review." *The Hastings Center* 15 (1). https://www.thehastingscenter.org/irb_article/a-study-to-evaluate-the-effect-of-investigator-attendance-on-the-efficiency-of-irb-review/.

TDR Global. 2025. "About—TDR Global Website Repository." TDR Global: Finding Experts and Building Collaboration. https://tdrgcommshub.org/about/.

TDR Global. 2017. "Lenore Manderson." News. TDR Newsroom, June 26. https://tdr.who.int/newsroom/feature-stories/item/lenore-manderson.

ten Have, Henk. 2022. *Bizarre Bioethics: Ghosts, Monsters, and Pilgrims*. Johns Hopkins University Press.

Thompson, Charis. 2013. *Good Science: The Ethical Choreography of Stem Cell Research*. Inside Technology. The MIT Press.

Thompson, Dennis F. 1993. "Understanding Financial Conflicts of Interest." *New England Journal of Medicine* 329 (8): 573–76. https://doi.org/10.1056/NEJM199308193290812.

Timmermans, Stefan, and Steven Epstein. 2010. "A World of Standards But Not a Standard World: Toward a Sociology of Standards and Standardization." *Annual Review of Sociology* 36 (1): 69–89. https://doi.org/10.1146/annurev.soc.012809.102629.

Torres, Cristina E. 2011. "Reflections on The FERCAP Experience: Moving Forward with Partnerships and Networks." In *FERCAP @ 10: In Commemoration of a Decade of Capacity Building in Ethical Health Research in the Asia-Pacific Region*, edited by Atoy M. Navarro and Cristina E. Torres, 43–54.

Traweek, Sharon, ed. 1992. *Beamtimes and Lifetimes: The World of High Energy Physicists*. 1st Harvard University Press pbk. ed. Harvard University Press.

Trnka, Susanna, and Catherine Trundle, eds. 2017. *Competing Responsibilities: The Politics and Ethics of Contemporary Life*. Duke University Press.

Tsing, Anna Lowenhaupt. 2005. *Friction: An Ethnography of Global Connection*. Princeton University Press.

Turnbull, David. 2000. *Masons, Tricksters and Cartographers: Comperative Studies in the Sociology of Scientific and Indigenous Knowledge*. Routledge.

Turner, Bryan S. 1992. "Preface to the 2nd Edition: Interpreting Emile Durkheim." In *Professional Ethics and Civic Morals*, by Émile Durkheim, 2nd ed. Taylor and Francis.

Tyler, Stephen A. 2010. "Post-Modern Ethnography: From Document of the Occult to Occult Document." In *Writing Culture: The Poetics and Politics of Ethnography*, edited by James Clifford and George E. Marcus, 122–40. University of California Press.

Ulrich, George. 2011. "Elucidating Ethics in Practice: Focus on Accountability." In *Evidence, Ethos and Experiment*, edited by P. Wenzel Geissler and Catherine Molyneux, 145–70. Berghahn Books. https://doi.org/10.1515/9780857450937-008.

United Nations Education, Scientific and Cultural Organization (UNESCO). 2005. "Universal Declaration on Bioethics and Human Rights." http://www.unesco.org / education/information/50y/nfsunesco/doc/hum-rights.htm.

Uyangoda, Jayadeva. 2010. "Sri Lanka in 2009: From Civil War to Political Uncertainties." *Asian Survey* 50 (1): 104–11. https://doi.org/10.1525/as.2010.50.1.104.

Valdez, Natali. 2023. "Studying Up from the Margins in a White-supremacist-cis-hetero-patriarchal-capitalist Culture1." *Medical Anthropology Quarterly* 37 (3): 190–203. https://doi.org/10.1111/maq.12765.

Vaughan, Diane. 1997. *The Challenger Launch Decision: Risky Technology, Culture, and Deviance at NASA*. University of Chicago Press. https://doi.org/10.7208/chicago/9780226346960.001.0001.

Vaughn, Sarah E. 2022. *Engineering Vulnerability: In Pursuit of Climate Adaptation*. Duke University Press. https://doi.org/10.1215/9781478022725.

Wagner, Caroline S., Irene Brahmakulam, Brian Jackson, Anny Wong, and Tatsuro Yoda. 2001. "Science and Technology Collaboration: Building Capacity in Developing Countries?" Prepared for the World Bank MR-1357.0-WN. Santa Monica, CA: RAND Corporation. https://www.rand.org/pubs/monograph_reports/MR1357z0.html.

Wahlberg, Ayo. 2022. "Assemblage Ethnography: Configurations Across Scales, Sites, and Practices: Post-Structuralism." In *The Palgrave Handbook of the Anthropology of Technology*, edited by Maja Hojer Bruun, Ayo Wahlberg, Rachel Douglas-Jones, et al., 125–44. Springer Nature Singapore. https://doi.org/10.1007/978-981-16-7084-8_6.

Wahlberg, Ayo. 2018. *Good Quality: The Routinization of Sperm Banking in China*. University of California Press.

Wahlberg, Ayo, Christoph Rehmann-Sutter, Margaret Sleeboom-Faulkner, et al. 2013. "From Global Bioethics to Ethical Governance of Biomedical Research Collaborations." *Social Science & Medicine* 98 (December): 293–300. https://doi.org/10.1016/j.socscimed.2013.03.041.

Wahlberg, Ayo, Dong Dong, Priscilla Song, and Zhu Jianfeng. 2021. "The Platforming of Human Embryo Editing: Prospecting 'Disease Free' Futures." *New Genetics and Society* 40 (4): 367–83. https://doi.org/10.1080/14636778.2021.1997578.

Walford, Tone, and Stine Krøjer. 2017. "Unruly Analogies, Uncontrolled Comparisons." In *Abstracts of the 116th Conference of the American Anthropological Association*, edited by American Anthropological Association, 301. Washington DC. https://openanthroresearch.org/index.php/oarr/preprint/view/48/87.https://openanthroresearch.org/index.php/oarr/preprint/view/48/87.

Wallerstein, Immanuel Maurice. 2011. *The Modern World-System I: Capitalist Agriculture and the Origins of the European World-Economy in the Sixteenth Century.* University of California Press. https://doi.org/10.1525/9780520948570.

Warlow, Charles. 2004. "Clinical Research under the Cosh Again." *BMJ* 329 (7460): 241–42. https://doi.org/10.1136/bmj.329.7460.241.

Weber, Max. 2014. *From Max Weber: Essays in Sociology.* Edited by H. H. Gerth and C. Wright Mills. Routledge. https://doi.org/10.4324/9780203759240.

Weingart, Peter. 2017. "How Robust Is 'Socially Robust Knowledge'?" In *Knowledge and Democracy: A 21st-Century Perspective*, 1st ed., edited by Nico Stehr. Routledge. https://doi.org/10.4324/9780203787687.

Wendland, Claire L. 2016. "Opening up the Black Box: Looking for a More Capacious Version of Capacity in Global Health Partnerships." *Canadian Journal of African Studies / Revue Canadienne Des Études Africaines* 50 (3): 415–35. https://doi.org/10.1080/00083968.2016.1266675.

West, Paige. 2016. *Dispossession and the Environment: Rhetoric and Inequality in Papua New Guinea.* Columbia University Press.

White, Elizabeth. 2011. "Protecting Human Subjects." Department of Energy Human Subjects Protection. https://web.archive.org/web/20120126051516/http://humansubjects.energy.gov/doe-resources/newsletter/HS21_ac.pdf.

WHO. 2023. "First WHO Global Clinical Trials Forum Puts Forward a Global Vision for Sustainable Clinical Research Infrastructure." *World Health Organization News.* November 29. https://www.who.int/news/item/29-11-2023-first-who-global-clinical-trials-forum-puts-forward-a-global-vision-for-sustainable-clinical-research-infrastructure.

WHO. 2022. "Seventy-Fifth World Health Assembly Agenda Item 16.2: Strengthening Clinical Trials to Provide High-Quality Evidence on Health Interventions and to Improve Resaerch Quality and Coordination." https://apps.who.int/gb/ebwha/pdf_files/WHA75/A75_R8-en.pdf.

WHO. 2024. *Women in Science: A Storytelling Showcase.* Geneva: World Health Organization.

WHO/TDR, ed. 2002. *Surveying and Evaluating Ethical Review Practices: A Complementary Guideline to the Operational Guidelines for Ethics Committees That Review Biomedical Research.* 6th ed. TDR/PRD/ETHOS/2002.1. Geneva: World Health Organization. https://doi.org/10.1017/CBO9780511550089.069.

Whyte, William H. Whyte. 1952. "Groupthink." *Fortune*, March 1. https://fortune.com/article/groupthink-fortune-1952/.

Widger, Tom, Noémi Tousignant, Michael Eddleston, et al. 2022. "Research as Development: Book Forum." *Medicine Anthropology Theory* 9 (2): 1–16. https://doi.org/10.17157/mat.9.2.6499.

Widler, Beat. 2012. Interview on *ClinPowerNews*. http://www.news.clinpower.com/201205-interview-dr-beat.html.

Widler, Beat, Artem Andrianov, and Maria Proupín-Pérez. 2015. "ICH GCP Goes Risk Based." *Applied Clinical Trials*. https://www.appliedclinicaltrialsonline.com/view/ich-gcp-goes-risk-based.

Wilhelm, Katherine, Shawn Shieh, Elizabeth Knup, et al. 2021. "What Future for International NGOs in China? | ChinaFile." *What Future for International NGOs in China?* (blog), November 24.

Willerslev, Rane, and Martin Holbraad. 2007. "Transcendental Perspectivism: Anonymous Viewpoints from Inner Asia." *Inner Asia* 9 (2): 329–45. https://doi.org/10.1163/146481707793646511.

Wilson, Duncan. 2011. "Creating the 'Ethics Industry': Mary Warnock, in Vitro Fertilization, and the History of Bioethics in Britain." *BioSocieties* 6 (2): 121–411. https://doi.org/10.1057/biosoc.2010.26.

Wilson, Duncan. 2012. "Who Guards the Guardians? Ian Kennedy, Bioethics and the 'Ideology of Accountability' in British Medicine." *Social History of Medicine* 25 (1): 193–211. https://doi.org/10.1093/shm/hkr090.

WMA, World Medical Association. 2024. "WMA Declaration of Helsinki—Ethical Principles for Medical Research Involving Human Participants." JAMA.

Woolgar, Steve, and Javier Lezaun. 2013. "The Wrong Bin Bag: A Turn to Ontology in Science and Technology Studies?" *Social Studies of Science* 43 (3): 321–40. https://doi.org/10.1177/0306312713488820.

World Health Organization. 2000. *Operational Guidelines for Ethics Committees That Review Biomedical Research*. https://doi.org/10.1017/CBO9780511550089.069.

World Health Organization. 2009. "Research Ethics Committees: Basic Concepts for Capacity-Building." *Comités d'éthique de La Recherche: Notions de Base Pour Le Renforcement Des Capacités*, 71.

World Health Organization. 2011. "Standards and Operational Guidance for Ethics Review of Health-Related Research with Human Participants." https://apps.who.int/iris/handle/10665/44783.

World Health Organization, ed. 2023. *WHO Tool for Benchmarking Ethics Oversight of Health-Related Research Involving Human Participants*. World Health Organization.

Yates, JoAnne, and Craig N. Murphy. 2019. *Engineering Rules: Global Standard Setting since 1880*. Johns Hopkins University Press.

Yates-Doerr, Emily. 2015. *The Weight of Obesity: Hunger and Global Health in Postwar Guatemala*. University of California Press.

Zhang, Joy Y., and Saheli Datta Burton. 2022. *The Elephant and the Dragon in Contemporary Life Sciences: A Call for Decolonising Global Governance.* Manchester University Press.

Zimmerman, Ann S. 2008. "New Knowledge from Old Data: The Role of Standards in the Sharing and Reuse of Ecological Data." *Science, Technology, & Human Values* 33 (5): 631–52. https://doi.org/10.1177/0162243907306704.

Zuckerman, Jeffrey, ed. 2022. *From Subject to Partner.* Center for Information and Study on Clinical Research Participation.

Index

Italicized page numbers indicate figures, illustrations, and photographs.

Anthropology of Policy

Cris Shore and Susan Wright, editors

Making Sanctuary Cities: Migration, Citizenship, and Urban Governance
Rachel Humphris
2024

Antinuclear Citizens: Sustainability Policy and Grassroots Activism in Post-Fukushima Japan
Akihiro Ogawa
2023

The Alternative University: Lessons from Bolivarian Venezuela
Mariya P. Ivancheva
2023

Village Gone Viral: Hidden Dimensions of Traveling Policy Models
Marit Tolo Østebø
2021

Wild Policy: Indigeneity and the Unruly Logics of Intervention
Tess Lea
2020

The Gray Zone: Sovereignty, Human Smuggling, and Undercover Police Investigation in Europe
Gregory Feldman
2019

Law Mart: Justice, Access, and For-Profit Law Schools
Riaz Tejani
2017

One Blue Child: Asthma, Responsibility, and the Politics of Global Health
Susanna Trnka
2017

The Orderly Entrepreneur: Youth, Education, and Governance in Rwanda

Catherine A. Honeyman

2016

Coercive Concern: Nationalism, Liberalism, and the Schooling of Muslim Youth

Reva Jaffe-Walter

2016

Fragile Elite: The Dilemmas of China's Top University Students

Susanne Bregnbæk

2016

Navigating Austerity: Currents of Debt along a South Asian River

Laura Bear

2015

Drugs, Thugs, and Diplomats: U.S. Policymaking in Colombia

Winifred Tate

2015

FSC
www.fsc.org
MIX
Papier | Fördert gute Waldnutzung
FSC® C083411

Kolibri 360 GmbH
Ferdinand-Jühlke-Straße 7
99095 Erfurt, Deutschland
produktsicherheit@kolibri360.de